Pediatric Psycho-Oncology

APOS CLINICAL REFERENCE HANDBOOKS

Psycho-Oncology: A Quick Reference on the Psychosocial Dimensions of Cancer Symptom Management, 2nd edition, Jimmie C. Holland, Mitch Golant, Donna B. Greenberg, Mary K. Hughes, Jon A. Levenson, Matthew J. Loscalzo, William F. Pirl

Pediatric Psycho-Oncology: A Quick Reference on the Psychosocial Dimensions of Cancer Symptom Management, 2nd edition, Lori Wiener, Maryland Pao, Anne E. Kazak, Mary Jo Kupst, Andrea Farkas Patenaude

Geriatric Psycho-Oncology: A Quick Reference on the Psychosocial Dimensions of Cancer Symptom Management, Jimmie C. Holland, Talia Weiss Wiesel, Christian J. Nelson, Andrew J. Roth, Yesne Alici

Pediatric Psycho-Oncology

A Quick Reference on the Psychosocial Dimensions of Cancer Symptom Management

SECOND EDITION

Edited by

Lori Wiener, PhD, DCSW

Maryland Pao, MD

Anne E. Kazak, PhD, ABPP

Mary Jo Kupst, PhD

Andrea Farkas Patenaude, PhD

Robert J. Arceci, MD, PhD

OXFORD

UNIVERSITY PRESS

OXFORD
UNIVERSITY PRESS

Oxford University Press is a department of the University of Oxford. It furthers the University's objective of excellence in research, scholarship, and education by publishing worldwide.

Oxford New York
Auckland Cape Town Dar es Salaam Hong Kong Karachi
Kuala Lumpur Madrid Melbourne Mexico City Nairobi
New Delhi Shanghai Taipei Toronto

With offices in
Argentina Austria Brazil Chile Czech Republic France Greece
Guatemala Hungary Italy Japan Poland Portugal Singapore
South Korea Switzerland Thailand Turkey Ukraine Vietnam

Oxford is a registered trademark of Oxford University Press in the UK and certain other countries.

Published in the United States of America by
Oxford University Press
198 Madison Avenue, New York, NY 10016

Library of Congress Cataloging-in-Publication Data
Quick reference for pediatric oncology clinicians
Pediatric psycho-oncology : a quick reference on the psychosocial dimensions of cancer symptom management/edited by Lori Wiener, Maryland Pao, Anne E. Kazak, Mary Jo Kupst, Andrea Farkas Patenaude; with the American Psycho-Social Oncology Society.—2nd edition.
p. ; cm.
Preceded by: Quick reference for pediatric oncology clinicians/senior editors, Lori Wiener, Maryland Pao. c2009. Includes bibliographical references and index.
ISBN 978–0–19–933511–4 (alk. paper)
I. Wiener, Lori, editor. II. Pao, Maryland, editor. III. Kazak, Anne E., editor. IV. Kupst, Mary Jo, editor. V. Patenaude, Andrea Farkas, editor. VI. American Psychosocial Oncology Society. VII. Title.
[DNLM: 1. Child. 2. Neoplasms—psychology. 3. Age Factors. 4. Family Relations. 5. Neoplasms—therapy. 6. Social Support. QZ 275]
RC281.C4
618.92'994—dc23
2014022636

This material is not intended to be, and should not be considered, a substitute for medical or other professional advice. Treatment for the conditions described in this material is highly dependent on the individual circumstances. And, while this material is designed to offer accurate information with respect to the subject matter covered and to be current as of the time it was written, research and knowledge about medical and health issues is constantly evolving and dose schedules for medications are being revised continually, with new side effects recognized and accounted for regularly. Readers must therefore always check the product information and clinical procedures with the most up-to-date published product information and data sheets provided by the manufacturers and the most recent codes of conduct and safety regulation. The publisher and the authors make no representations or warranties to readers, express or implied, as to the accuracy or completeness of this material. Without limiting the foregoing, the publisher and the authors make no representations or warranties as to the accuracy or efficacy of the drug dosages mentioned in the material. The authors and the publisher do not accept, and expressly disclaim, any responsibility for any liability, loss or risk that may be claimed or incurred as a consequence of the use and/or application of any of the contents of this material.

9 8 7 6 5 4 3 2 1
Printed in the United States of America
on acid-free paper

This book is dedicated to all children and families affected by pediatric cancer. Those we have worked with have taught us what we are now sharing with others in this volume.

LW
MP
AEK
MJK
AFP
RJA

Contents

Foreword

I vividly recall, as a second-year medical school student, accompanying my clinical advisor to visit a 2-year-old child who had been hospitalized with acute leukemia. My advisor was a relatively newly appointed faculty member in pediatric hematology-oncology—a field very much in its infancy at that time. The suffering of the child and family was apparent even to me, a novice medical student, and I wondered how anyone could pursue a career focusing on children with such a catastrophic disease. Although I was touched by the sensitive way in which my advisor interacted with the child and his family, I was still frightened by the likely life-threatening illness that this child faced and how he and his family would cope with its consequences.

Only a few years later, as a newly minted intern in pediatrics at the same children's hospital where my clinical advisor had trained me, I found myself drawn to the care of the very children toward whom I had such a worried reaction as a young medical student. In the few short years that had intervened, incredible progress had been made in the care of children with acute leukemia. The role of combination chemotherapy and the prospect for preventing central nervous system relapse with prophylactic radiation therapy was being defined and providing hope. I found myself drawn to the excitement of working in a field of medicine that was changing rapidly and where research could impact patient outcomes in meaningful ways. Having been educated in a medical school that had defined the biopsychosocial model of care, I also appreciated the importance of combining psychosocial care with medical treatment. In many ways, this challenging area of medicine brought together all my interests and passions—basic and clinical research, challenging multisystem medical disease management, along with interdisciplinary psychosocial care and intervention. I don't think I ever questioned whether a child diagnosed with cancer should receive psychosocial support; I believed that this was necessary for every child and family to have comprehensive care.

Over the decades that have followed my early entry into the field of pediatric oncology, I have witnessed, over and over again, the impact of serious disease on the child, adolescent, and young adult. In tandem, the impact of a serious childhood disorder on the parents, siblings, grandparents, relatives, and the community of friends is also abundantly apparent. It is implausible to think that any child or family facing the diagnosis of cancer will be unaffected emotionally and psychologically. Regardless of one's background, resources, social strata, professional status or knowledge, every child and every family requires help and support. No amount of inner strength or resilience can cope with the impact of cancer and its treatment without psychosocial support. From my perspective, psychosocial support is as important as medical care and treatment—both are needed to successfully manage catastrophic disease. I was fortunate to witness this over and over again during the many years that I worked at the National Cancer Institute where we formed a team with social workers, psychologists, recreation therapists, and others to bring our respective skills and knowledge into a compassionate unison on behalf of the children and families we treated. I have long viewed the management of fears and feelings of children, adolescents—no matter how resistant—and young adults, about their illness and its consequences, and the ability to support the child within the family constellation and community not as ideal care (even though it is) but as the standard of care for the child with cancer.

Coping with cancer requires the ability to face the prospect of death along with numerous physical and emotional alterations. Learning how to cope with these challenges is a prerequisite to survival and should be part of every program of care for children with cancer (and I believe adults with cancer as well).

Since I began, much research has been brought to bear on many important aspects of caring for children with cancer including developmental and educational needs, impact on family, and the adverse psychological and social sequelae of cancer and its therapy. Many psychosocial specialists and researchers have dedicated their lives and careers to caring for children and families with cancer and catastrophic diseases. Their work has contributed as much to the quality survival of children as has the medical care that has been administered. Every pediatric oncologist must be conversant in the psychosocial dimensions of cancer management delineated in this book. I am honored to provide a personal introduction and affirmation of this important book.

Philip A. Pizzo, MD
David and Susan Heckerman Professor of Pediatrics,
Microbiology, and Immunology
Stanford University School of Medicine
Stanford, California
February, 2014

Preface

We are pleased to provide the second edition of this comprehensive reference book written to provide pediatric oncologists, pediatric nurse practitioners and nurses, psychologists, psychiatrists, and social workers with an overview of the many facets that comprise excellent psychosocial care for children and adolescents living with cancer and their family members. It is not meant to be an exhaustive reference; rather, we aim to provide helpful recommendations and best-practice models for management of the emotional reactions of children undergoing cancer treatment and of the psychological, cognitive, and social outcomes for children with cancer and of the emotional burdens of pediatric cancer care on siblings and parents.*

This book is unique in covering a broad range of topics in pediatric psychosocial oncology in a handbook format geared toward answering specific clinical questions. An international group of experts in each area have written chapters to help clinicians review, anticipate, and respond to emotional issues that often arise in the context of treating pediatric cancer patients. The chapters may also help pediatric oncologists and nurses recognize when it may be best to refer patients to their behavioral health colleagues. We hope it will be useful for those who are establishing pediatric oncology services or adding psychosocial components to existing clinics to recognize the range of ways in which psychological services are important for the provision of comprehensive care to children and families.

All the chapters have been updated since the first edition, and they cover a wide range of topics including psychological aspects of particular pediatric cancers and their treatments; how to talk to a child and family at critical times during the disease course; new information in the area of genomics and genetic testing; individual, family, educational, psychological and psychiatric interventions; and how to assist the international family. This second edition includes additional clinically relevant chapters on stem cell transplantation, social media, and electronic psychosocial interventions. Each chapter recognizes the necessity of embracing an interdisciplinary approach to ensure that each child with cancer has the best opportunity for a satisfying, productive life and, when cure is not possible, that the period of time prior to, at the time of, and following death occurs with as much dignity as possible for the child and family.

We have assembled the handbook in concise, practical, and highly readable brief chapters. The "bullet point" format is to facilitate a quick read. We anticipate most clinicians will turn to specific chapters for guidance on managing the psychosocial care of their patients. Some readers, however, may read this book more comprehensively. Such readers may find that similar issues such as diagnosis, treatment completion, and survivorship are addressed in multiple chapters. Each chapter stands on its own, but we have cross-referenced places in other chapters where similar issues are dealt with in depth to avoid unnecessary repetition.

We recognize that not every child and family will have access to a full range of psychosocial services. We have described state-of-the-art care as practiced in cancer centers that have the greatest resources, and we acknowledge that providers elsewhere will know how best to adapt these principles to their own circumstances, possibly through developing referral connections to trusted mental health colleagues in their community.

We hope this book conveys and extends the warm spirit of collegiality and mutual respect that exists in many centers and regions between pediatric oncology clinicians and mental health professionals who have productively worked together over the past 30 years.

We recognize that children are cared for by adults with many different relationships to them. We use the term *parents* to refer to all adult caregivers who have parenting responsibilities.

The pharmacological dosage information in this handbook has been carefully reviewed. However, the drug manufacturers' current indications, dosage information, and drug interaction warnings should be consulted prior to prescribing any drug listed in this work.

Lori Wiener, PhD, DCSW
Maryland Pao, MD
Anne E. Kazak, PhD, ABPP
Mary Jo Kupst, PhD
Andrea Farkas Patenaude, PhD
Robert J. Arceci, MD, PhD

Acknowledgments

The editors thank those who support access of psychosocial support services to all patients and families coping with cancer.

We especially acknowledge the support of Vicki Sardi-Brown and Peter Brown who established the Mattie Miracle Cancer Foundation, which focuses on improving psychosocial care and on the development of psychosocial standards of care for children with cancer.

Jimmie C. Holland, MD, is widely recognized as the founder of "psychooncology". She is also the driving force behind the creation of the first and second editions of *Pediatric Psycho-Oncology: A Quick Reference on the Psychosocial Dimensions of Cancer Symptom Management*. While Dr. Holland's recent research focus has been geriatric oncology, she has consistently challenged clinicians and researchers to investigator and focus on the needs of children with cancer. We will be forever be indebted to Dr. Holland for her insight, wisdom, perseverance, and commitment to the needs of children with cancer and their families and for helping to pave the road for the field of Pediatric Psychooncology to develop, expand, and thrive.

Contributors

Allistair Abraham, MD
Attending, Division of Blood and Marrow Transplantation
Center for Cancer and Blood Disorders
Children's National Health System
Assistant Professor of Pediatrics
The George Washington University Medical Center
Washington, D.C.

Robert J. Arceci, MD, PhD
Director
Children's Center for Cancer and Blood Disorders
Director of the Ron Matricaria Institute of Molecular Medicine
Phoenix Children's Hospital
Department of Child Health
University of Arizona College of Medicine
Phoenix, Arizona

Sarah R. Brand, PhD
Instructor of Psychology
Harvard Medical School
Staff Psychologist
Department of Psychosocial Oncology and Palliative Care
Dana Farber Cancer Institute
Boston, Massachusetts

Joanna Breyer, PhD
Assistant Professor of Psychiatry
Harvard Medical School
Pediatric Psychosocial Unit
Dana-Farber Cancer Institute
Boston, Massachusetts

Ronald T. Brown, PhD
President
University of North Texas at Dallas
Dallas, Texas

William M. Bukowski, PhD
Research Chair in Psychology
Concordia University
Montreal, Quebec

Anu Chittenden, MS, CGC
Genetic Counselor
Center for Cancer Genetics and Prevention
Dana-Farber Cancer Institute
Boston, Massachusetts

Todd Dalberg, DO
Division of Pediatric Hematology-Oncology
Oregon Health and Science University
Doernbecher Children's Hospital
Portland, Oregon

Brian P. Daly, PhD
Assistant Professor of Psychology
Drexel University
Philadelphia, Pennsylvania

Mary Lynn Dell, MD, DMin
Department of Psychiatry
Nationwide Children's Hospital
Columbus, Ohio

Jeffrey S. Dome, MD, PhD
Professor of Pediatrics
George Washington University
School of Medicine and Health Sciences
Thomas Willson and Lenore Williams McKnew Professor of Pediatric Oncology
Chief, Divisions of Hematology and Oncology
Children's National Medical Center
Washington, D.C.

Dennis Drotar, PhD
Professor of Pediatrics
University of Cincinnati
Clinical Psychologist, Behavioral Medicine and Clinical Psychology
Cincinnati Children's Hospital
Cincinnati, Ohio

Jennifer S. Ford, PhD
Clinical Psychologist
Department of Psychiatry and Behavioral Sciences
Memorial Sloan-Kettering Cancer Center
New York, New York

Sarah Friebert, MD
Director of Pediatric Palliative Care
Akron Children's Hospital
Akron, Ohio

Debra L. Friedman, MD
Associate Professor of Pediatrics
Vanderbilt University School of Medicine
Vanderbilt-Ingram Cancer Center
Monroe Carell Jr. Children's Hospital at Vanderbilt
Nashville, Tennessee

Terry J. Fry, MD
Center for Cancer Research
National Cancer Institute
National Institutes of Health
Bethesda, Maryland

Martha A. Grootenhuis, PhD
Pediatric Psychosocial Department
Emma Children's Hospital
Academic Medical Center
University of Amsterdam
Amsterdam, the Netherlands

Daniel H. Grossoehme, DMin, MS
Chaplain
Division of Pulmonary Medicine
Assistant Professor of Pediatrics
University of Cincinnati
Cincinnati, Ohio

Kristina K. Hardy, PhD
Neuropsychology Division
Children's National Medical Center
The George Washington University School of Medicine
Washington, D.C.

Pamela S. Hinds, PhD, RN, FAAN
Department of Pediatrics
The George Washington University
Department of Nursing Research and Quality Outcomes
Children's National Medical Center
Washington, D.C.

Marilyn J. Hockenberry, PhD, RN, PNP-BC, FAAN
Bessie Baker Professor of Nursing
Duke University School of Nursing
Durham, North Carolina

Lisa M. Horowitz, PhD, MPH
Staff Scientist and Clinical Psychologist
National Institute of Mental Health
National Cancer Institute
Bethesda, Maryland

Mary Jo Kupst, PhD
Emeritus Professor of Pediatrics
Medical College of Wisconsin
Milwaukee, Wisconsin

Ernest R. Katz, PhD
Adjunct Professor of Clinical Pediatrics and Psychology
Keck School of Medicine and the Dornsife College
University of Southern California
University Center of Excellence in Developmental Disabilities
Children's Hospital of Los Angeles
Founder, School Transition and Re-Entry Service
Children's Center for Cancer and Blood Diseases
Los Angeles, California

Anne E. Kazak, PhD, ABPP
Center for Healthcare Delivery Science
Nemours Pediatric Health System
Wilmington, Delaware
Professor
Department of Pediatrics
Sidney Kimmel Medical School of Thomas Jefferson University
Philadelphia, Pennsylvania

Julia A. Kearney, MD
Child Psychiatrist and Pediatrician
Department of Psychiatry and Behavioral Sciences
Memorial Sloan-Kettering Cancer Center
New York, New York

Elliot J. Krane, MD
Professor of Anesthesiology
Perioperative and Pain Medicine
Stanford University Medical Center
Professor of Pediatrics
Lucile Salter Packard Children's Hospital
Stanford, California

Marguerite S. Lederberg, MD
Psychiatrist
Department of Psychiatry and Behavioral Sciences
Memorial Sloan-Kettering Cancer Center
New York, New York

Jennifer M. Levine, MD, MSW
Assistant Professor of Pediatrics
Columbia University Medical Center
New York, New York

Avi Madan-Swain, PhD
Associate Professor of Pediatrics
University of Alabama at Birmingham
Children's Hospital of Alabama
Birmingham, Alabama

David Malkin, MD
Professor of Pediatrics and Medical Biophysics
University of Toronto
The Hospital for Sick Children
Toronto, Ontario

D. Richard Martini, MD
Division Chief of Behavioral Health
Department of Pediatrics
University of Utah School of Medicine
Director of Psychiatry and Behavioral Health
Primary Children's Medical Center
Salt Lake City, Utah

Hilary McClafferty, MD, FAAP
Assistant Director of the Integrative Medicine Fellowship
Arizona Center for Integrative Medicine
University of Arizona
Tucson, Arizona

Anna T. Meadows, MD
Emeritus Professor of Pediatrics and Medicine
University of Pennsylvania School of Medicine
The Children's Hospital of Philadelphia
Philadelphia, Pennsylvania

Melinda Merchant, MD, PhD
Pediatric Oncology Branch Clinical Director
Center for Cancer Research
National Cancer Institute
Bethesda, Maryland

Travis Mickelson, MD
Assistant Professor of Pediatrics
University of Utah
Salt Lake City, Utah

Robert B. Noll, PhD
Professor of Pediatrics
University of Pittsburgh School of Medicine
Children's Hospital of Pittsburgh
Pittsburgh, Pennsylvania

Diana E. Nora, BS
National Institute of Mental Health
National Cancer Institute
Bethesda, Maryland

Kevin C. Oeffinger, MD
Director, Adult Long-Term Follow-Up Program
Memorial Sloan-Kettering Cancer Center
New York, New York

Ahna L. H. Pai, PhD
Associate Professor of Pediatrics
University of Cincinnati
Clinical Psychologist, Behavioral Medicine and Clinical Psychology
Cincinnati Children's Hospital
Cincinnati, Ohio

Maryland Pao, MD
Clinical Director and Deputy Scientific Director
National Institute of Mental Health
Bethesda, Maryland

Andrea Farkas Patenaude, PhD
Associate Professor of Psychology
Harvard Medical School
Director, Psychology Research and Clinical Services
Center for Cancer Genetics and Prevention
Dana-Farber Cancer Institute
Boston, Massachusetts

Sean Phipps, PhD
Chair & Member, Department of Psychology
St. Jude Children's Research Hospital
Memphis, Tennessee

Rebecca A. Prengler, MD
National Institute of Mental Health
National Cancer Institute
Bethesda, Maryland

Maria E. Radulovic, CMI-Spanish
Department of Social Work
National Institutes of Health
Bethesda, Maryland

Steven K. Reader, PhD
Nemours Center for Healthcare Delivery Science
Assistant Professor
Department of Pediatrics
Sidney Kimmel Medical School of Thomas Jefferson University
Philadelphia, Pennsylvania
Division of Behavioral Health
Nemours Alfred I. duPont Hospital for Children
Wilmington, Delaware

Cheryl C. Rodgers, PhD, RN, CPNP
Assistant Professor of Nursing
Duke University School of Nursing
Durham, North Carolina

Marilyn A. Rosen, MLS
University of Rochester Medical Center
Rochester, New York

Julia H. Rowland, PhD
Director, Office of Cancer Survivorship
National Cancer Institute
Bethesda, Maryland

Olle Jane Z. Sahler, MD
Professor of Pediatrics, Psychiatry, Medical Humanities, and Oncology
University of Rochester Medical Center
Rochester, New York

Lisa A. Schwartz, PhD
Psychologist
University of Pennsylvania School of Medicine
The Children's Hospital of Philadelphia
Philadelphia, Pennsylvania

Jaclyn Schienda, ScM, CGC
Genetic Counselor
Center for Cancer Genetics and Prevention
Dana-Farber Cancer Institute
Boston, Massachusetts

Aziza Shad, MD
Amey Distinguished Professor of Neuro-Oncology and Childhood Cancer
Georgetown University
Lombardi Comprehensive Cancer Center
Georgetown University Hospital
Washington, D.C.

Nirali N. Shah, MD
Pediatric Oncology Branch
Center for Cancer Research
National Cancer Institute
National Institutes of Health
Bethesda, Maryland

Charles A. Sklar, MD
Director
Long-Term Follow-Up Program
Department of Pediatrics
Memorial Sloan-Kettering Cancer Center
New York, New York

Giselle Saulnier Sholler, MD, MSc
Department of Pediatric Hematology-Oncology
Helen DeVos Children's Hospital
Grand Rapids, Michigan

Barbara Sourkes, PhD
Professor of Pediatrics
Stanford University Medical Center
Lucile Salter Packard Children's Hospital
Stanford, California

Rachel A. Tunick, PhD
Instructor of Psychology
Harvard Medical School Staff Psychologist
Department of Psychiatry and Children's Hospital Primary Care Center
Boston Children's Hospital
Boston, Massachusetts

Katherine E. Warren, MD
National Cancer Institute
Pediatric Oncology Branch
Bethesda, Maryland

Alan S. Wayne, MD
Professor of Pediatrics
Keck School of Medicine
University of Southern California
Director
Children's Center for Cancer and Blood Diseases
Head, Division of Hematology, Oncology and Blood & Marrow Transplantation
Children's Hospital Los Angeles
Los Angeles, California

Lori Wiener, PhD, DCSW
Co-Director
Behavioral Science Core
Director
Psychosocial Support and Research Program
Pediatric Oncology Branch, Center for Cancer Research
National Cancer Institute, National Institutes of Health
Bethesda, Maryland

Matthew Wright, MD
Chief of Hospital Medicine
Western Regional Medical Center
Goodyear, Arizona

Lonnie Zeltzer, MD
Professor of Pediatrics, Anesthesiology, and Psychiatry and Biobehavioral Sciences
David Geffen School of Medicine
University of California
Los Angeles, California
UCLA Mattel Children's Hospital
UCLA Jonsson Comprehensive Cancer Center
Los Angeles, California

Introduction

Jimmie C. Holland

It is a pleasure to write the Purpose and Overview for the second edition of the *Pediatric Oncology Handbook* relating to the psychiatric and psychosocial care of the child with cancer. The first edition was published in 2009 by the American Psychosocial Oncology Society. This second edition is being published by the Oxford University Press as part of its series of handbooks for psychiatric and psychosocial care of the adult, child, and elder with cancer. Because these handbooks depend strongly on tables and rapid learning formats, they are ideal not only for the busy clinic staff but also for teaching students, residents, and fellows in pediatric oncology and its subspecialties. Every child at every visit presents psychological and social issues that, if handled well, result in enhanced trust, reduced distress, and greater adherence to treatment. If handled poorly, the converse too often results in greater distress, distance from the staff, and poorer adherence. The consequences are too great to be neglected as we progress to truly patient-centered care.

The psychological care of children with cancer has for far too long lacked both standards of quality and clinical practice guidelines to assure that pediatric staff take care of the whole child with the optimal tools available. This volume goes a long way to assuring that this goal is reached. The editors are five outstanding clinical investigators in pediatric psycho-oncology. They have chosen authors to write on specific critical areas of clinical care: how to talk to parents and children; psychological and social problems by site of cancer; management of common psychological and physical symptoms; psychotherapeutic approaches; cognition problems, their impact and treatment; school issues; spiritual and religious issues. Taken together, these chapters contribute greatly to the development of the first practice guidelines for psychosocial care of children with cancer. This is a goal that we can all celebrate as a benchmark of progress.

Jimmie C. Holland, MD Wayne E. Chapman
Chair in Psychiatric Oncology Department of Psychiatry and Behavioral Sciences
Memorial Sloan-Kettering Cancer Center, New York, New York
February, 2014

Section I

Cancers of Childhood

Chapter 1

Leukemias and Lymphomas

Nirali N. Shah and Alan S. Wayne

Leukemia is the most common pediatric cancer diagnosis, comprising approximately 25% of all childhood malignancies.[1] Lymphomas account for about 15% of pediatric cancer. In general, cure rates for leukemias and lymphomas in childhood exceed 75%. However, the outcome varies between subtypes and prognostic groups, and hematologic malignancies remain the most common cause of cancer-related mortality in pediatrics.[2]

Although leukemias and lymphomas are highly curable in pediatrics, given the intensive nature of therapy that these children receive, they are at risk for a multitude of acute and late effects associated with both the therapy and the underlying disease (Table 1.1).[3–5] Diagnosis and treatment confer significant physical, neurocognitive, psychological, and social risks that can have life-long impact. Accordingly, children and adolescents with leukemia and lymphoma should receive systematic and serial neurocognitive and psychosocial assessments during and after treatment as part of comprehensive multidisciplinary care. This chapter will focus specifically on these particular issues.

Epidemiology and Treatment

Acute lymphoblastic leukemia (ALL) accounts for about 75% and acute myelogenous leukemia (AML) about 20% of pediatric leukemia, whereas chronic myelogenous leukemia (CML) and juvenile myelomonocytic leukemia (JMML) are infrequent (Figure 1.1),[6,7] with Hodgkin disease slightly more prevalent than non-Hodgkin lymphoma (NHL). There are three predominant subtypes of NHL in pediatrics, each occurring with approximate equal frequency: lymphoblastic (LBL), large cell, and Burkitt lymphoma.

Treatment regimens, which are specific to the disease subtype and risk-adapted based on clinicopathologic prognostic features, in most cases consist of combination chemotherapy (Table 1.2). Initial treatment phases are commonly more intensive, with the goal of inducing and consolidating a remission. Such "induction" and "consolidation" chemotherapy is usually administered in an inpatient setting. Individuals with ALL require long-term low-dose outpatient chemotherapy ("maintenance" or "continuation"). The duration of therapy is also subtype specific and may be quite prolonged (e.g., 2–3 years for ALL and LBL). Central nervous system (CNS) involvement is common in ALL, AML, LBL, and Burkitt lymphoma, and CNS-directed

Table 1.1 Common Acute and Late Effects for Patients Diagnosed with and Treated for Leukemia or Lymphoma

Effect	Risk Factors	Monitoring
Cardiomyopathy	Anthracyclines (e.g., doxorubicin) (cumulative dose) Cyclophosphamide (high-dose) Radiation (thoracic) Younger age	Electrocardiogram Echocardiogram
Pulmonary dysfunction	Bleomycin (cumulative dose) Busulfan Radiation (thoracic) Stem cell transplantation	Oxygen saturation Pulmonary function tests Imaging studies
Endocrinopathies	Alkylators (e.g., cyclophosphamide) (cumulative dose) Radiation (CNS, glandular) Corticosteroids Stem cell transplantation	Growth Sexual development & fertility Hormone levels
Altered body appearance and composition (e.g., alopecia, Cushing's, obesity), Metabolic syndrome	Corticosteroids (cumulative dose) Systemic chemotherapy Stem cell transplantation Radiation Reduced physical activity High caloric intake Female sex	Growth and development Body mass index Lipid profile
Infection (e.g., opportunistic, bacterial, fungal, viral)	Systemic chemotherapy Corticosteroids Stem cell transplantation Hodgkin lymphoma Central venous catheter	Blood counts Surveillance for infection Prophylactic interventions for prevention of infectious complications during periods of highest risk
Cytopenias with need for transfusion and associated complications (e.g., transfusion-transmitted infection; iron overload)	Systemic chemotherapy Stem cell transplantation	Blood counts Surveillance for bleeding
Neurocognitive dysfunction, Neuropsychologic dysfunction, Leukoen-cephalopathy	Intrathecal chemotherapy (e.g., Methotrexate, Cytarabine, Corticosteroids) Radiation (CNS) Female sex Younger age Environmental/Familial/Social	Neurodevel-opmental, Psychosocial, Cognitive, Educational, and Vocational assessments

(continued)

Table 1.1 (Continued)

Effect	Risk Factors	Monitoring
CNS hemorrhage, Stroke	L-asparaginase Hyperleukocytosis Radiation (CNS)	Neurologic examination Imaging studies
Neuropathies	Vinca alkaloids (cumulative dose) Cranial nerve infiltration	Neurologic examination
Ophthalmologic: Cataracts, Glaucoma, Visual impairment	Corticosteroids (cumulative dose) Stem cell transplantation Radiation (eye) Cranial nerve infiltration Orbital infiltration	Visual acuity Ophthalmologic examination
Osteopenia, Osteonecrosis	Corticosteroids (cumulative dose) Stem cell transplantation Caucasians Adolescents	Bone mineral density Imaging studies
Secondary malignancy	Alkylators (e.g., cyclophosphamide) (cumulative dose) Epipodophyllotoxins (e.g., etoposide) Stem cell transplantation Radiation	Complete blood count Imaging studies

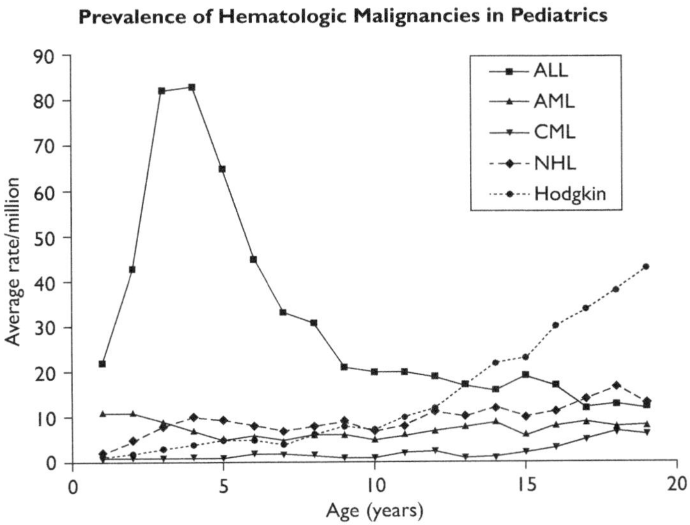

Figure 1.1 Age-Related Prevalence. Data from: Gloeckler L, Percy C, Bunin GR. Introduction. In: Cancer Incidence and Survival among Children and Adolescents: United States SEER Program 1975–1995, NIH Publication 1999; (99-4649): 1–16.

Table 1.2 General Approach to Treatment: Treatment Is Stratified Based on Diagnostic Subtype and Clinicopathologic Prognostic Risk Factors

Diagnosis	Therapy
ALL & LBL	Treatment phases (excluding mature B-cell) • Induction chemotherapy • Consolidation/Re-induction chemotherapy • Maintenance chemotherapy, total treatment duration 2–3 years • CNS treatment: intrathecal chemotherapy; +/- XRT if CNS involvement Mature B-ALL: as per Burkitt lymphoma regimens
AML	Treatment phases (excluding promyelocytic) • Induction chemotherapy • Consolidation chemotherapy • CNS treatment: intrathecal chemotherapy; +/- XRT if CNS involvement • Matched-sibling donor SCT (higher risk subtypes) Promyelocytic: Include all-*trans*-retinoic acid during induction and maintenance
JMML	Allogeneic SCT
CML	Tyrosine kinase inhibitors (e.g., imatinib mesylate) Allogeneic SCT
Burkitt lymphoma	Chemotherapy CNS treatment: intrathecal chemotherapy; +/- XRT if CNS involvement
Large cell lymphoma	Chemotherapy
Hodgkin lymphoma	Chemotherapy +/- local XRT

therapy is required for all individuals with those diagnoses. Allogeneic stem cell transplantation (SCT) is commonly utilized for individuals with the highest risk features (e.g., relapse). Radiation therapy (XRT) is infrequently employed in pediatric hematologic malignancies. Its use is reserved for local control of active disease involving the CNS or testes, certain cases of lymphoma, and for pretransplant conditioning (total body irradiation).

Neurocognitive and Psychosocial Concerns

Because disease prevalence is age related (Figure 1.1), the risks of long-term side effects, or late effects, are influenced by the state of organ development at the time of diagnosis and during treatment. Patients with leukemia and lymphoma are at particularly high risk for long-standing neurocognitive and neuropsychologic dysfunction due, in part, to the intensive therapy that these children receive. This is especially notable in those patients receiving CNS-directed therapy.[8–10] More recent retrospective evaluations of cohorts of patients treated for childhood ALL have demonstrated impairment rates of up to 60% across various neurocognitive domains in adult survivors, likely related to a combination of intensive intrathecal methotrexate and CNS radiation therapy.[10,11] Girls and younger children are at greatest risk of neurocognitive toxicities (Table 1.3).[8,9] As these impairments are often persistent and significant, ongoing monitoring of neurocognitive and psychological function is needed well into adulthood.[11] (See Chapter 18, Cognitive Sequelae.)

Table 1.3 Common Neurocognitive and Psychosocial Effects

Effect	Intervention
Neurocognitive dysfunction • IQ • Memory • Executive functions • Problem solving • Organizational skills • Visual perceptual and motor function • Information processing	Educational approaches (e.g., individualized education plans, accommodations, special services, assistive technologies, targeted learning and "re-training" approaches, selective environment) Compensatory techniques (e.g., organizational tools, environmental supports, occupational therapy) Vocational training
Neuropsychological dysfunction • Attention, concentration Risky behaviors Adjustment (school, work, relationships) • Social isolation • Adherence	Mental health specialist, neuropsychologist Behavioral therapy Behavioral therapy Support groups Social work and/or school counselor support Psychosocial service consultation for psychotherapy, cognitive behavioral therapy Pharmacologic approaches
Psychiatric manifestations • Anxiety • Depression • Post-traumatic stress	Mental health specialist Individual and group therapy Pharmacologic approaches
School absenteeism	Homebound schooling School re-entry program
Financial concerns • Healthcare expenses • Unemployment • Parental loss of work • Lack of insurance	Social work assessment Referral to local and national resources
Healthcare concerns • Complex multidisciplinary care needs • Inadequate insurance	Coordinated oncologic care followed by cancer survivorship care Social work support

The diagnosis and treatment of leukemias and lymphomas not only impacts the affected child, but also parents, siblings, extended family members, and their communities.[12] (See Chapter 24, Impact of Cancer on Family and Siblings.) In addition to the direct psychological effects that the diagnosis of cancer confers, there are substantial psychosocial consequences of the demands of treatment and associated toxicities (Tables 1.1 and 1.3).[13] Specific to ALL therapy, for instance, the use of steroids may lead to a Cushingoid appearance with altered body image, in addition to a sequale of medical complications including but not limited to the development of obesity, metabolic syndrome, and osteoporosis.

Prolonged school absenteeism can be anticipated during induction and consolidation chemotherapy and after stem cell transplantation, and the ability to arrange for intermittent school attendance is often restricted due to concerns about infection during periods of neutropenia and especially after bone marrow transplant. Homebound schooling can be arranged, but may further contribute to the sense of isolation due to reduced direct interaction with peers. Videoconferencing and other innovative strategies of communication that allow improved integration of the affected child into the school system may prove especially effective in patients with leukemia or lymphoma. (See Chapter 27, School and Peer Relationships, and Chapter 28, School and Academic Planning.) Maintenance therapy for ALL, which usually begins 9–12 months after the start of treatment, is often a good time for children to re-enter the school system and return to their usual routine.

Adolescents and young adults (AYA) are at particularly high risk for adverse consequences, for both medical and psychosocial issues.[14] The AYA population generally has worse outcomes, and may be at higher risk of relapse.[15] A specific emphasis on medication adherence, which may be especially challenging during the long periods of ALL maintenance therapy and also posttransplant, is an important consideration for which innovative strategies of monitoring may be indicated.[16] (See Chapter 16, Psychosocial Issues for Transplant Patients and Donors, and Chapter 17, Medication Adherence.) After completion of therapy, the AYA population often has significant barriers to obtaining healthcare during survivorship follow-up and monitoring. Specific attention to obtaining resources and medical insurance is needed to optimize their long-term care and overall quality of health. (See Chapter 33, Pediatric Cancer Survivors.)

Summary

Although leukemias and lymphomas are highly curable in pediatrics, diagnosis and treatment confer significant physical, psychological, and social risks that can have life-long impact.

- Children and adolescents with leukemia and lymphoma should receive systematic and serial neurocognitive and psychosocial assessments during and after treatment as part of comprehensive multidisciplinary care.

- Long-term follow-up is essential to monitor for possible relapse, treatment- and disease-associated toxicities, and secondary malignancies.
- Recommended guidelines for healthcare providers and patients/families are available from a number of sources (e.g., http://www.survivorshipguidelines.org).

References

1. Gloeckler L, Percy C, Bunin GR. Introduction. In: *Cancer Incidence and Survival among Children and Adolescents: United States SEER Program 1975-1995*. NIH Publication 99-4649. Bethesda, MD: National Institute of Health; 1999: 1–16.
2. Gloeckler Ries L, Mortality CC. In: Reis LAG SM, Gurney JG, et al. eds. *Cancer Incidence and Survival among Children and Adolescents: United States SEER Program 1975-1995. National Cancer Institute, SEER Program.* NIH Pub No. 99-4649. Bethesda, MD: National Cancer Institute; 1999: 165–170.
3. Oeffinger KC, Mertens AC, Sklar CA, et al. Chronic health conditions in adult survivors of childhood cancer. *N Engl J Med.* 2006;355(15):1572–1582.
4. Pui CH, Cheng C, Leung W, et al. Extended follow-up of long-term survivors of childhood acute lymphoblastic leukemia. *N Engl J Med* 2003;349(7):640–649.
5. Leung W, Hudson MM, Strickland DK, et al. Late effects of treatment in survivors of childhood acute myeloid leukemia. *J Clin Oncol.* 2000;18(18):3273–3279.
6. Pui CHe. *Childhood Leukemias*. 3rd ed. Cambridge, UK: Cambridge University Press; 2012.
7. Smith MA, Gloeckler Ries LA, Gurney JG, Ross J. Leukemia. In: Reis LAG SM, Gurney JG, et al., eds. *Cancer Incidence and Survival among Children and Adolescents: United States SEER Program 1975-1995*. National Cancer Institute, SEER Program. NIH Pub. No. 99-4649. Bethesda, MD: National Cancer Institute; 1999: 17–34.
8. Butler RW, Mulhern RK. Neurocognitive interventions for children and adolescents surviving cancer. *J Pediatr Psychol.* 2005;30(1):65–78.
9. Nathan PC, Patel SK, Dilley K, et al. Guidelines for identification of, advocacy for, and intervention in neurocognitive problems in survivors of childhood cancer: a report from the Children's Oncology Group. *Arch Pediatr Adolesc Med.* 2007;161(8):798–806.
10. Duffner PK, Armstrong FD, Chen L, et al. Neurocognitive and neuroradiologic central nervous system late effects in children treated on pediatric oncology group (POG) P9605 (standard risk) and P9201 (lesser risk) acute lymphoblastic leukemia protocols (ACCL0131): a methotrexate consequence? A report from the children's oncology group. *J Pediatr Hematol Oncol.* 2014;36(1):8–15.
11. Krull KR, Brinkman TM, Li C, et al. Neurocognitive outcomes decades after treatment for childhood acute lymphoblastic leukemia: a report from the st jude lifetime cohort study. *J Clin Oncol.* 2013;31(35):4407–4415.
12. Buchbinder D, Casillas J, Krull KR, et al. Psychological outcomes of siblings of cancer survivors: a report from the Childhood Cancer Survivor Study. *Psychooncology* 2011;20(12):1259–1268.
13. Zebrack BJ, Zeltzer LK, Whitton J, et al. Psychological outcomes in long-term survivors of childhood leukemia, Hodgkin's disease, and

non-Hodgkin's lymphoma: a report from the childhood cancer survivor study. *Pediatr.* 2002;110(1 Pt 1):42–52.

14. Zebrack B, Isaacson S. Psychosocial care of adolescent and young adult patients with cancer and survivors. *J Clin Oncol.* 2012;30(11):1221–1226.
15. Keegan TH, Tao L, Derouen MC, et al. Medical care in adolescents and young adult cancer survivors: what are the biggest access-related barriers? *J Cancer Surviv.* 2014;8(2):282–292.
16. Rohan JM, Drotar D, Alderfer M, et al. Electronic monitoring of medication adherence in early maintenance phase treatment for pediatric leukemia and lymphoma: Identifying patterns of nonadherence. *J Pediatr Psychol.* 2013; Epub ahead of print.

Chapter 2

Neuroblastoma

Giselle Saulnier Sholler

Neuroblastoma is the most common malignant solid tumor of childhood, and may be diagnosed as early as the prenatal period (by fetal ultrasound) or as late as young adulthood (Table 2.1). Most patients are from 3 months of age to 6 years.[1,2] Children may present with symptoms related to an abdominal mass, back or bone pain with limping, malaise, anemia, and occasionally orbital ecchymoses or skin nodules. Diagnosis is by surgical biopsy, or by bone marrow biopsy and urine sample for tumor markers (catecholamines). The child's treatment, which depends on the age, stage, and tumor biology, may range from biopsy only followed by observation for regression (low risk) to surgery, high dose chemotherapy, stem cell transplant, and immune therapies for advanced disease (high risk). Children diagnosed at less than one year of age usually have early stage disease with good outcome (survival may exceed 80–90%) and require minimal therapy. Children diagnosed after 12–18 months of age often have disease that has spread and require extensive therapy with lower chance of survival.[3,4]

Therapy

Large studies have shown that patients treated on clinical trials tend to have better survival. Most children will be eligible for such trials. These clinical trials (often called "protocols"), which include standard therapies as well as a novel component, are designed to improve survival. Sometimes protocols involve a randomization between standard therapy and standard therapy plus experimental therapies. During the protocol consent discussion between physicians and family, the parents will require time and professional help in order to understand the therapies and side effects (Tables 2.2 and 2.3). Parents should be informed that, if they decline to consent, they will be given the best known therapy with full medical staff support. Treatment of side effects is also an important component of treatment (Table 2.4). In some instances, in disorders with a particularly poor prognosis, discussions of palliative care are initiated at the time of diagnosis.

Table 2.1 Specific Neuroblastoma Syndromes

Perinatal neuroblastoma	• Neuroblastoma may be detected as a suprarenal mass by fetal ultrasound before birth, or in the newborn. • Current practice is to inform parents that most of these infants do not need treatment and to observe with repeated radiological scans.
Stage IVS (IV = Four and S = Special)	• Infants have small primary adrenal tumors but with liver infiltration and/or cells in the marrow cavity and/or in pale skin nodules. • Encourage parents that these infants do well in more than 90% of cases. • This unique kind of tumor shrinks over about 6 months without treatment, although rare cases may need surgical intervention or chemotherapy because an enlarged liver may compromise breathing. • Explain to parents that some patients have disease that may progress initially, and "watching" the tumor shrink may be stressful.
Opsoclonus-Myoclonus (neurological syndrome of 'dancing' eye movements and/or muscle jerks with dis-coordination almost always associated with early Stage I-II tumors)	• It is very likely their child will survive; this neurological syndrome can improve with chemotherapy and immunotherapy with prednisone and gammaglobulin, but some children can have life-long neurological complications.
Spinal Cord compression by tumor	• If treated rapidly, the nerve damage improves over time with surgery, radiation, or chemotherapy. • Patients may have residual weakness or paralysis.
Horner's Syndrome (unilateral facial paralysis from neck tumor)	• This mild asymmetry of the face may be permanent.
Profuse diarrhea secondary to increased hormone (VIP) secretion	• This syndrome abates with chemotherapy.

Table 2.2 Common Questions Asked by Parents During the Diagnostic Period

Question	Parent Education and Management Suggestions
What caused the tumor?	• Neuroblastoma occurs in all populations throughout the world. • Provide parents information that the cause is currently unknown. • Recent studies have linked an inherited gene, ALK, with neuroblastoma in approximately 7% of patients. Children may be tested for this.
What about environment/ diet?	• Environmental studies have not found a cause.

(continued)

Question	Parent Education and Management Suggestions
Was my child born with the disease?	• There is evidence that occasionally neuroblastoma may start in the fetus, but no links have been found to maternal health.
Could the cancer have been found earlier?	• Timing of diagnosis has not been shown to change the outcome. • High-risk neuroblastoma is a rapidly arising tumor in children greater than one year at diagnosis. It is often not present long before diagnosis.
What will the diagnostic testing be like for my child?	• Diagnostic testing by several different radiologic procedures are required. These often require sedation so the child will be able to remain still. The child may be hungry and irritable beforehand and when he or she wakes up. Biopsy of the tumor and bone marrow will be done under sedation and may require pain medication afterwards.
Will my child need surgery?	• The child may require a central venous line placement for chemotherapy. • Surgery to remove all or part of a tumor may be needed. The child's pain will be treated hour by hour with medicine and he or she will be up and about usually in 1–3 days depending on the extent of surgery.
Will I be able to continue working?	• The impact of intensive treatments should be discussed with parents, particularly with regard to support available to the family and employment options. • One parent may be required to take time away from work to be with the child throughout treatment. • Offer to call, write letters to employers, and assist with family medical leave forms. • Assist with communication with the child's school. It may be possible for the child to keep up with schoolwork in hospital if hospital educators are present.
What about my other child(ren)?	• Suggest the parent(s) ask family and friends for help, shared parenting if possible (weekdays, weekends, week nights). • Encourage the involvement, understanding, and frequent presence of siblings. • Refer siblings to sibling support programs within the hospital if available or within the community.
Will my child die?	• At diagnosis, the therapy given is expected to cure the child. • Support with encouragement that survival is the goal and therapies continually improve. • It is important to remain aware that some tumors will be resistant to therapy and not all children will survive; this will only be known months to years after the initial diagnosis.

Table 2.3 Concerns Surrounding Initiation of Treatment

Concern	Parent Education and Management Suggestions
Will the chemotherapy cause immediate sickness, vomiting and/or pain?	• Provide information that many children play and have no side effects as the drugs infuse. • Supportive medicines are given to prevent nausea before it occurs and can be adjusted for each child as needed. • Nausea or pain may develop over days, but will be treated to minimize or omit their symptoms.
What will happen when we go home?	• Children will not be discharged until it is considered safe. Some patients may require IV nutrition and/or pain medication, which may be able to be given at home. • Some children will require daily subcutaneous shots with G-CSF to help boost the immune system. Nurses can help teach parents how to administer injections. • Due to risk of infections, lifestyle adjustments will be necessary. Fevers can be life threatening and parents need to be instructed to call their physician immediately if a fever occurs. • Most children will resume normal activities, including eating, and many return to school as their energy rebounds.
Should I make my child eat? Should he/she follow a certain diet or take vitamins?	• Certain vitamins may interact with chemotherapy and it is important to encourage parents to discuss all supplements with their physician before taking them. • Chemotherapy may change the child's taste preferences. Encourage parents to have their child try different foods to find those he/she likes to eat. Encourage children to help choose foods to eat and eating times.
What should I be concerned about at home?	• Caution that the parent should call the medical-care team at any time for any fever or any new symptoms. • Parents should call if they are worried about their child for any reason.
How quickly will the tumor shrink?	• Most children may have fewer symptoms from the cancer as early as the first few weeks after chemotherapy, suggesting improvement. • Radiology scans and other repeat tests are generally scheduled 2–3 months later, when future therapies need to be determined and scheduled.

Table 2.4 Common Chemotherapy Side Effects

Side Effect	Parent Education and Management Suggestions
Vincristine: Constipation Peripheral neuropathy Pain	• Parents should keep track of stool frequency and consistency. • Therapy with prescribed laxative medications should be given. • Numbness, tingling, or mild weakness in the hands or feet is possible and usually resolves over time. • Pain is reversible and will subside over several days to a week if Vincristine is decreased or omitted. • Inform parents that Tylenol should not be given unless they have spoken with the child's physician and only after a temperature check, since it may mask the presence of fever and infection. • Opiates may be prescribed if pain is significant.
Platinum: Hearing Loss	• Hearing loss can increase over time with recurrent exposures of this drug. • Patients will be monitored with hearing tests to prevent significant loss, but some children will need hearing aids.
Retinoic Acid	• Side effects such as dry, chapped lips can be treated topically.

Bone Marrow Transplant (BMT)

Bone Marrow Transplant includes very high dose chemotherapy with stem cell rescue for Stage IV and high-risk Stage III patients, given as one or two transplants successively (Table 2.5).

Therapeutic Options for the Child Who Relapses

There is currently no standard therapy for children who relapse. Explore options with the family taking into consideration those that are most suitable for the child and family's expectations:

- New chemotherapy with standard drugs.
- Experimental therapies, including Phase I and II trials, should also be considered if part of a clinical trial.
- Radiation therapy to sites of symptomatic masses or to bone disease to help with pain and symptoms.
- Nonstandard holistic therapies chosen from outside of the medical center (see Chapter 21, Integrative Oncology).
- No therapy with curative goal—Supportive care to manage symptoms and promote quality time with family including family trips and time for increased sibling involvement (see Chapter 11, Pain, and Chapter 30, Integrating Palliative Care).

Table 2.5 Concerns Surrounding BMT

Concern	Parent Education and Management Suggestions
Fear of "high dose" therapy	• Children will experience similar side effects as with standard chemotherapy, although older patients may have more nausea-vomiting during therapy. Other side effects, such as mucositis, may be more severe.
Fear of the early weeks after stem cell infusion when the child has very low blood cells	• Patients will be given almost daily transfusions, antibiotics, and will be given IV nutrition as well as opiates for mucositis mouth pain. • The child may prefer to rest in bed most of the day, but many patients feel better in the third week. • Gently inform parents that fatalities are rare but may occur.
Distress with isolation in specially filtered room, boredom, inability to have visitors, exhaustion	• Shared parent-family "shifts" may help to give caregivers a break. • A planned daily schedule (washing up, mouth care, out-of-bed-to-chair, TV time, book time, craft time, etc.) is helpful. • Daily phone calls or e-mails to and from family and friends are helpful. • Creating a free, personalized webpage through programs such as Care Pages or Caring Bridge can help families keep others abreast of their child's progress.
Antineuroblastoma antibody therapy posttransplant	• Side effects of pain and numbness during infusion will be treated aggressively.

Symptom Relief for the Child Who Is Dying

- Children with neuroblastoma may experience worsening bone pain, fever-infections, massive liver enlargement, lung infiltration, or sometimes bony growths on scalp and trunk. This may occur over weeks to months.
- Reassure family that aggressive pain and symptom control will be provided and involvement with a hospice team is recommended.
- Decision for continuation of transfusions is individual. Transfusions can help alleviate some side effects such as fatigue from anemia and bleeding due to low platelet counts, but it may become difficult and painful to transport child to the hospital and the decision to stop transfusions is acceptable. A balance of the advantages and disadvantages are usually different for each family.
- Communicate openly with parents and encourage honest discussions with relatives, siblings, and the patient, if age appropriate.
- Encourage sibling involvement, even if distressing, to alleviate future survival guilt.
- Integrate palliative care principles. (See Chapter 30, Integrating Palliative Care).

References

1. American Cancer Society. *Cancer Facts and Figures*. Atlanta, GA: Author; 2008.
2. Bernstein ML, et al., A population-based study of neuroblastoma incidence, survival, and mortality in North America. *J Clin Oncol*. 1992: 10(2):323–329.
3. Brodeur GM, et al., Revisions of the international criteria for neuroblastoma diagnosis, staging, and response to treatment. *J Clin Oncol*. 1993: 11(8):1466–1477.
4. Park JR, Eggert A, Caron H. Neuroblastoma: biology, prognosis, and treatment. *Pediatr Clin North Am*. 2008;55(1):97–120.

Chapter 3

Wilms Tumor

Jeffrey S. Dome

Pediatric kidney tumors comprise approximately 7% of cancers in children and adolescents.[1] The vast majority are Wilms tumor, though other tumor types such as renal cell carcinoma, clear cell sarcoma of the kidney, malignant rhabdoid tumor, congenital mesoblastic nephroma, and renal sarcomas are occasionally encountered. Wilms tumor is historically important because it was one of the first malignancies to be treated with a multidisciplinary approach involving surgeons, pediatric oncologists, and radiation oncologists. With multimodality therapy, cure rates have risen to 85–90%.[2] Additionally, biological studies of Wilms tumor have provided a paradigm for our understanding cancer genetics.[2] Although the majority of patients with Wilms tumor are cured, patients and families face significant psychosocial challenges at diagnosis, during treatment, and after completion of therapy (Table 3.1). The total care of a patient involves a multidisciplinary approach that includes family support measures to optimize the quality of life.

Diagnosis of Wilms Tumor

- The average age of a child at the time of Wilms tumor diagnosis is about 3.5 years, although older children and adults may develop the disease.[3]
- In North America, there is a slight predisposition to Wilms tumor in girls compared to boys.
- The tumor presents as an abdominal mass and is often discovered incidentally by parents giving their child a bath or by a healthcare provider during a routine physical exam.
- Children with Wilms tumor usually appear healthy but may have abdominal pain, fever, or hematuria.
- Physical examination reveals high blood pressure in about 25% of patients.
- Once an abdominal mass is detected, patients undergo an abdominal ultrasound and computed-tomography (CT) scan.
- The most common sites of spread for Wilms tumor are the lymph nodes, lung, and liver.
- Wilms tumor can also migrate through blood vessels and grow into the renal vein, inferior vena cava, and, occasionally, the heart.

- Based on this pattern of spread, Doppler ultrasound of the abdominal veins and CT scan of the chest have become a routine part of the initial evaluation.
- Wilms tumor cannot be distinguished from other kidney tumors on the basis of imaging studies alone—the diagnosis must be made by obtaining a tissue sample.
- The Children's Oncology Group (COG), based in North America, advocates surgical resection at the time of diagnosis in order to yield the most accurate staging information. The International Society of Pediatric Oncology (SIOP), based in Europe, recommends several weeks of pre-operative chemotherapy with the aim of decreasing tumor size to facilitate the surgery.

Table 3.1 Medical and Psychosocial Considerations throughout Wilms Tumor Therapy

Phase of Therapy	Medical Considerations	Psychosocial Considerations
Diagnosis	• Radiology studies (x-rays, ultrasounds, CT scans) to evaluation extent of disease • Surgery to remove the tumor or biopsy to establish the diagnosis • Placement of central catheter to administer chemotherapy	Parents: • Difficulty accepting and adjusting to the diagnosis • Guilt associated with not making the diagnosis sooner • Guilt about what caused the tumor and whether it could have been prevented • Questions about risks to other family members
On Treatment	• Favorable Wilms tumor: 19–31 weeks of outpatient chemotherapy; radiation therapy for stage III/IV disease • Anaplastic Wilms tumor: 25–36 weeks of inpatient and outpatient chemotherapy; radiation therapy for all patients	*For both favorable and anaplastic Wilms tumor* Child: • Disruption to the patient's schooling and activities • Hair loss and other changes in appearance, affecting the patient's image and self-esteem Parents: • Disruption to the parents' jobs and the normal family routine • Financial concerns from costly treatment and absence from work
Completion of Therapy	• Radiology studies and physical exam at the end of therapy and every 3–6 months for 4 years • Monitoring for late effects of treatment	• Acclimation back to normal routine • Anxiety about tumor recurrence • Anxiety about long-term effects of therapy

Parental Questions and Concerns

Guilt

After overcoming the initial shock of the diagnosis of Wilms tumor, it is very common for families to experience feelings of guilt. They may scrutinize recent events and question whether aches, behavioral changes, or other symptoms should have tipped them off to the diagnosis sooner. It is important for clinicians to apprise families of certain facts to assuage guilty emotions.

- It is very unlikely that the tumor could have been detected earlier.
- Because Wilms tumor affects only one in 10,000 children, it is understandable that primary-care providers would not consider Wilms tumor in the differential diagnosis for common childhood ailments.
- Studies estimate that Wilms tumors can double in size every two weeks, so even large tumors are undetectable up until a few weeks before the diagnosis is rendered.

Was the tumor preventable?

- A case-control study found an association with the paternal occupations of vehicle mechanics, auto body repairmen, and welders, though no unifying exposure could be established.[4]
- On the maternal side, small studies suggested possible associations with cigarette smoking, coffee/tea drinking, exposure to sex hormones, vaginal infections, and the use of hair coloring products during pregnancy, though none of these factors were confirmed by a subsequent case-control study.[5]
- Even if the risk for Wilms tumor increases with certain occupations or exposures, the chance of developing the disease remains exceptionally small.

Siblings

Families worry about the siblings of the affected child, though only 1.5% of patients with Wilms tumor have an affected relative.[6] Included in this 1.5% are distant relatives, so it is even less likely for a sibling to be affected. Although inborn genetic alterations that predispose to Wilms tumor have been identified, genetic testing is not routinely recommended for patients or siblings. Testing is generally reserved for patients who have clinical features of genetic syndromes or a family history of Wilms tumor.[7]

Prognosis

A common pitfall of healthcare professionals is to assure families that "if you could choose any cancer, Wilms tumor is the best one to have." Given the excellent prognosis for favorable histology (nonanaplastic) Wilms tumor, this is true to some extent. However, anaplastic Wilms tumor, malignant rhabdoid tumor, and renal cell carcinoma carry considerably worse prognoses than favorable histology Wilms tumor. Because at least 15% of children have "unfavorable histology" kidney tumors, providers should refrain from conveying optimistic statistics until a final diagnosis is rendered.

Prognostic Factors

Several clinical and biological prognostic factors are used to determine the level and intensity of Wilms tumor therapy. The most powerful prognostic indicators are tumor stage and histology.

Tumor Stage

- Stage I tumors are localized to the kidney and removed completely during surgery with no residual disease.
- Stage II tumors demonstrate invasion of blood vessels or tissues surrounding the kidney, but are completed removed during surgery without residual disease.
- Stage III tumors have tumor involvement of local lymph nodes, tumor spillage in the abdominal cavity, or residual tumor remaining after surgery.
- Stage IV tumors have spread to distant sites.
- Stage V is a special designation for bilateral Wilms tumor, involving both kidneys. Advanced-stage tumors (stages III–V) require more chemotherapy and radiation therapy than low-stage tumors (I–II). However, even with advanced stage, the majority of patients with Wilms tumor are cured.

Tumor Histology

- About 8% of Wilms tumors contain large and irregular cells that are termed "anaplastic." Anaplastic Wilms tumors have considerably poorer prognosis than tumors without anaplasia (called "favorable histology"), with survival rates of only 50%.[8]

Genetic Biomarkers

- A genetic change in the tumor tissue called loss of heterozygosity (LOH) at chromosomes 1p and 16q is associated with increased risk of relapse.[9] Recently completed COG studies assessed whether augmentation of therapy improves outcome for patients whose tumors contain LOH. The results are not yet available.
- Gain of chromosome 1q in the tumor tissue has also been shown to be associated with increased risk of relapse.[10] Future COG studies will use 1q status to guide treatment.

Treatment

The dramatic advances in Wilms tumor therapy are a testimony to the efforts of large international cooperative groups such as the National Wilms Tumor Study Group (merged into the COG in 2002) and SIOP. In order to expand upon past successes, it is recommended that all children be treated as part of a clinical trial.

The selection of chemotherapy is based on tumor stage and histology. The most widely used drugs for Wilms tumor are vincristine, dactinomycin, doxorubicin, cyclophosphamide, etoposide, ifosfamide, and carboplatin. In general, only vincristine and dactinomycin are required for patients with stage I or II favorable histology Wilms tumor. Patients with stages III and IV favorable histology Wilms tumor receive vincristine, dactinomycin, and doxorubicin, along with radiation to affected areas. Patients with anaplastic Wilms tumor require the aforementioned therapy plus additional drugs such as cyclophosphamide, carboplatin, and etoposide.

Impact of Wilms tumor therapy on the Family

- Chemotherapy regimens for favorable histology Wilms tumor are given on an outpatient basis and last 19–31 weeks. Patients are evaluated by their oncologist once a week and are often able to attend school and maintain their usual activity. The most common acute side effects are hair loss, nausea, vomiting, constipation, abdominal pain, and neuropathies such as difficulty walking (Table 3.2). Blood clots and infections related to the presence of a central venous catheter may also occur.
- The treatment of anaplastic Wilms tumor is more disruptive to families. Every three weeks, children must receive 2–5 consecutive days of chemotherapy that is administered over several hours in the inpatient hospital setting, although some centers with extended clinic hours give this treatment in the outpatient clinic. The major side effect of therapy for anaplastic Wilms tumor is low blood counts, which places patients at risk for bleeding and infection. Patients are often admitted to the hospital for fevers.
- For both favorable histology and anaplastic Wilms tumor, the inconvenience of frequent clinic visits and the acute toxicities of treatment pose formidable psychosocial challenges. Patients miss school and other activities, which can affect grades and interfere with goals and aspirations.
- Changes in the child's appearance may affect self-esteem and interactions with peers. Hair loss is particularly concerning for adolescents, but it may be less of a concern for preschool and school-age patients.
- The impact on the family should not be underestimated. Parents typically have multiple absences from work, which can lead to financial pressure, especially if medical insurance does not fully cover the expenses of treatment.
- Siblings also are affected because parents become preoccupied with the patient and may not prioritize the needs of siblings. It is important to engage them in the treatment process. Some oncology centers have special programs for siblings to promote a sense of inclusion.

Completion of Therapy

The end of treatment is a time of mixed emotions for patients and families. On one hand, they welcome a return to normalcy. On the other hand, they feel nervous about the decreased frequency of doctor visits and worry about the prospect of relapse.

Table 3.2 Short and Long-Term Toxicities of Wilms Tumor Treatment

Drug	Short-term Toxicities	Long-term Toxicities
Vincristine	Hair loss, constipation, jaw pain, abdominal pain, drooping of eyelid, loss of reflexes, muscle weakness, foot drop with difficulty walking, fluid retention,* seizures,* burning of skin if drug escapes the vein	
Dactinomycin	Nausea, vomiting, hair loss, low blood counts predisposing to bleeding and infection, diarrhea, liver damage,* burning of skin if drug escapes the vein	
Doxorubicin	Nausea, vomiting, hair loss, low blood counts predisposing to bleeding and infection, mouth sores, temporary red discoloration of urine	Decreased heart function, heart failure,* irregular heart rhythm*
Etoposide	Nausea, vomiting, hair loss, low blood counts predisposing to bleeding and infection, mouth sores, allergic reactions	leukemia*
Cyclophosphamide	Nausea, vomiting, hair loss, low blood counts predisposing to bleeding and infection, inflammation of the bladder that causes pain or blood in the urine, fluid retention,* blurred vision*	Infertility, second cancer*
Carboplatin	Nausea, vomiting, hair loss, low blood counts leading to higher risk for bleeding and infection	Hearing loss
Ifosfamide	Nausea, vomiting, hair loss, low blood counts predisposing to bleeding and infection, inflammation of the bladder, sleepiness, confusion or altered behavior, weakness, seizures,* coma,* kidney damage	Infertility, second cancer*
Radiation therapy	Red or brown discoloration of skin, nausea, vomiting, low blood counts leading to higher risk for bleeding and infection, liver or lung damage	Decreased height, infertility, premature births and low birth weight in children of female Wilms tumor survivors, second cancer in area of radiation*
Other		Kidney failure (most common in patients with bilateral Wilms tumor)*

* Indicates rare side effect.

- Most Wilms tumor recurrences occur within two years of diagnosis, with the risk of recurrence decreasing as time elapses.
- After therapy, patients with Wilms tumor typically are evaluated with physical exams and radiology studies every 3 months for 2 years, every 6 months for another 2 years, and then yearly.
- The days or weeks leading up to these visits are commonly anxiety ridden for parents and sometimes the patients themselves.
- Although unease about recurrence never disappears completely, it dissipates with time.
- See Chapter 33, Pediatric Cancer Survivors.

Late Effects

It is uncommon for Wilms tumor survivors treated with only vincristine and dactinomycin to have late effects (Table 3.2). However, survivors treated with anthracyclines, cyclophosphamide, ifosfamide, carboplatin, etoposide, and radiation therapy may have serious complications related to therapy, including second cancers, heart failure, infertility, issues related to pregnancy, and kidney failure (Table 3.2).[11] It is ideal for Wilms tumor survivors to receive life-long follow-up in a clinic with expertise in the area of long-term follow-up for childhood cancer.

References

1. Howlader N, Noone A, Krapcho M, et al. SEER Cancer Statistics Review, 1975-2008, 2011 [cited; Available from: http://seer.cancer.gov/csr/1975_2008/</csr/1975_2008/>
2. Fernandez C, Geller JI, Ehrlich PF, et al. Renal tumors. In: Pizzo PA, Poplack, D.G., eds. *Principles and Practice of Pediatric Oncology*. Philadelphia, PA: Lippincott Williams & Wilkins; 2011.
3. Breslow N, Olshan A, Beckwith JB, Green DM. Epidemiology of Wilms tumor. *Med Pediatr Oncol*. 1993;21:172–181.
4. Olshan A, Breslow N, Daling JR, et al. Wilms Tumor and paternal occupation. *Cancer Res*. 1990;50:3212–3217.
5. Olshan A, Breslow N, Faletta JM, et al. Risk factors for Wilms Tumor; report from the National Wilms Tumor Study. *Cancer*. 1993;72:938–944.
6. Breslow NE, Olson J, Moksness J, Beckwith JB, Grundy P. Familial Wilms' tumor: a descriptive study. *Med & Pediatr Oncol*. 1996;27:398–403.
7. Dome JS, Huff V. Wilms Tumor Overview. In: Pagon RA, Adam MP, Bird TD, et al., eds. *GeneReviews*. Seattle, WA: University of Washington; 2013.
8. Dome JS, Cotton CA, Perlman EJ, et al. Treatment of anaplastic histology Wilms' tumor: results from the fifth National Wilms' Tumor Study. *J Clin Oncol*. 2006;24:2352–2358.
9. Grundy PE, Breslow NE, Li S, et al. Loss of heterozygosity for chromosomes 1p and 16q is an adverse prognostic factor in favorable-histology Wilms tumor: a report from the National Wilms Tumor Study Group. *J Clin Oncol*. 2005;23:7312–7321.

10. Gratias EJ, Jennings LJ, Anderson JR, Dome JS, Grundy P, Perlman EJ. Gain of 1q is associated with inferior event-free and overall survival in patients with favorable histology Wilms tumor: A report from the Children's Oncology Group. *Cancer.* 2013;119:3887–3894.
11. Sadak KT, Ritchey ML, Dome JS. Paediatric genitourinary cancers and late effects of treatment. *Nature Rev Urol.* 2013;10:15–25.

Chapter 4

Retinoblastoma

Debra L. Friedman and Anna T. Meadows

Retinoblastoma is a rare malignant tumor of the retina, a thin layer of nerve tissue in the back of the eye that is responsible for vision. When the tumor is limited to the orbit, most children can be cured. However, if it has spread to other organs, it is difficult to treat and a cure may not be possible. This is a disease of very young children, and it has genetic implications. Potential loss of vision and its developmental implications, as well as the increased risk of future cancers in a subset of patients, requires consideration of long-term psychosocial impact on affected children and their parents.

Epidemiology[1–4]

- Retinoblastoma is the most common intraocular malignancy of childhood, occurring in 1 in 20,000 live births.
- Retinoblastoma tumors result from changes or mutations in both copies of the RB1 gene, a tumor suppressor gene located on chromosome 13q14.
- Approximately 40% of cases are hereditary. These patients have a germline mutation in the RB1 gene, which is present in every cell of the body. Most (85%) of these are new spontaneous mutations (sporadic), whereas the remaining 15% have a positive family history (familial). Postconception, a second somatic mutation occurs in the remaining RB1 gene in one or more retinoblasts resulting in tumorigenesis. Generally, these patients present with bilateral disease and multiple tumors in each eye in the first year of life. All children with bilateral disease have the germline form.
- The remaining 60% of cases are nonhereditary, presenting with unilateral and unifocal disease in the second and third years of life. These patients inherit two normal copies of the RB1 gene. Postconception, two somatic mutations occur, one in each copy of the RB1 gene in a retinoblast causing tumor formation.
- About 15% of unilateral cases will also have the germline form, but in the absence of a positive family history, those cases cannot be identified without genetic screening. (See Chapter 7, Hereditary Cancer Syndromes.)
- Genetic testing is available, which is becoming much more accurate, but it should be accompanied by counseling regarding the results.

Table 4.1 Psychosocial Considerations of Retinoblastoma[5–11]

Risk for impaired psychosocial well-being	Screening and interventions; Evidence-based treatments are limited and need more research.
Life-threatening experience of cancer (although cure following intraocular disease is almost universal)	Screening evaluation of psychosocial supports of the child and family by social work or psychology.
Adverse effects from chemotherapy, radiation therapy and surgery	• Symptom control for side effects of therapy—nausea, emesis, pain, decreased nutritional intake. • Assist patients and family to manage the effects of the cancer and its treatment, including need for hospitalizations, surgeries and examinations under anesthesia, complications of therapy, potential loss of the eye or vision.
Loss of an eye in those treated with enucleation	Counseling to help the child/family prepare for and cope with the loss of an eye is critical. Prepare child and family for surgery, for obtaining a prosthesis and the need to be refitted as the child grows.
Challenges related to impaired vision in children. Although few children with retinoblastoma become completely blind, vision may be impaired in ways that can affect development and school performance	• Working collaboratively with social work, referral for services to assist with impaired vision; neuropsychological testing for educational problems (see Chapter 18, Cognitive Sequelae). • Recommend that parents obtain an Individualized Education Plan (IEP) or a 504 plan through the school district (see Chapter 18, School and Academic Planning), and access services for visually impaired individuals at the local or state level as needed. • Assessment for child and family counseling.
Cosmetic changes and body image disturbance	Supportive care for anxiety; counseling for body image concerns
Continued risk and need for surveillance for second cancers	Supportive care for anxiety related to recurrence risk and development of second cancers; expert genetic counseling regarding the risk for siblings and offspring.
Increased familial risks of retinoblastoma in siblings and offspring • Questions about genetic factors and risk	All families of children with retinoblastoma should have genetic counseling in order to clarify the potential role of heredity and to determine which children with unilateral disease carry the mutation. (See Chapter 8, Genetic Counseling for Hereditary Cancers.)

Clinical Considerations

Presentation[12]

- Leukocoria.
- Strabismus.

- Decreased visual acuity.
- Inflammatory changes.
- Hyphema.
- Vitreous hemorrhage.

Diagnosis

- Screening performed during well-child check-ups by eliciting red reflexes in the eye.
- Definitive diagnosis made by ophthalmologists and oncologists using a combination of an examination performed while under anesthesia (EUA), retinal camera (RetCam) imaging, ultrasound, CT or MRI, and laboratory studies.[12]

Treatment[13–15]

- Systemic chemotherapy.
- External beam radiotherapy.
- Local plaque radiotherapy.
- Local ophthalmic therapy, such as cryotherapy and thermotherapy.
- Local administration of chemotherapy—subtenon, intravitreous, and most recently selective intra-arterial.
- Enucleation.

Posttreatment Management[16–18]

- Pediatric oncologists and ocular ophthalmologists follow these patients for disease recurrence using examination, imaging and lab studies.
- Children with enucleations are referred to prosthetics for artificial eye production.
- Services for blind or visually impaired children are accessed as early as possible for help with developmental challenges and emotional adjustment.
- Visual acuity is assessed at least annually.
- Patients are followed for long-term effects of chemotherapy and radiotherapy, namely growth and development.
- Individuals with the germline form of retinoblastoma are at a very increased risk for development of second malignancies and require lifelong surveillance for this.
- Both patients and their parents are at risk for adverse psychosocial consequences (Table 4.1).

References

1. Broaddus E, Topham A, Singh AD. Incidence of retinoblastoma in the USA: 1975–2004. *Br J Ophthalmol.* 2009;93(1):21–23.
2. Broaddus E, Topham A, Singh AD. Survival with retinoblastoma in the USA: 1975–2004. *Br J Ophthalmol.* 2009;93(1):24–27.
3. Clark RD, Mansfield NC. Retinoblastoma: Genetic testing and counseling. In: Singh AD, Damato BE, Pe'er J, Murphree AL, Perry JD, eds. *Clinical Ophthalmic Oncology.* Philadelphia, PA: Saunders Elsevier; 2007:441–446.

4. Murphree AL, Singh AD. Heritable retinoblastoma: The RB1 cancer predisposition syndrome. In: Singh AD, Damato BE, Pe'er J, Murphree AL, Perry JD, eds. *Clinical Opththalmic Oncology*. Philadelphia, PA: Sanders Elsevier; 2007:428–433.
5. van Dijk J, Grootenhuis MA, Imhof SM, Cohen-Kettenis PT, Moll AC, Huisman J. Coping strategies of retinoblastoma survivors in relation to behavioural problems. *Psychooncology*. 2009;18(12):1281–1289.
6. van Dijk J, Huisman J, Moll AC, et al. Health-related quality of life of child and adolescent retinoblastoma survivors in the Netherlands. *Health Qual Life Outcomes*. 2007;5:65. PMCID: 2219958.
7. van Dijk J, Imhof SM, Moll AC, Ringens PJ, Cohen-Kettenis PT, Rijmen F, Huisman J. Quality of life of adult retinoblastoma survivors in the Netherlands. *Health Qual Life Outcomes*. 2007;5:30. PMCID: 1894785.
8. van Dijk J, Oostrom KJ, Huisman J, Moll AC, Cohen-Kettenis PT, Ringens PJ, Imhof SM. Restrictions in daily life after retinoblastoma from the perspective of the survivors. *Pediatr Blood Cancer*. 2010;54(1):110–115.
9. van Dijk J, Oostrom KJ, Imhof SM, Moll AC, Schouten-van Meeteren AY, Bezemer PD, Huisman J. Behavioural functioning of retinoblastoma survivors. *Psychooncology*. 2009;18(1):87–95.
10. Weintraub N, Rot I, Shoshani N, Pe'er J, Weintraub M. Participation in daily activities and quality of life in survivors of retinoblastoma. *Pediatr Blood Cancer*. 2011;56(4):590–594.
11. Sheppard L, Eiser C, Kingston J. Mothers' perceptions of children's quality of life following early diagnosis and treatment for retinoblastoma (Rb). *Child Care Health Dev*. 2005;31(2):137–142.
12. Abramson DH, Beaverson K, Sangani P, et al. Screening for retinoblastoma: Presenting signs as prognosticators of patient and ocular survival. *Pediatrics*. 2003;112(6, Pt. 1):1248–1255.
13. Jubran, RF, Villablanca JG, Meadows AT. Chemotherapy for retinoblastoma: An overview. In: Singh AD, Damato BE, Pe'er J, Murphree AL, Perry JD, eds. *Clinical ophthalmic oncology*. Philadelphia, PA: Saunders Elsevier; 2007:449–453.
14. Murphree AL. Local therapy, brachytherapy and enucleation. In: Singh AD, Damato BE, Pe'er J, Murphree AL, Perry JD, eds. *Clinical Ophthalmic Oncology*. Philadelphia, PA: Sanders Elsevier; 2007:454–461.
15. Shields CL, Shields JA. Retinoblastoma management: advances in enucleation, intravenous chemoreduction, and intra-arterial chemotherapy. *Curr Opin Ophthalmol*. 2010;21(3):203–212.
16. Fletcher O, Easton D, Anderson K, Gilham C, Jay M, Peto J. Lifetime risks of common cancers among retinoblastoma survivors. *J Natl Cancer Inst*. 2004:96(5):357–363.
17. Marees T, Moll AC, Imhof SM, de Boer MR, Ringens PJ, van Leeuwen FE. Risk of second malignancies in survivors of retinoblastoma: more than 40 years of follow-up. *J Natl Cancer Inst*. 2008;100(24):1771–1779.
18. Yu CL, Tucker MA, Abramson DH, Furukawa K, Seddon JM, Stovall M, Fraumeni JF, Jr., Kleinerman RA. Cause-specific mortality in long-term survivors of retinoblastoma. *J Natl Cancer Inst*. 2009;101(8):581–591. PMCID: 2669101.

Chapter 5

Sarcomas and Other Solid Tumors

Melinda Merchant and Matthew Wright

Sarcoma is derived from the Greek word for flesh and refers to a malignancy that arises in bone (osteosarcoma), muscle (rhabdomyosarcoma), or other soft tissues of the body (e.g., Ewing sarcoma or synovial sarcoma).[1,2] Pain and swelling are common symptoms that may lead to diagnosis of sarcoma. Extremity sarcomas can cause palpable masses even if small; however, sarcomas that develop in the pelvis or thorax will often grow to a larger size before detection so that patients may have multiple medical visits prior to an actual diagnosis. The exact treatment of sarcomas will be dependent on the histology and molecular biology of the biopsy sample as well as the stage of disease. The presence of metastatic disease indicates high risk, whereas the low- and intermediate-risk definitions are determined by cooperative group treatment studies. Cancers of liver (hepatoblastoma) or head and neck (nasopharyngeal carcinoma) that are not covered in specific chapters also undergo treatments similar to sarcomas. These therapies may cause both physical and psychological dysfunction and require a comprehensive plan for support services.

Therapy

The treatment of children with solid tumors requires the teamwork of experts from many disciplines. In addition to pediatric oncologists, surgeons, orthopedic oncologists, and radiation oncologists, important contributors to this team include physical or occupational therapists, child-life specialists, child psychologists and psychiatrists. Although some low risk nonrhabdomysarcoma soft tissue sarcomas may be treated with surgery alone, the majority of pediatric solid tumors require multi-agent chemotherapy regimens. The roadmap for treatment of intermediate or high-risk tumors often calls for months of therapy. Aggressive therapies for solid tumors can present psychosocial challenges for patients and families both during and after active treatment. An understanding of the range of local and systemic implications of these therapies as well as the potential complications will enable the multidisciplinary team to provide medical and psychological support for the child, caregivers, and siblings or extended family (Table 5.1).

Table 5.1 Common Treatments for Pediatric Solid Tumors

Treatment	General Principles	Education or Management Suggestions
General Surgery	• En bloc resections with wide margins. • If negative margins cannot be achieved at resection, postoperative radiation therapy is often recommended. • Abdominal surgery for pediatric solid tumors. • Surgical tumor debulking, radiation, or intraperitoneal chemotherapy may be considered for certain tumors.	• Curative intent for most situations means that aggressive surgical options may be considered. • Key points of discussion prior to surgery should include expected outcome and impact on function.
Limb salvage surgeries	• Surgical resection preserving the effected limb using an endoprosthesis allows for wide surgical resections that avoid amputations. • Local control has been shown to be similar to earlier studies where amputation was the mainstay. • Optimizing the function of a limb following limb salvage surgery requires commitment to intensive physical therapy, both in the postsurgical time period and also in the transition to survivorship. • Patients must be counseled regarding a lifelong risk for infection, which could result in loss of the prosthesis and amputation. All fevers should be promptly evaluated and treated empirically until culture results are negative.	• Provide time to prepare psychologically for the procedure.[6] • Provide opportunities to discuss the multiple consequences of the procedure (functional expectations, pain, disability, deformity, changes in appearance).[1] • Discussion with other patients who have received similar procedures may be helpful. • Adjuvant chemotherapy can impair post surgical recovery and wound healing to a greater extent than post amputation, but long-term psychological adjustment and function may be improved. • Limb salvage surgery does not guarantee postsurgical function at the same level of the natural extremity; therefore, expectations need to be clearly spelled out at the time of informed consent for surgery. • Physical and occupational therapy, often with the assistance of a social worker, child psychologist, or recreation therapist, should be engaged following surgery and chemotherapy in order to obtain and maintain goal function.[7] • Need for future revisions may provoke anxiety especially if significant complications surrounding initial surgery. Consideration should be given for posttraumatic stress-like reactions and treatment.

Amputation	• Amputation may be recommended when functional outcome or cancer control is expected to be better than that achieved with limb salvage or radiation.
	  • Involvement of nerves or vessels.
	  • Tumors of the distal lower extremity can be resected with good function following a below the knee amputation (BKA).
	• Amputation may also be recommended for palliation of intractable pain.
		• Provide adequate time to prepare psychologically for the procedure.[6]
		• Sometimes helpful for patients to discuss outcomes with another amputee. Also consider books/stories/movies by or about other amputees.
		• Some families find it difficult to comprehend amputation as a viable option and will need several sessions to discuss and process the recommendation. Social work, psychology, or recreation therapy may be helpful in preparing for surgery and support postsurgery.
		• Phantom pain can be an issue post-op for which multidisciplinary assistance is needed.

Radiation	• Radiation is a curative option for many sarcomas when full resection is not possible. • Short-term effects of irradiation can include fatigue, nausea, skin rash or breakdown, colitis, pericarditis, or inflammation of other tissues in the radiation field. • Radiation given while continuing chemotherapy may add to delays in count recovery. • Long-term effects may include permanent tightening and discoloration of the irradiated skin, lymphedema, cataracts, growth discrepancies, and risk for fracture. • Irradiated tissues have a limited ability to heal and are at risk for second malignancies.	• Early introduction to a radiation oncologist if radiation planned. • Simulation requires time in scans, and team should consider cognitive behavioral measures to help with pain and/or anxiety that may arise. • If radiation to brain, consider neuropsychiatric testing and follow-up assessments (See Chapter 18, Cognitive Sequelae). • Consider ovarian transposition for ovarian protection if planned abdominal/pelvic radiation.[8]

(continued)

Table 5.1 (Continued)

Treatment	General Principles	Education or Management Suggestions
Chemotherapy	• Nausea remains a common side effect, but nausea and vomiting can often be controlled with current anti-emetic regimens. • Alopecia or hair loss is common with most front line chemotherapies. • Myelosuppression leads to a heightened risk for infection and the need for prolonged hospitalization. • Specific side effects: • Vincristine or other vinca alkyloids: Reversible constipation, neuropathy with weakness of foot flexors. • Platinum: Irreversible hearing loss. • Alkylators and other high dose therapies: Irreversible infertility may occur in a fraction of patients (related to cumulative dose). Early menopause may occur in female patients following typical treatment for pediatric sarcoma.[9] • Doxorubicin and other anthracyclines: cardiotoxicity, thus frequent monitoring is important during and after treatment.[10]	• Hair loss occurs at approximately 2–3 weeks post initiation of myelosuppressive chemotherapy. This is often a trying time especially for teens and young women. Consultation with wig maker, donation of long hair prior to loss, support groups or cutting hair as it starts to come out in clumps can be helpful to patients and families. • During times of cytopenias, patients are encouraged to avoid crowds, and this may limit social interactions. • Fertility conversations are necessary prior to induction treatment. Males may delay start of therapy for sperm banking. Some trials exist for ovarian tissue harvest, but most often chemotherapy cannot be delayed for the necessary hormone treatments. (See Chapter 13, Fertility and Sexuality.)

Care of solid tumors in pediatrics generally requires a combination of surgery or radiation to control the local site of the tumor plus chemotherapy to treat micrometastatic disease, even if obvious metastases are not visible on the scans. The chemotherapy agents used in the treatment of pediatric solid tumors are generally given in multiagent regimens and often as part of a clinical trial to improve on the standard of care. It is important to inform the patients and their families about possible side effects and recommended surveillance for the acute and long-term toxicities of these regimens. Some toxicities such as hair loss are reversible, whereas other adverse effects, such as hearing loss and neuropathy, may be permanent or take longer to resolve. The systemic chemotherapy may delay healing and also causes repeated cycles of neutropenia with infectious risk plus the possible chronic side effects of cardiac toxicity, infertility, renal toxicity, among others. Treatment for solid tumors has also been found to increase the risk of developing chronic health problems such as heart disease and secondary malignancies.[3]

Patients treated for pediatric sarcomas can be particularly challenging. Local control of bone and soft tissue sarcomas requires surgery that has an impact on the function and appearance of the affected limb or site of disease. Limb salvage surgeries or amputations have medical, functional, and psychological impact on the patient and caregivers. Survivors of bone sarcomas have been reported to have a higher rate of medically significant chronic conditions, including severe musculoskeletal conditions, than survivors of any other pediatric malignancies. The stresses associated with treatment and tumor-induced changes in body image, loss of fertility, and impact on future independence can be especially acute in the adolescent and young adult population where sarcomas can have their peak occurrence.

Successful treatment and survivorship care for patients with pediatric solid tumors requires a comprehensive approach that builds trust between caregivers, the patients, and their families (Table 5.2). Psychosocial support should be provided in order to assist in the treatment-related challenges in a manner that respects the autonomy of the individual and encourages patients to be active participants in their care (Table 5.3).[4,5]

Strategies for Recurrent Disease

Although some low-risk tumors can be salvaged if there is a recurrence, the majority of sarcomas and other solid tumors do not have a standard second line therapy for relapsed disease. Prognosis depends on presence of metastases and time that patient was free of disease. Several of the sarcomas such as Ewing sarcoma and synovial sarcoma can have late relapses (>5–10 years). In general, the strategy to treat such recurrent disease will be balanced with priorities for care and quality of life. Options include a range from standard chemotherapy, to clinical trials of experimental therapies, to supportive care aimed at palliation of symptoms.

Table 5.2 Transition to Survivorship

Issue	General Principles	Education or Management Suggestions
End of therapy	• Active therapy changes to more passive follow-up. • Readdress any physical therapy or disability needs. • Transition primary care back to primary caregiver.	• Can be anxiety provoking as shift from regular visits and provider support to more independence. • Consider occupational therapy consult or follow-up with neuropsychology team.
Follow-up scans	• Surveillance scans for identification of disease status. • Most often more frequent in initial year post therapy.	• Provide supportive environment to acknowledge anxiety that comes with scans.
Health maintenance	• Side effects may include increase risk for metabolic syndrome.[11] • Sarcoma patients at risk of more sedentary life style after treatment.	• Provide primary-care team with survivorship care plan so that anticipatory guidance can be given.
Transition to independence	• Especially for older adolescents, this may also be a time of transition from parent responsibility for medical issues to patient taking on more responsibility.	• Help emerging young adult to learn how to maintain medical care and advocate for themselves (See Chapter 33, Pediatric Cancer Survivors).

Table 5.3 Medical Situations in Which Anticipatory Psychosocial Support May Be Helpful

Vascular access • Central venous catheters • Psychosocial support should be considered in introducing concept of line placement, access, and regular care of dressing changes plus flushing of lines. • Child-life/psychosocial provider involvement with dolls for medical role play. • Needle sticks required for peripheral blood draws or port-a-cath access. • Topical numbing with anesthetic cream to needle stick site 20–30 minutes prior to planned blood draw. • Child-life assistance for distraction and to model helpful tactics.
Consent and start of treatment • Establish trust and open communication. • Include the patient in assent and guardian for consent in language that is developmentally appropriate. • Clearly identify standard therapy and any experimental questions being asked as part of the recommended therapy in a clinical trial or as per a clinical trial. • Identify team members available for assistance in specific areas of support services.

(continued)

Table 5.3 (Continued)

Compliance • Include the patient in decision making and allow the patient as much autonomy as possible. • Establish cues to help the patient remember to take medicine (e.g., every morning when brushing teeth). • If concern for noncompliance, may require a patient or family meeting to set clear guidelines and expectations for compliance. • May consider a contract with the patient for critical elements of care.
Nutritional problems due to chemotherapy, changes in taste, or mucositis • Involve support of dietician/nutritionist. • Consider appetite stimulants. • Anticipate high-risk situations for mucositis to consider prophylactic treatment with palifermin or early consideration of G-tube feeds if unlikely to be able to take oral foods for some time. May also require parenteral nutrition if unable to feed through gut. • Intravenous hydration and opiates for pain relief.
Changes in bowel habits • Diarrhea: can be infectious requiring IV hydration and antibiotics. • Constipation: stool softeners, laxatives. • Some children may have aversion to discussing such bodily habits and psychosocial support is helpful in facilitating these important regular medical discussions.
Risk of infection • Importance of central-line-care training. • Use of universal precautions. • Especially during times of neutropenia, families are counseled about the need to notify medical care team urgently for potentially serious infections when they have an elevated temperature, chills, new pain, new rashes, diarrhea. • Possible need for isolation and importance of adhering to guidelines. Important for patient and family to understand rationale for isolation. Social support while isolated.
Depression, Withdrawal • Involve child-life specialists to encourage play with children. • Consult child psychologists, psychiatrists, social workers. • Consider cognitive behavioral techniques (CBT), antidepressants.
Disability • Where possible, peer support groups to discuss sources of anxiety, depression, anger. • Wellness counseling to emphasize cosmetic approaches to improve appearance, use of wigs, etc. • Psychological counseling to discuss stress associated with altered physical appearance, both temporary and/or permanent. • Psychological counseling to discuss issues related to sexual activity, sexual function, intimacy. • Occupational and vocational counseling to discuss impact on future job decisions and to educate regarding opportunities.

Summary

- Patients with pediatric solid tumors require good clinical care that incorporates teamwork by physicians, surgeons, nurses, social workers, psychologists, psychiatrists, as well as occupational, physical, and vocational therapists, dieticians, and child-life specialists.
- Systemic therapy with chemotherapy can cause dramatic changes in body image and overall well-being as well as risk for future chronic health issues.
- Sarcomas require intensive procedures to accomplish local control of the tumor, leaving many patients with decreased function.
- Optimal care for this population requires clear, consistent, and empathic communication from the entire healthcare team so that the patients and their families confront the psychological and psychosocial challenges as effectively as possible.

References

1. Link M, Gebhardt M, Meyers P. Osteosarcoma. In: Poplack P, ed. *Principles and Practice of Pediatric Oncology*. 5th ed. Philadelphia, PA: Lippincott, Williams & Wilkins; 2005: 1051–1090.
2. Merchant MS, Mackall CL. Current approach to pediatric soft tissue sarcomas. *Oncologist*. 2009;14(11):1139–1153.
3. Oeffinger KC, Mertens AC, Sklar CA, et al. Chronic health conditions in adult survivors of childhood cancer. *N Engl J Med*. 2006;355(15):1572–1582.
4. Horowitz ME, Fordis M, Krause S, McKellar J, Poplack DG. Passport for care: implementing the survivorship care plan. *J Oncol Pract*. 2009;5(3):110–112.
5. Kurt BA, Armstrong GT, Cash DK, et al. Primary care management of the childhood cancer survivor. *J Pediatr*. 2008;152(4):458–466.
6. Kusch M, Labouvie H, Ladisch V, Fleischhack G, Bode U. Structuring psychosocial care in pediatric oncology. *Patient Educ Couns*. 2000;40(3):231–245.
7. Robert RS, Ottaviani G, Huh WW, Palla S, Jaffe N. Psychosocial and functional outcomes in long-term survivors of osteosarcoma: a comparison of limb-salvage surgery and amputation. *Pediatr Blood Cancer*. 2010;54(7):990–999.
8. Martin JR, Kodaman P, Oktay K, Taylor HS. Ovarian cryopreservation with transposition of a contralateral ovary: a combined approach for fertility preservation in women receiving pelvic radiation. *Fertil Steril*. 2007;87(1):189 e5–e7.
9. Sklar CA, Mertens AC, Mitby P, et al. Premature menopause in survivors of childhood cancer: a report from the childhood cancer survivor study. *J Natl Cancer Inst*. 2006;98(13):890–896.
10. Longhi A, Ferrari S, Bacci G, Specchia S. Long-term follow-up of patients with doxorubicin-induced cardiac toxicity after chemotherapy for osteosarcoma. *Anticancer Drugs*. 2007;18(6):737–744.
11. Hoffman KE, Derdak J, Bernstein D, et al. Metabolic syndrome traits in long-term survivors of pediatric sarcoma. *Pediatr Blood Cancer*. 2008;50(2):341–346.

Chapter 6

Tumors of the Central Nervous System

Katherine E. Warren

Tumors of the central nervous system (CNS) are the most common solid tumors of childhood, with approximately 4,000 children diagnosed with a malignant or nonmalignant CNS tumor each year.[1] Pediatric CNS tumors are a heterogeneous group of diseases, varying in their histology, location, biology, prognosis, and treatment approach. Overall 5-year survival for children with CNS tumors is now over 70%,[1,2] but this is highly dependent on tumor type. For example, children with pilocytic astrocytomas have an estimated 5-year survival of >95%,[1] whereas median survival for children with the brainstem tumor, diffuse intrinsic pontine glioma (DIPG), is less than one year, and long-term survivors are rare. Compared to other childhood cancer survivors, those children who do survive CNS tumors have poor health-related quality of life and are at greatest risk for neuropsychological dysfunction and difficulties with psychosocial adjustment.[3–5]

The effects of the disease, treatment choice, and psychologic impact depend on the age of the child, tumor type, rate of growth, tumor location, and prognosis.

- Symptoms may be due to the tumor itself (e.g., destruction of neurons), from local effects of tumor (e.g., mass effect on surrounding tissue, hydrocephalus from obstruction, increased intracranial pressure), and from the treatment (e.g., residual deficits after surgery; long-term effects from radiation and chemotherapy).
- Location of the tumor is important because it defines the area of the brain involved and the subsequent function affected (Table 6.1), and many times determines if surgical resection can be performed.
- In adults, the majority of brain tumors are supratentorial, thereby exerting direct destructive or mass effect on the lobes of the cerebral cortex (i.e., frontal, temporal, parietal, and occipital). In contrast, childhood brain tumors are frequently located infratentorially in the posterior fossa, with major effects on the cerebellum and brainstem.

Psychological effects may manifest at varying times during the course of the disease. Some may have acute effects from anxiety around the initial diagnosis or from the primary medical treatment.

Table 6.1 Effects from Tumor or Treatment Based on Location

Location	Major Effects
Supratentorial	Motor, sensory, memory, and vision/visual field abnormalities; personality, emotion, and behavior changes
Thalamic	Mental status, personality, and memory changes; tremor
Hypothalamus, pituitary	Visual changes, endocrine abnormalities, obesity, sleep disturbance
Posterior fossa	Gait and coordination abnormalities, papilledema from obstruction, cranial neuropathies, torticollis, personality changes
Brainstem	Gait and coordination abnormalities, cranial neuropathies, pyramidal signs, ataxia, motor dysfunction, headache; vision, hearing, speech abnormalities; personality changes

- Initial management of children presenting with symptoms from CNS tumors involves glucocorticoids for those with evidence of significant edema (commonly those with malignant tumors and poor prognosis), anticonvulsants for those presenting with, or at risk of, seizure, and placement of a shunt to relieve hydrocephalus in those presenting with signs and symptoms of obstruction.
- Each of these therapies can cause symptoms: steroids are associated with mood and personality changes, difficulty sleeping, and rapid changes in appearance, whereas anticonvulsant therapy and shunt placement can add to cognitive dysfunction.[6,7]

A recommended approach to treatment of the tumor itself takes histology, grading, prognosis, and patient age into consideration (Boxes 6.1 and 6.2). For all tumor types, the guiding principle for treatment is risk versus benefit; the potential of long-term toxicities must be balanced with adequate treatment of the tumor.

- Modalities for treatment of CNS tumors include surgery, radiation and chemotherapy.[3] In general, low-grade tumors are surgically resected when possible, and chemotherapy is administered for some tumor types and in cases in which complete resection is not possible (Box 6.3).
- Malignant tumors are initially managed with surgical resection if feasible, followed by radiation therapy, and sometimes adjuvant chemotherapy. Preferably, radiation therapy is avoided or delayed in young children and those with neurofibromatosis.

Almost all survivors of pediatric CNS tumors will have long-term effects from the tumor and its treatment (Box 6.4, Table 6.2). These long-term effects can include physical, medical, psychological, social, and neurocognitive issues. Effects can vary even among patients treated similarly. We do

Box 6.1 Points on Classification of CNS Tumors

- Tumors are described by (a) tumor cell type, (b) location, (c) degree of differentiation, and, recently (d) genomics.
- Tumors are classified as benign or malignant based on histologic criteria (generally the World Health Organization, WHO, classification system), but all intracranial tumors are potentially lethal because of confinement within the cranium and involvement of critical structures, such as the brainstem.
  - Low-grade tumors are usually slow-growing, well-circumscribed, and noninfiltrative lesions that rarely spread to other locations within the CNS, and are associated with an indolent course.
  - High-grade lesions grow rapidly, are more diffuse and infiltrative, frequently disseminate throughout the neuroaxis, have rapid onset of symptoms, and a fulminant course.

Box 6.2 Most Common Pediatric CNS Tumors

- Astrocytomas (Gliomas).
  - Low-grade (WHO Grade I and II; include optic pathway gliomas, which are typically not biopsied).
  - High-grade (WHO Grade III and IV; include Diffuse Intrinsic Pontine Gliomas, which are typically not biopsied).
- Embryonal tumors (including medulloblastomas, primitive neuroectodermal tumors).
- Ependymomas.
- Neuronal/mixed glioneuronal tumors.
- Craniopharyngiomas.
- Germ-cell tumors.
- Choroid plexus tumors.

not yet know why some children are more susceptible to adverse effects than others, but a number of factors, including tumor characteristics, treatment, host, environmental and psychosocial factors, can influence outcome.[7]

- It is estimated that approximately 75% of brain tumor survivors will need special education services at some point during their schooling,[8] and early identification and intervention is key.
- It is important to discuss potential long-term effects during the initial-treatment conversation and consent, but these should be re-addressed during the course of treatment and at follow-up visits, as treatment-related effects can be acute, subacute, and chronic, and change over time.

Box 6.3 Common Treatment Modalities for Pediatric CNS Tumors

- Surgery.
    - Biopsy: establish a histologic diagnosis.
    - Partial resection/debulking: establish a diagnosis, reduce symptoms.
    - Total resection: establish diagnosis, reduce symptoms, improve prognosis, cure.
- Radiation Therapy.
    - Focal.
    - Whole ventricle.
    - Whole brain.
    - Craniospinal.
- Chemotherapy: used as adjuvant therapy or in younger children to delay/avoid XRT. Its role differs by tumor type and grade.
    - Oral.
    - Intravenous.
    - Intrathecal.

Box 6.4 Psychiatric and Psychologic Issues

Neurocognitive/Learning Issues Common in Children Treated for CNS Tumors[7,8,12]

- Overall cognitive decline.
- Slowed processing speed.
- Difficulty with attention.
- Poor short-term memory.
- Visual-motor integration.
- Academic problems, e.g., math.
- Executive dysfunction (e.g., problems with planning, problem-solving, task switching).

School Issues and Resources[13]

- Special/individualized education plans (IEPs).
- Frequent absences.
- School-based speech/physical/occupational therapy.
- Hearing and vision adaptive technologies.
- Need for accommodations for physical disabilities, including incontinence.

Emotional and Social Issues in Children Diagnosed with CNS Tumors[4–6,14]

- Global distress/anxiety.
- Irritability.
- Emotional lability.
- Depression.
- Suicide ideation.
- Body image concerns.
- Somatization.
- Low self-esteem.
- Tendency to be more socially withdrawn than peers.
- Social sensitivity-isolation.
- Fewer friends.
- Decreased social competency.
- Poor eye contact.
- Lower rates of employment.
- Lower rates of independent living.
- Lower rates of marriage.

Table 6.2 Medical Late Effects of Treatment of CNS Tumors[15–17]

Medical Issue	Recommended Screening
General • Secondary malignancies (esp. skin cancer, meningiomas, secondary high-grade gliomas, thyroid cancer) • Chronic fatigue	• Laboratory and diagnostic imaging per COG late effects guidelines
Endocrine dysfunction • Growth hormone deficiency • Precocious or delayed puberty • Panhypopituitarism • Hypothyroidism • Metabolic syndrome • Decreased sex hormones • Premature ovarian failure • Diabetes insipidus • Infertility	• Minimum yearly neuro-endocrine evaluation for those at risk • Neuro-endocrine evaluations every 3–6 months for those with existing endocrine issues
Ophthalmologic issues • Cataracts • Esotropia/exotropia • Vision loss/blindness • Incomplete lid closure	• Yearly ophthalmology exam with visual field testing for those who receive radiation to brain/eyes
Auditory/Hearing Issues • Tinnitus • Hearing loss • Vertigo	• Yearly audiology evaluation until at least 5 years off treatment
Physical alteration/deformity • Permanent alopecia/visible scars • Micro or macrocephaly • Scoliosis • Short stature • Facial or truncal asymmetry • Obesity/anorexia	• Yearly physical examination, referral to appropriate specialists (plastic surgery, orthopedics, etc.)
Neurologic Issues • Seizures • Stroke • Ataxia/movement disorders • Paralysis • Peripheral neuropathies • Chronic headaches/pain • Focal weakness • Sensory deficits • Encephalopathies	• Yearly detailed neurologic exam for those at risk • As medically indicated for those with active issues

(continued)

Table 6.2 (Continued)

Medical Issue	Recommended Screening
Other Medical Issues (common with other childhood cancer survivors) • Renal dysfunction • Pulmonary dysfunction • Cardiac dysfunction • Infertility • Fatigue/sleep disturbances	• Screening tests per COG late effects screening guidelines

- Routine longitudinal neuropsychological testing for survivors of pediatric tumors is not yet the standard of care in many centers,[9] although a number of pediatric neuro-oncology programs perform neurocognitive assessments, and an increasing number of cancer centers have pediatric oncology survivorship clinics, including clinics specifically designed toward survivors of CNS tumors.
- The Children's Oncology Group recommends that survivors of high-risk CNS tumors undergo neurocognitive testing when they transition from active treatment into a survivorship program, even if there are no specific complaints, to identify subtle issues and to serve as a baseline for future testing.[7] In general, patients should be re-evaluated if there is worsening academic performance, acute changes, or identification of new difficulties.[7]

In addition to the well-known neurocognitive late effects, medical late effects are significant.

- Survivors of CNS tumors who have received radiation therapy are at increased risk of a second malignancy within the CNS, with a cumulative incidence of 7.1% at 25 years from diagnosis in patients.[10]
- Those who survive childhood CNS tumors have a mortality rate 13 times higher than that for an age- and gender-matched population.[10]
- It is, therefore, important to establish long-term medical, neurocognitive, psychological, and medical follow-up of survivors in a pediatric or adult clinic to maximize their overall functioning and quality of life.

It is well documented that survivors of childhood CNS tumors face a number of life challenges, with social, emotional, psychological, and medical late effects of therapy (Box 6.4). It is clear that these effects are interrelated, and the whole patient must be comprehensively assessed and monitored. There are a number of excellent books and Web resources, such as the CureSearch website (www.curesearch.com) and the Children's Oncology Group's Long-Term Follow-up Guidelines[11] now available as excellent resources to clinicians and parents alike to provide answers to many of the questions that arise regarding late effects in brain tumor survivors.

References

1. Kohler B, Ward E, Mccarthy B, et al. Annual report to the nation on the status of cancer, 1975–2007, featuring tumors of the brain and other nervous system. *J Natl Cancer Inst.* 2011;103:714–736.
2. Smith M, Seibel N, Altekruse S, et al. Outcomes for children and adolescents with cancer: challenges for the twenty-first century. *J Clin Oncol.* 2010;28(15):2625–2634.
3. Ellenberg L, Liu Q, Gioia G, et al. Neurocognitive status in long-term survivors of childhood CNS malignancies: a report from the Childhood Cancer Survivor Study. *Neuropsychol.* 2009;23(6):705–717.
4. Zeltzer L, Recklitis C, Buchbinder D, et al. Psychological status in childhood cancer survivors: a report from the Childhood Cancer Survivor Study. *J Clin Oncol.* 2009;27:2396–2404.
5. Fuemmeler B, Elkin T, Mullins L. Survivors of childhood brain tumors: behavioral, emotional, and social adjustment. *Clin Psychol Rev.*2002;22(4):547–585.
6. Bromley R, Leeman B, Baker G, et al. Cognitive and neurodevelopmental effects of antiepileptic drugs. *Epilepsy Behav.* 2011;22:9–16.
7. Ullrich N, Embry L. Neurocognitive dysfunction in survivors of childhood brain tumors. *Semin Pediat Neurol.* 2012;19:35–42.
8. Nathan P, Patel S, Dilley K, et al. Guidelines for identification of, advocacy for, and intervention in neurocognitive problems in survivors of childhood cancer: a report from the Children's Oncology Group. *Arch Pediatr Adoles Med.* 2007;161(8):798–806.
9. Robinson K, Kuttesch J, Champion J, et al. A quantitative meta-analysis of neurocognitive sequelae in survivors of pediatric brain tumors. *Pediatr Blood Cancer.* 2010;55:525–531.
10. Armstrong G, Liu Q, Yasui Y, Huang S, et al. Long-term outcomes among adult survivors of childhood central nervous system malignancies in the Childhood Cancer Survivor Study. *J Natnl Cancer Inst.* 2009;101(13):946–958.
11. Children's Oncology Group. *Long-Term Follow-Up Guidelines for Survivors of Childhood, Adolescent, and Young Adult Cancers.* Arcadia, CA: CureSearch Children's Oncology Group; 2007.
12. Reimers T, Ehrenfels S, Mortensen E, et al. Cognitive deficits in long-term survivors of childhood brain tumors: identification of predictive factors. *Med Pediatr Oncol.* 2003;40(1):26–34.
13. Mitby P, Robison L, Whitton J, et al. Utilization of special education services and educational attainment among long-term survivors of childhood cancer: a report from the childhood cancer survivor study. *Cancer.* 2003;97(4):1115–1126.
14. Vannatta K, Gerhardt C, Wells R, Noll R. Intensity of CNS treatment for pediatric cancer: prediction of social outcomes in survivors. *Pediatr Blood Cancer.* 2007;49(5):716–722.
15. Anderson D, Rennie K, Ziegler R, Neglia J, Robison L, Gurney J. Medical and neurocognitive late effects among survivors of childhood central nervous system tumors. *Cancer.* 2001;92(10):2709–2719.

16. Packer R, Gurney J, Punyko J, et al. Long-term neurologic and neurosensory sequelae in adult survivors of a childhood brain tumor: childhood cancer survivor study. *J Clin Oncol*. 2003;21(17):3255–3261.

17. Gurney J, Kadan-Lottick N, Packer R, et al. Endocrine and cardiovascular late effects among adult survivors of childhoodbrain tumors: Childhood Cancer Survivor Study. *Cancer*. 2003;97:663–673.

Section II

Hereditary Cancers

Chapter 7

Hereditary Cancer Syndromes

David Malkin

The combined approach of astute clinical observation and ever-improving molecular tools has resulted in the characterization of an increasing number of cancer predisposition syndromes (CPSs). Identification of molecular alterations provides risk information for the individual tested, as well as for both affected and unaffected relatives in these families. All members of the healthcare team for patients with cancer (and family members with CPSs) should familiarize themselves with these syndromes and have a basic understanding of the clinical course, the genetic basis, the diagnostic possibilities and preventive and therapeutic intervention options. Hereditary cancers touch more areas of a patient's life and family than a childhood cancer diagnosis usually does. Although most parents of children with cancer can be reassured that it is highly unlikely that their other children will be at increased risk for cancer, this is not the case when the cancer is part of a hereditary syndrome. Thus, genetic counseling and attention to psychosocial concerns of parents and children with hereditary cancers is paramount.

Molecular Basis of Hereditary Cancer Predisposition in Children

Although CPSs account for less than 10% of childhood tumors,[1] genes identified through study of these syndromes are involved not only in the pathogenesis of inherited cancers but also in their common sporadic counterparts. Furthermore, more thorough evaluation of family history and recognition of CPSs by oncologists and other practitioners, as well as ongoing discovery of cancer susceptibility genes with use of next generation sequencing technologies will increase the actual proportion of genetically based childhood tumors. CPSs are generally associated with alterations in one of three classes of genes: tumor suppressor genes (TSG), oncogenes, and DNA stability genes (Table 7.1).[2] Tumor suppressor genes normally control cell proliferation by either inhibiting progression through the cell cycle or promoting apoptosis (programmed cell death). Inactivation of both alleles of a TSG by mutation or deletion causes uncontrolled proliferation, thereby contributing to tumorigenesis. In contrast, oncogenes normally potentiate cell proliferation, so mutation of one allele is sufficient to produce uncontrolled cell growth. Inactivation of DNA stability or repair genes permits cells that harbor damaged DNA to divide, potentially leading to malignant

Table 7.1 Inherited Cancer Predisposition Syndromes and the Involved Genes (Adapted from Vogelstein et al.)[2]

Syndrome	Major Tumor Types	Mode of Inheritance	Gene
Tumor Suppressor Genes			
Familial attenuated polyposis	colon, thyroid, stomach, intestine	dominant	*APC*
Attenuated polyposis	colon	dominant	*AXIN2*
Familial gastric carcinoma	stomach	dominant	*CDH1* (E-Cadherin)
Simpson-Golabi-Behmel syndrome	embryonal tumors	X-linked	*GPC3*
Familial cylindromatosis	pilotrichomas	dominant	*CYLD*
Hereditary multiple exostoses	bone	dominant	*EXT1,2*
Gorlin syndrome	skin, medulloblastoma	dominant	*PTCH*
Medulloblastoma predisposition	skin, medulloblastoma	dominant	*SUFU*
Hereditary leiomyomatosis	leiomyomas	dominant	*FH*
Familial paraganglioma	paragangliomas, pheochromocytomas, gastrointestinal stromal tumors (GIST)	dominant	*SDHA, AF2,B, C, D; MAX,*
Von Hippel-Lindau syndrome	kidney	dominant	*VHL*
Li-Fraumeni syndrome	breast, sarcoma, adrenal, brain	dominant	*TP53*
Familial Wilms tumor	Wilms tumor	dominant	*WT1*
Peutz-Jeghers syndrome	intestinal, ovarian, pancreatic	dominant	*STK11 (LKB1)*
Cowden syndrome	hamartoma, glioma, uterus	dominant	*PTEN*
Tuberous sclerosis	hamartoma, kidney	dominant	*TSC1, TSC2*
Familial malignant melanoma	melanoma, pancreas	dominant	*CDKN2A (p16INK4A, p14ARF)*
Familial malignant melanoma	melanoma	dominant	*CDK4*
Hereditary retinoblastoma	eye	dominant	*RB1*
Neurofibromatosis type 1	neurofibroma	dominant	*NF1*
Juvenile polyposis	gastrointestinal	dominant	*BMPR1A*
Multiple endocrine neoplasia type I	parathyroid, pituitary, islet cell, carcinoid	dominant	*MEN1*
Juvenile polyposis	gastrointestinal	dominant	*SMAD4 (DPC4)*

(continued)

Table 7.1 (Continued)

Syndrome	Major Tumor Types	Mode of Inheritance	Gene
Birt-Hogg-Dube syndrome	renal, hair follicle	dominant	*BHD*
Hyperparathyroidism Jaw-tumor syndrome	parathyroid, jaw fibroma	dominant	*HRPT2*
Neurofibromatosis type 2	meningioma, acoustic neuroma	dominant	*NF2*
DICER1 syndrome	Pineoblastoma, pituitary blastoma, cystic nephroma, pleuropulmonary blastoma, Sertoli-Leydig cell tumor, Wilms tumor, multinodular goiter	Dominant	*DICER1*
Oncogenes			
Familial gastrointestinal stromal tumors	gastrointestinal stromal tumors	dominant	*KIT*
Hereditary papillary renal cell carcinoma	kidney	dominant	*MET*
Familial gastrointestinal stromal tumors	gastrointestinal stromal tumors	dominant	*PDGFRA*
Multiple endocrine neoplasia type II	thyroid, parathyroid, adrenal	dominant	*RET*
Stability Genes			
Attenuated polyposis	colon	recessive	*MUTYH*
Ataxia telangiectasia	leukemias, lymphomas, brain	recessive	*ATM*
Bloom syndrome	leukemias, lymphomas, skin	recessive	*BLM*
Hereditary breast cancer	breast, ovary	dominant	*BRCA1, BRCA2*
Fanconi anemia	leukemias, head&neck, gynecological system	recessive	*FANCA, C, D2, E, F,G*
Nijmegen breakage syndrome	lymphomas, brain	recessive	*NBS1*
Rothmund-Thomson syndrome	bone, skin	recessive	*RECQL4*
Werner syndrome	bone, brain	recessive	*WRN*
HNPCC	colon, uterus	dominant	*MSH2, MLH1, MSH6, PMS2*
Biallelic mismatch repair syndrome	Colon, brain, lymphoma	Dominant	*MSH2, MLH1, MSH6, PMS2*
Xeroderma pigmentosum	Skin	recessive	*XPA, C; ERCC2-5; DDB2*

transformation of those cells.[2] Examples of prototype childhood cancers will be used to highlight the breadth of tumors that arise from molecular changes in these genes.

Retinoblastoma

Retinoblastoma (RB) is a malignant tumor of the eye that originates from developing cells of the retina (see Chapter 4, Retinoblasoma). Retinoblastoma has an incidence of 1 in 15,000, with 90% arising in children under 3 years of age,[3] and it occurs in either a sporadic or a hereditary form. Knudson proposed the "two-hit-hypothesis" based on the patterns of inheritance of RB that established the basis for discovery of TSGs[4] wherein the inactivation of both alleles of the causally associated gene is necessary for tumor development.

Patients with Sporadic RB

- Usually have unilateral tumors and are older (median age 22 months) at diagnosis.[5]
- Both alleles are inactivated in the somatic cell leading to unifocal and later onset.

Patients with Hereditary RB

- Often develop bilateral or multifocal tumors and are younger (median age 11 months) at diagnosis.[5]
- In hereditary tumors, one mutated allele is inherited through the germline, and the second one is inactivated by a somatic event, often a gene deletion.

The *RB1* gene was initially localized to chromosome 13 (13q14)[6] and was the first TSG to be cloned.[7] Loss of function of both alleles of *RB1* in tumor specimens[8] and the presence of germline mutations in hereditary RB[9] validated Knudson's "two-hit-hypothesis." The *RB1* gene is mutated or deleted in all retinoblastomas, as well as a wide spectrum of other tumors.[10] The retinoblastoma protein, pRB, serves as the "molecular switch" that controls the passage of cells through division and proliferation.[11,12] Loss of this regulatory function allows uncontrolled proliferation, thereby contributing to tumorigenesis.

Risk of Developing Retinoblastoma

- An individual that inherits a germline *RB1* mutation carries a 90% risk of developing RB; however, due to a high rate of new mutations, the family history is often negative.
- The risk of transmitting the mutated gene to the offspring is 50%.
- Genetic testing of a proband can improve clinical management and facilitate the genetic counseling of other family members (cf. genetic counseling section, later).
- For an individual at risk, a positive result will reinforce the necessity of surveillance for early diagnosis and treatment, whereas negative results will prevent the risks and costs of the examinations.

- Because retinoblastoma patients have very high rates of second malignancies, careful, lifelong screening is necessary, with consequent anxieties for patients and family members.
- The use of genetic testing for preimplantation diagnosis has been reported.[16]

Li-Fraumeni Syndrome

Li-Fraumeni Syndrome (LFS) is associated with germline mutations in the *TP53* TSG. Classical LFS is defined by a proband with a sarcoma diagnosed before 45 years of age who has a first degree relative with any cancer under 45 years of age, and a first- or second-degree relative with any cancer under 45 years of age or a sarcoma at any age.[17,18] For families with similar patterns of cancer that did not meet the definition of LFS, the term Li-Fraumeni-like syndrome (LFS-L) was suggested.[19]

Li-Fraumeni-like Syndrome (LFS-L)

- A proband with a characteristic LFS tumor (sarcoma, brain tumor, breast cancer, adrenocortical carcinoma) before 36 years and at least one first or second degree relative with a characteristic LFS tumor (other than breast cancer if the proband is affected by breast cancer) before 46 years.
- A proband with multiple primary tumors two of which are characteristic LFS tumors and the first of which occurred before 36 years, whatever the family history.
- A proband with adrenocortical carcinoma, choroid plexus carcinoma or anaplastic rhabdomyosarcoma, whatever the age of onset and family history.[20,21]
- Over 50% of sporadic human tumors harbor somatic *TP53* mutations,[22] and transgenic mice carrying mutant *TP53* alleles develop a wide spectrum of malignancies.[23] The *p53* protein is a component of an extensive cell cycle control network that is "switched-off" under physiologic conditions. In response to cellular stresses that induce DNA damage, activated *p53* can induce apoptosis, cell-cycle arrest, DNA damage repair, senescence, and differentiation.[24] Loss of *p53* function contributes to tumor development.

Prevalence of Germline Mutations in *TP53*

- Account for >75% of cases of LFS[20,25–27] and occur in children with classical LFS tumors in the absence of a family history of cancer: adrenocortical carcinoma—50–80%;[28] osteosarcoma—10%;[29] rhabdomyosarcoma—10%.[30]
- Only 1–2% of women with familial, early onset, or bilateral breast cancer harbor germline *TP53* mutations,[31] although up to 7% of women with very early onset breast cancer (i.e., <30 years) harbor germline *TP53* mutations, suggesting a different role of p53 in the pathogenesis of these tumors.[32]
- The overall lifetime risk of cancer in patients with LFS is high (80–90% with a risk as high as 40% within the first two decades,[33] with high probability of developing multiple, primary tumors), yet the variable

expressivity, penetrance, and diversity of the tumor spectrum render clinical surveillance and genetic testing a difficult task.
- Once an individual is diagnosed with LFS and the *TP53* mutation is identified, predictive testing for yet unaffected relatives is possible. However, in contrast to RB, with the advent of feasible and effective clinical surveillance for early tumor detection, recommendations for *TP53* testing in both at-risk children and adults (as defined by the LFS criteria) have been established (see NCCN).[34,35]

Multiple Endocrine Neoplasia

The multiple endocrine neoplasias (MEN)—MEN type 1, MEN type 2A, and MEN type 2B—define a constellation of tumors of the endocrine system.[36]

MEN 1

- Caused by mutations in a TSG, termed *MEN1*.[37]
- The most common features are parathyroid adenomas, pancreatic islet cell tumors, and pituitary adenomas.
- By age fifteen, 28% of mutation carriers show clinical or biochemical evidence of disease[38] making direct mutation analysis of the *MEN1* gene justified at an early age in documented *MEN 1* families.
- Clinical and laboratory screening guidelines for the management of these patients and families have been published.[39]

MEN 2A

- Caused by mutations in the RET proto-oncogene.
- Associated with medullary thyroid carcinoma, parathyroid adenoma, and pheochromocytoma (adrenal gland tumor).
- Biochemical screening for early cancer detection is complex.
- May need to consider prophylactic thyroidectomy (by age of 5 years) and ongoing screening for pheochromocytoma and parathyroid disease.

MEN 2B

- Caused by mutations in the RET proto-oncogene.
- Characterized by onset of tumors in early infancy, ganglioneurinoma of the gastrointestinal tract, and skeletal abnormalities.
- Biochemical screening for early cancer detection is complex.
- May need to consider prophylactic thyroidectomy (by 1 year of age) and ongoing screening for pheochromocytoma and parathyroid disease.

Constitutional mutations in the RET proto-oncogene are found in families with *MEN 2A* and *2B* and, in addition, a wider range of somatic mutations is found in patients with nonhereditary medullary thyroid carcinoma.[40,41] The pattern of mutations seen in *MEN 2* families does not follow the "two-hit-hypothesis" for tumor suppressor genes: the RET proto-oncogene is not inactivated and there is no loss of the second allele in the tumors. Thus, the predisposition to cancer in families with *MEN 2* is based on the inheritance of an activating mutation in the RET proto-oncogene. Because the risk of developing medullary thyroid carcinoma is virtually 100% in mutation carriers, all children with a confirmed RET mutation should receive a prophylactic thyroidectomy by the age of 5 years (*MEN 2A*) or 1 year (*MEN 2B*), respectively.[42] In addition, mutation carriers need lifelong screening for pheochromocytoma and parathyroid disease.

Fanconi Anemia

Fanconi Anemia (FA) is one of the CPSs caused by mutations in DNA repair/stability genes. It is a rare disease characterized by a wide variety of congenital abnormalities; bone marrow failure; chromosome instability; cellular hypersensitivity to DNA crosslinking-agents such as mitomycin C and cisplatin; and increased predisposition to cancer, mainly leukemias and squamous cell carcinoma of the head and neck or gynecologic system.[43] At least 11 "complementation" groups are known, and the genes for 8 of these have been cloned.[44] Recently, it has been shown that one of these genes *FANCD1* actually is *BRCA2*,[45] a gene associated with breast and ovarian cancer susceptibility. Although the function of the *FANC* genes and their protein products is not completely clear, they are associated with other chromosome stability genes that are activated in the presence of DNA damage.[45,46]

Diagnosis of Fanconi Anemia

- Confirmed by the demonstration of increased chromosomal breakage in response to mitomycin C in cell culture; the test can be used to screen asymptomatic siblings.
- Hematological abnormalities usually develop in early childhood (median age of onset 7 years) and cumulative risk of bone marrow failure is 84% by the age of 20 years, followed by a 52% risk of leukemia by 40 years.[45,48]
- Patients that are cured of hematological complications are still at risk to develop solid malignancies.[45,48,49]
- Chromosomal breakage studies can be carried out on amniotic cells, chorion villus cells, or fetal blood, and can, therefore, be used for prenatal diagnosis.[50]
- Preimplantation genetic diagnosis has been offered to parents to select an embryo that is unaffected, and human leukocyte antigen (HLA) identical to the previously born affected sibling with the aim of performing stem cell transplantation using umbilical cord blood. This procedure has been successfully performed, but raises ethical controversies as well.[51,52]

Conclusion

Many genes play important roles in the development of sporadic cancers, and their identification and functional characterization have led to better understanding of cancer biology and potential new therapeutic targets. It is likely that as more CPSs are characterized and more "cancer genes" are identified, causal associations between the two will continue to develop. The emerging age of cancer genetics and cancer genomics will, therefore, have enormous impact on the management of all cancer patients.

References

1. Narod SA, Stiller C, Lenoir GM. An estimate of the heritable fraction of childhood cancer. *Br J Cancer.* 1991;63(6):93–999.
2. Vogelstein B, Kinzler KW. Cancer genes and the pathways they control. *Nat Med.* 2004;10(8):789–799.
3. Ross JA, Severson RK, Pollock BH, Robison LL. Childhood cancer in the United States. A geographical analysis of cases from the Pediatric Cooperative Clinical Trials groups. *Cancer.* 1996;77(1):201–207.
4. Knudson AG Jr. Mutation and cancer: statistical sudy of retinoblastoma. *Proc Natl Acad Sci USA.* 1971;68(4):820–823.
5. Lohmann DR, Gallie BL. Retinoblastoma: Revisiting the model prototype of inherited cancer. *Am J Med Genet, Part C, Seminars in Medican Genetics.* 2004;129C(1):23–28.
6. Cavenee WK, Dryja TP, Phillips RA, et al. Expression of recessive alleles by chromosomal mechanisms in retinoblastoma. *Nature.* 1983;305(5937):779–784.
7. Friend SH, Bernards R, Rogelj S, et al. A human DNA segment with properties of the gene that predisposes to retinoblastoma and osteosarcoma. *Nature.* 1986;323(6089):643–646.
8. Fung YK, Murphree AL, T'Ang A, Qian J, Hinrichs SH, Benedict WF. Structural evidence for the authenticity of the human retinoblastoma gene. *Science.* 1987;236(4809):1657–1661.
9. Dunn JM, Phillips RA, Becker AJ, Gallie BL. Identification of germline and somatic mutations affecting the retinoblastoma gene. *Science.* 1988; 241(4874):1797–1800.
10. Horowitz JM, Park SH, Bogenmann E, et al. Frequent inactivation of the retinoblastoma anti-oncogene is restricted to a subset of human tumor cells. *Proc Natl Acad Sci USA.* 1990;87(7):2775–2779.
11. Nurse P. A long twentieth century of the cell cycle and beyond. *Cell.* 2000;100(1):71–78.
12. Weinberg RA. The retinoblastoma protein and cell cycle control. *Cell.* 1995;81(3):323–330.
13. Musarella MA & Gallie BL. A simplified scheme for genetic counseling in retinoblastoma. *J Pediatr Ophthalmol Strabismus,* 1987;24(3):124–125.
14. Richter S, Vandezande K, Chen N, et al. Sensitive and efficient detection of RB1 gene mutations enhances care for families with retinoblastoma. *Am J Hum Genet.* 2003;72(2):253–269.
15. Cohen JG, Dryja TP, Davis KB, Diller LR, Li FP. RB1 genetic testing as a clinical service: A follow-up study. *Med Pediatr Oncol.* 2001;37(4):372–378.
16. Girardet A, Hamamah S, Anahory T, et al. First preimplantation genetic diagnosis of hereditary retinoblastoma using informative microsatellite markers. *Mol Hum Reprod.* 2003;9(2):111–116.
17. Li FP, Fraumeni JF Jr. Soft-tissue sarcomas, breast cancer, and other neoplasms. a familial syndrome? *Ann Intern Med.* 1969;71(4):747–752.

18. Li FP, Fraumeni JF Jr, Mulvihill JJ, et al. A cancer family syndrome in twenty-four kindreds. *Cancer Res.* 1988;48(18):5358–5362.

19. Varley JM, Evans DG, Birch JM. Li-Fraumeni syndrome—A molecular and clinical review. *Br J Cancer.* 1997;76(1):1–14.

20. Chompret A, Abel A, Stoppa-Lyonnet D, et al. Sensitivity and predictive value of criteria for p53 germline mutation screening. *J Med Genet. 2001*;38(1):43–47.

21. Hettmer S, Archer NM, Somers GR. Anaplastic rhabdomyosarcoma in *TP53* germline mutation carriers. *Cancer. 2014* Apr 1;120(7):1068–1075.

22. Nigro JM, Baker SJ, Preisinger AC, et al. Mutations in the p53 gene occur in diverse human tumour types. *Nature.* 1989;342(6250):705–708.

23. Lavigueur A, Maltby V, Mock D, Rossant J, Pawson T, Bernstein A. High incidence of lung, bone, and lymphoid tumors in transgenic mice overexpressing mutant alleles of the p53 oncogene. *Mol Cell Biol.* 1989;9(9):3982–3991.

24. Vousden KH, Lu X. Live or let die: Rhe cell's response to p53. *Nature Rev Cancer.* 2002;2(8):594–604.

25. Malkin D, Li FP, Strong LC, et al. Germ line p53 mutations in a familial syndrome of breast cancer, sarcomas, and other neoplasms. *Science.* 1990;250 (4985):1233–1238.

26. Birch JM, Hartley AL, Tricker KJ, et al. Prevalence and diversity of constitutional mutations in the p53 gene among 21 Li-Fraumeni families. *Cancer Res.* 1994;54(5):1298–1304.

27. Kleihues P, Schäuble B, zur Hausen A, Estève J, Ohgaki H. Tumors associated with p53 germline mutations: a synopsis of 91 families. *American J Pathol.* 1997;150(1):1–13.

28. Wagner J, Portwine C, Rabin K, Leclerc JM, Narod SA, Malkin D. High frequency of germline p53 mutations in childhood adrenocortical cancer. *J Natl Cancer Inst.* 1994;86(22):1707–1710.

29. McIntyre JF, Smith-Sorensen B, Friend SH, et al. Germline mutations of the p53 tumor suppressor gene in children with osteosarcoma. *J Clin Oncol.* 1994;12(5):925–930.

30. Diller L, Sexsmith E, Gottlieb A, Li FP & Malkin D. Germline p53 mutations are frequently detected in young children with rhabdomyosarcoma. *J Clin Invest.* 1995;95(4):1606–1611.

31. Borresen AL, Andersen TI, Garber J, et al. Screening for germ line TP53 mutations in breast cancer patients. *Cancer Res.* 1992;52(11):3234–3236.

32. Malkin D. The role of p53 in human cancer. *J Neuro-Oncol.* 2001;51(3):231–243.

33. Le Bihan C, Moutou C, Brugieres L, Feunteun J, Bonaiti-Pellie C. ARCAD: A method for estimating age-dependent disease risk associated with mutation carrier status from family data. *Genet Epidemiol.* 1995;12(1):13–25.

34. American Society of Clinical Oncology. Statement of the American Society of Clinical Oncology: Genetic testing for cancer susceptibility, Adopted on February 20, 1996. *J Clin Oncol.* 1996;14(5):1730–1736.

35. American Society of Clinical Oncology. American Society of Clinical Oncology policy statement update: Genetic testing for cancer susceptibility. *J Clin Oncol.* 2003;21(12):2397–2406.

36. Pang JT, Thakker RV. Multiple endocrine neoplasia type 1 (MEN1). *Eur J Cancer.* 1994;30A(13):1961–1968.

37. Chandrasekharappa SC, Guru SC, Manickam P, et al. Positional cloning of the gene for multiple endocrine neoplasia-type 1. *Science*. 1997;276(5 311):404–407.

38. Bassett JH, Forbes SA, Pannett AA, et al. Characterization of mutations in patients with multiple endocrine neoplasia type 1. *Am J Hum Genet*. 1998;62(2):232–244.

39. Brandi ML, Gagel RF, Angeli A, et al. (2001). Guidelines for diagnosis and therapy of MEN type 1 and type 2. *J Clin Endocrinol Metabol*. 2001;86(12):5658–5671.

40. Gardner E, Papi L, Easton DF, et al. Genetic linkage studies map the multiple endocrine neoplasia type 2 loci to a small interval on chromosome 10q11.2. *Hum Mol Genet*. 1993;2(3):241–246.

41. Mulligan LM, Ponder BA. Genetic basis of endocrine disease: Multiple endocrine neoplasia type 2. *J Clin Endocrinol Metabol*. 1995;80(7):1989–1995.

42. Skinner MA, DeBenedetti MK, Moley JF, Norton JA, Wells SA Jr. Medullary thyroid carcinoma in children with multiple endocrine neoplasia types 2A and 2B. *J Pediatr Surg*. 1996;31(1):177–181.

43. Alter BP, Greene MH, Velazquez I, Rosenberg PS. Cancer in Fanconi anemia. *Blood*. 2003;101(5):2072.

44. Levitus M, Rooimans MA, Steltenpool J, et al. Heterogeneity in Fanconi anemia: Evidence for 2 new genetic subtypes. *Blood*. 2004;103(7):2498–2503.

45. Wagner JE, Tolar J, Levran O, et al. Germline mutations in BRCA2: Shared genetic susceptibility to breast cancer, early onset leukemia, and Fanconi anemia. *Blood*. 2004;103(8):3226–3229.

46. D'Andrea AD. The Fanconi road to cancer. *Genes Dev*. 2003;17(16):1933–1936.

47. Venkitaraman AR. A growing network of cancer-susceptibility genes. *N Engl J Med*. 2003;348(19):1917–1919.

48. Tischkowitz MD, Hodgson SV. Fanconi anaemia. *J Med Genet*. 2003;40(1):1–10.

49. Alter BP. Cancer in Fanconi anemia, 1927–2001. *Cancer*. 2003;97(2):425–440.

50. Auerbach AD, Sagi M, Adler B. Fanconi anemia: Prenatal diagnosis in 30 fetuses at risk. *Pediatrics*. 1985;76(5):794–800.

51. Damewood MD. Ethical implications of a new application of preimplantation diagnosis. *JAMA*. 2001;285(24):3143–3144.

52. Verlinsky Y, Rechitsky S, Schoolcraft W, Strom C, Kuliev A. Preimplantation diagnosis for Fanconi anemia combined with HLA matching. *JAMA*. 2001; 285(24):3130–3133.

Chapter 8

Genetic Counseling for Hereditary Cancer in Childhood

Anu Chittenden and Jaclyn Schienda

Genetic Counseling

The National Society of Genetic Counselors[1] defines genetic counseling as "the process of helping people understand and adapt to the medical, psychological, and familial implications of genetic contributions to disease. This process integrates:

- Interpretation of family and medical histories to assess the chance of disease occurrence or recurrence.
- Education about inheritance, testing, management, prevention, resources and research.
- Counseling to promote informed choices and adaptation to the risk or condition." (p. 52)

The foundation of genetic counseling is obtaining a good family and medical history. Tools are available to help families obtain an accurate history (Table 8.1). The health history generated will be valuable for them to share with all their healthcare providers and is essential for providing a useful differential diagnosis. However, there is no substitute for clinicians spending time reviewing the history directly with the individual or family. The health history is critical in determining the likelihood of a hereditary cancer syndrome being present in the pediatric patient or family.

- In the case of a suspected hereditary condition in a child, assessment of developmental delay, growth, birthmarks, congenital defects, and other medical problems is important.
- If there is a question of a cancer or related diagnosis in a relative, it is helpful to obtain medical records (in particular, pathology reports) or, if these are unavailable, death-certificate information.
- For patients who were adopted or who know little of their family history because of family circumstances, pursuit of this information can be difficult if not impossible. In these situations, whatever information the family can provide is useful.
- If there is concern about the possibility of hereditary susceptibility, referrals can be made to genetics specialists.

Table 8.1 Online Guidelines for Compiling a Family Medical History	
The US Surgeon General—My Family Health Portrait	https://familyhistory.hhs.gov/
The National Society of Genetic Counselors	http://www.nsgc.org/About/FamilyHistoryTool/tabid/226/Default.aspx
The American Medical Association	http://www.ama-assn.org//ama/pub/physician-resources/medical-science/genetics-molecular-medicine/family-history.page
North Shore University Health System	http://www.northshore.org/genetics/mygenerations/
Mayo Clinic	http://www.mayoclinic.com/health/medical-history/HQ01707
March of Dimes	http://www.marchofdimes.com/pregnancy/your-family-health-history.aspx
Centers for Disease Control	http://www.cdc.gov/Features/FamilyHistory/

Genetic counseling for hereditary pediatric cancer susceptibility disorders is a complex undertaking at different levels. The compilation of a good medical and family history is the first step in providing a good risk assessment and evaluation. Before undergoing any type of testing, the provider must assess and discuss the risks, benefits, and limitations of the testing for the child and the family and weigh these appropriately (Box 8.1).

- Is there an immediate medical benefit to the child and/or family?
- Is there any psychological benefit to the child and/or family?
- If there is no immediate medical benefit to the child, are the reasons for pursuing testing sufficient?
- Is the child old enough to participate in the conversation and give informed assent?
- Is this the right time to undergo testing (i.e., is it necessary for decision-making at this stage, or can this test be put off)?
- What is the cost of the testing, will it be covered by insurance, and is the family able and willing to pay for it?
- What is the accuracy of the testing and what does the process involve?
- How long will it take to get results?
- What are the possible ramifications for insurability or employment in the future?
- Has the family been given all the necessary information and provided sufficient time in which to make an informed decision?
- What are the potential psychological consequences of a positive, negative, or indeterminate genetic test result in the context of this family?

- Are there alternatives to testing that should be considered (e.g., noninvasive screening)?
- Can testing lead to unforeseen consequences (e.g., discovering nonpaternity)?

If these issues have been considered, and the decision to go forward with testing is made together with the family, then genetic testing has the potential to be a powerful tool in arming the family with knowledge to aid them in early detection and/or prevention of disease.

Box 8.1 Genetic Testing Considerations

When to test[3]

- A child has a clinical diagnosis, and the testing may be done to confirm the diagnosis.
- There is a known hereditary susceptibility in the family and the chance of developing disease (also known as penetrance) is high, especially if the disease can present in childhood and treatment to reduce morbidity and mortality is available.
- There is a suspected hereditary susceptibility in the child or the family, and testing is done to help determine whether this is actually present[2] (see p. 53).

Informed consent for genetic testing in minors[3]

- Most groups do not advocate genetic testing in children without a clear medical benefit to the child or the family[2] (see pp. 53 and 54).
- The age of the child may be important in determining the type of consent that is required, so that the older the child is, the more involved the child should be in the consent process. For certain conditions, there may be resources to help the child understand the condition in age-appropriate language.
- Even with evidence of clear medical benefit, testing for these patients should take into consideration the psychosocial risks and benefits for the child and the family.

Finances, logistics, laboratories

- Tests are often expensive and may not always be covered by insurance. Families may have to pay high out of pocket costs for these types of tests, which can be financially burdensome.
- Although most genetic testing is done through a blood or cheek swab sample, occasionally samples from tumors or other tissue also need to be sent (e.g., retinoblastoma testing may require both blood and tumor specimens for analysis).

(continued)

Box 8.1 (Continued)

- There are limited numbers of laboratories that offer specific types of gene testing and many of them do not work directly with insurance companies.
- Genetic Testing Registry (http://www.ncbi.nlm.nih.gov/gtr/) is an invaluable website resource for a comprehensive listing of laboratories that offer genetic testing. Laboratories are listed that perform both research and clinical testing.
  - It is important to distinguish between the two types of testing since laboratories that provide testing through research may not be CLIA-certified (regulations to promote good laboratory practices and to assure reliable laboratory results and documentation/records) or have a definite time frame in which results will be returned, if at all.
  - Testing that is performed in a research laboratory may have to be confirmed in a clinical lab before results can be returned to the patient or family; on the other hand, researchers may be interested in looking at other genes over time, so the family may have the benefit of their expertise and continued analysis.
  - The sensitivity and specificity of different methods of gene testing need to be considered, as does the laboratory's support of clinicians ordering the tests.

Interpretation of testing

- Testing has become increasingly complicated with the advent of multigene panels and even whole exome or whole genome sequencing. Tests may take weeks or months to complete and interpretation of test results is not always straightforward.
- These types of tests can often result in variants of uncertain clinical significance, when laboratories do not have enough information to determine whether the specific genetic alteration is actually harmful to the gene (e.g., if the alteration is rare and the gene is recently discovered, there may be little information to help guide the laboratory). The results can sometimes lead to further testing of other family members to try to clarify the significance of these results.
- In some cases, the test result cannot be clarified for an indefinite amount of time, leaving families in limbo about whether a particular syndrome is present or who in the family may be at risk for having the syndrome.

Genetic discrimination

- Although there are no reported cases of genetic discrimination associated with hereditary cancer susceptibility to date, families may express concern about future insurability for children, especially if a child is presymptomatic.

(continued)

Box 8.1 (Continued)

- Federal legislation through the Genetic Information Non-Discrimination Act (GINA) prohibits health insurers and employers from treating genetic test results like a preexisting condition. Please see the NIH fact sheet for more information on the specifics of this legislation (http://report.nih.gov/nihfactsheets/ViewFactSheet.aspx?csid=81).
- Other types of insurers, such as private life insurers, do not face the same legislative mandates as health insurers, so individuals may be charged higher premiums or denied coverage because of a genetic predisposition to cancer.

Table 8.2 Finding a Genetic Counselor or Oncologist Specializing in Genetics

The National Society of Genetic Counselor's Find a Counselor tool	http://www.nsgc.org/resourcelink.cfm (by specialty and location)
The National Cancer Institute's Cancer Genetics Services tool	http://www.cancer.gov/search/geneticsservices/ (by disease and location)
The American Society of Clinical Oncology's Find an Oncologist tool	http://www.plwc.org/

Who Provides Genetic Counseling?

- Genetic counselors are generally Masters-level healthcare professionals with specialized training in genetics, education, and counseling.
- Clinical geneticists are typically physicians who have completed a fellowship in genetics. Both genetic counselors and geneticists must be board-eligible or board-certified in their respective fields.
- Other types of providers such as oncologists, through the American Society of Clinical Oncology (ASCO), and nurses, through the International Society of Nurses in Genetics (ISONG), may obtain genetics training through courses, conferences, and clinical experience.
- Individuals who provide genetic counseling services for patients and families with a possible hereditary pediatric cancer susceptibility syndrome usually have specific expertise in clinical cancer genetics.
- There are many ways to find individuals who provide genetic counseling or risk-assessment services (Table 8.2). If appropriate providers are not available within the local area, specialist consultations may be able to be arranged via phone or teleconference.

References

1. National Society of Genetic Counselors. Genetic counseling as a profession. Chicago, IL: NSGC; 2005. http://www.nsgc.org/about/definition.cfm. Accessed Sept 9, 2008.

2. Ross LF, Moon MR. Ethical issues in genetic testing of children. *Arch Pediatr Adolesc Med*. 2000;154(9):873–879.

3. Committee on Bioethics, Committee on Genetics, and, the American College of Medical Genetics and Genomics Social, Ethical, and Legal Issues Committee. *Pediatrics*. 2013;131;620–622.

Chapter 9

Psychosocial Aspects of Pediatric Hereditary Cancer Syndromes

Andrea Farkas Patenaude

The psychological issues aroused by the diagnosis of a child or adolescent with a cancer that is found to be part of a hereditary syndrome arouse even more complex and far-reaching feelings than those that occur around the diagnosis of a sporadic cancer. The diagnosis of a hereditary cancer syndrome begins a never-ending cycle of anxiety, wariness, medicalization of one's life experience, and concern about other living relatives and future generations.[1] Children with some hereditary cancers will be at increased risk for second or even third or fourth cancers.[2,3] They may also have significant nonmalignant features of the syndrome, with which their cancer is associated, that affect their physical appearance or functioning. Although initially both children with hereditary and nonhereditary cancers and their families are focused on getting life-saving treatment for the child, the feelings associated with the etiology of the cancer and the likelihood that other risks lurk beyond the cancer and its late effects are particularly challenging for hereditary cancer family members to cope with over a prolonged period following treatment. As it is now hypothesized that one-quarter to one-third of pediatric cancers may be hereditary in origin,[4] attention to these issues becomes more salient. This section illustrates some of the unique emotional and medical challenges faced by members of hereditary cancer families. See Boxes 9.1 and 9.2.

Research about how children with hereditary cancers feel about their circumstance has shown differential responses to genetic testing:

- Testing children and adults for *APC* mutations predisposing them to familial adenomatous polyposis (FAP), a precursor of colon cancer has shown mixed results in terms of resulting levels of anxiety or depression. Although most individuals have not had general distress levels above those of the general population, more cancer-related distress is typical and there is greater disruption to quality of life in individuals with FAP who have undergone surgery.[10] Clinically significant increases in anxiety were found at some follow-up points in mutation-negative children with mutation-positive siblings.[11] Future

Box 9.1 Diagnostic Difficulty: Finding Answers

Uncertainty

- Diagnosis of hereditary childhood cancer is often difficult to make.
- It may require extra tests on the child, gathering of extensive family medical history,[5] seeing a range of nononcology specialists, and may take a great deal of time.
- Parents may find attempting to answer physicians' questions about symptoms, which appear initially unrelated to the current condition, difficult.
- Parents may not be sure what answer they wish for from the genetic tests; a positive test provides an explanation for why their child developed cancer but with it come associated risks for the ill child and for other family members.

Challenge

- Diagnosis of the hereditary nature of one's illness often occurs together or in close proximity to the child's cancer diagnosis, further straining parents' emotional resources.
- Dealing with the emotional adjustment of knowing one's child has cancer, discussing and preparing for the child's treatment, arranging home care for other children, and informing family members of the diagnosis are all magnified in difficulty with the diagnosis of hereditary disease.
- Parents may be overwhelmed thinking of future risks the child faces, especially those of possible additional cancers.
- Identification of the underlying hereditary etiology may change treatment or even limit available treatment options.

Challenges

- Medical specialists may disagree about whether a hereditary syndrome is truly present when the child's symptoms meet clinical criteria but there is not a definitive test. Treatment may also be difficult to plan when the definitive testing does not occur, as when parents are unwilling to have the child tested for social or economic reasons Additionally, providers may disagree about the value of new screening protocols for unaffected children who carry or may carry deleterious mutations.
- Direct to consumer testing (DTC) companies say they refuse testing known to be from minors, but they sometimes unknowingly receive samples from minors sent by parents eager to learn if their children carry mutations that the parents are known to have. DTC testing can be accessed without going through a medical provider, but the results can be confusing to parents who should contact knowledgeable genetic counselors or geneticists prior to DTC testing or when results are returned to help them interpret the results.[6,7]
- Incidental and often unwanted information about mutations or variations in genes not originally considered as related to the child's

(continued)

Box 9.1 (Continued)

condition can be found during genomic studies, panel testing (testing of a number of genes at once) or from DTC testing. Parents should be told about this possibility and be queried in advance about whether they want to receive these results. It can be upsetting and confusing to receive such previously unwanted and often difficult to interpret information. Professional interpretation is critical to determine if the variants found provide any meaningful information. These issues are particularly complex in the context of tested children where the potential benefits of acquired information must be weighed against a host of ethical concerns about the children's rights to an "open future," the right to make decisions about nonessential genetic or genomic testing when they reach the age of maturity.[8,9]

Secrecy

- Some relatives may not be open to discussing family cancer history.
- Searching through family records or talking with family members about the health histories of relatives, living and dead, may reveal family secrets that can sometimes place additional burden on parents.
- Difference in openness about talking about the hereditary cancer within the nuclear family or in different branches of the family may lead to the creation of "secrets," with some family members being told not to talk to others about the hereditary cancer because that branch of the family doesn't want to know or is being kept in the dark about it. This can be very difficult for children who are told not to talk to cousins or siblings.

longitudinal research would be of great value in ascertaining the trajectory of the impact of FAP on affected individuals and families.

- Young adult survivors of hereditary retinoblastoma differ from survivors with nonhereditary retinoblastoma only in that they rate their general health as less good. This is likely a realistic evaluation of their high risk of secondary malignancies and their more frequent experience of bilateral disease and visual impairment than those with sporadic retinoblastoma. Both groups experience poorer quality of life in mental health domains, associated with early experiences of bullying in childhood and visual impairment.[12]
- Studies in adults indicate that family constellations of genetic test results may predict emotional distress following testing rather than an individual's own test score alone.[13] This suggests that a child who tests negative and who has a mutation-positive sibling may have a far different emotional reaction to learning his/her test results than a child who tests negative when all the siblings are negative.

Box 9.2 Coping with Hereditary Cancer

Guilt

- Parents feel guilty if they are told that they have passed on a genetic alternation that resulted in their child having an increased chance of developing cancer, even if they were unaware of the hereditary syndrome at the time the child was conceived.

Fear

- Fear for who else in the family may be affected, including sometimes fear for parents' own health and implications of their own vulnerability in their ability to care for their children may be immobilizing for some parents.

Blame

- Identification of the relationship between a child's cancer and genes inherited through one side of the family can lead to placing blame on the other parent.

Anger

- Parents may experience intense anger and may ask questions such as, "How did this happen to our family?" "How can it be possible to bear even more of a burden than most parents of children with sporadic cancers?"

Disbelief

- One or both parents may refuse to believe the doctors about the hereditary cause for the child's cancer; this may cause disharmony within the couple or between the parents and the staff.

Loneliness

- Even among parents of children with cancer, the parents of children with hereditary cancers are a minority and have concerns that set them apart from other parents.

Frustration

- Little is known by pediatricians and often even by some specialists about hereditary cancers, which can add to parental frustration.
- Parents sometimes feel they have to educate the professionals about the hereditary syndrome their child has.
- Sometimes there is nothing more specific recommended to detect early cancers in a vulnerable child than seeking prompt medical advice.
- Yearly scans on at-risk children (see later) may offer some parents a more active way to search for early cancers in their at-risk children, but they may also lead to false positive results, additional testing, and increased anxiety.
- Insurance companies may not understand the child's condition and need for extensive follow-up, which differs from that of other children with similar cancers, adding frustration and stress on parents.

Talking about Hereditary Cancer—Children's Developmental Understanding

- Children's first understanding of illness has to do with contagion, the fear of getting diseases from direct contact with others. Such feelings persist as an emotional component even in adults who understand that certain diseases are not contagious. For school-age and younger children, explain that childhood cancer is not contagious; one can't catch it from being close to someone who has had cancer. If more than one person in the child's family has had cancer, this may be difficult for them to accept.
- Young children often believe that getting sick, especially getting a serious illness like cancer, may be due to bad behavior, such as doing something one was told by parents not to do. This, too, is important to ascertain and to correct if present.
- Cancer is a very common word on television and in general discussion today. Even very young children age 4 years or older have some idea that cancer is a serious illness that can kill people. Research has shown that it is important to speak honestly, simply, and openly to children about their cancer. For example, explaining that cancer is due to changes in cells in their bodies which make it difficult for their bodies to function normally, but which can often be cured with special treatments. Asking children about their beliefs about why kids get cancer can often elicit their misconceptions, which can then be addressed and corrected.
- Children do not typically understand that cancer can be many different diseases. They may connect a grandparent's death from cancer with their own disease and assume that all cancers are fatal. Thus, drawing distinctions between different types of cancer and different potential outcomes may be very important.
- Although children are often familiar with the idea of diseases "running in the family" from mid-childhood on, the concept of a hereditary cancer may be more difficult to understand. Point out that many families have diseases that are more common in them than they are in the general population, but that not all families can find out information that can help them to find the disease early and treat it successfully. Differentiate contagion and behavioral causes from the known genetic cause for cancer in hereditary cancer families.
- Children may find it difficult to understand why they got cancer and their sibling(s) did not if the cancer is due to inherited factors. Adolescents and some older children may have learned about dominant and recessive genes in school and can be reminded of how this results in not everyone in the family having the same characteristics. Younger children's thoughts should be solicited and errors due to misconceptions corrected. They can simply be told that different children inherit different characteristics like hair and eye color and that the parent doesn't make those choices, they just happen when the baby is created.

- Children who do understand the hereditary risks for cancer in their family may become quite worried about cancer recurring or occurring in a parent, themselves or developing in siblings. These are difficult issues and may require reassurance that everyone is being appropriately checked so that cancers will be caught early and hopefully treated successfully. Reassure the child that nothing will be hidden. Being honest about how everyone in the family is doing can also decrease anxiety.

Identity, Childbearing and Hereditary Cancer

Mutation carriers may face many complex feelings, including fears about possibly passing on deleterious mutations in their decisions about whether to have children. These decisions touch on feelings about the individual's own identify and self-value. Members of hereditary cancer families may come to very different conclusions about this matter, and there is the potential for relatives with different views to be judgmental about those with differing views. The possible range of feelings about whether it is fair for mutation carriers to become parents is evident in the following paraphrases:

- "I want to have kids like everyone else. If my parents had decided not to have kids because they might pass on this bad gene, I would never have been born. And here I am, 30 years of age and glad I am alive. And maybe doctors will find better answers that will cure cancer or at least this type of cancer by the time my kids are older."
- "I don't feel right having children when I know what misery these genes can bring. I watched how sick my mother was and I have been through chemo and everything and I don't want to bring a child into the world for that kind of life." (Composite quotes to illustrate range of preferences about childbearing among those at hereditary cancer risk.)

The increasingly utilized option of pre-implantation genetic diagnosis (PGD) is available for parents with an identified mutation. This approach, which can prevent the birth of a child with the deleterious mutation, is, however, expensive and, for some, morally unacceptable.[4]

Genetic Testing of Children

See Chapter 8 on Genetic Counseling for Hereditary Cancer in Childhood.

Testing children who are potentially at increased hereditary risk for developing cancer may allow for initiation of preventive or diagnostic efforts, guided by the test result. Testing of affected children with a cancer, which can be part of a hereditary cancer syndrome, is not ethically controversial. Some examples are:

- Children in families with strong hereditary history of retinoblastoma are often tested within their first year of life to determine if they should have their eyes screened regularly, since retinoblastoma is usually diagnosed at very young ages.

- A child with cancer who is suspected of having Li-Fraumeni Syndrome (LFS) in whom testing would help guide treatment. The child, if positive for *p53*, would be less likely to be treated with radiation, since individuals with LFS are very sensitive to radiation and are more likely than the average patient to develop secondary cancers following radiation.[2]

However, testing of unaffected children, in whom there is not a clear preventive strategy that would follow from knowing the child's test results, is more controversial.

- Some parents simply want to know if their children are at risk in hopes that children's negative results will reduce their anxiety and guilt.
- Parents also want to know children's results to help them know when to pursue medical evaluation of symptoms, which, in a noncarrier, would not be an indication of serious illness.
- Other parents fear that testing would only make noncarrier children feel guilty that they do not have the burden to bear and would make no difference in the child's medical care.
- The risk/benefit ratio of testing unaffected siblings of children with deleterious mutations changes as improvements arise in screening approaches. There has been growing acceptance of proactive screening of unaffected children at risk for Li-Fraumeni syndrome, a relatively rare but highly penetrant cancer predisposition syndrome.[14,15] It is hoped that children who are old enough to understand that they are being tested will have an opportunity to ask a knowledgeable professional questions they may have about the testing. Older adolescents (above age 14) may want to take part in the decisions about testing and screening.
- The most common genetic testing is done in adults for hereditary breast-ovarian cancer due to mutations in the *BRCA1/2* genes. Testing in childhood for *BRCA1/2* mutations is not recommended since screening is not advised until the mid-20s.[16]
- There are few known connections between mutations in *BRCA1/2* and childhood cancers.[17] However, if a childhood cancer occurs in a family in which the mother or other relatives have had breast cancer, especially if the diagnosis of breast cancer occurred at an earlier-than-usual age, there may be concern raised about hereditary cancer, given widespread media coverage of *BRCA1/2* genetic testing. If the childhood cancer were a sarcoma, leukemia, or a brain tumor, genetic counseling in such cases might be recommended to look for *p53* mutations indicating the presence of Li-Fraumeni syndrome.

Genetic or genomic testing for conditions that are not determined by single gene mutations may be less clearly predictive of risk. In that scenario, very careful genetic counseling to describe the risks and benefits of testing and limitations in the predictive value of the result should occur. These discussions should include talking about the fact that nonspecific findings can be frustrating and subject to misunderstanding. See Box 9.3.

Box 9.3 Lifetime Issues with Hereditary Cancers

Independence and Hereditary Cancer—"It's not hypochondriasis; it's hereditary"

- All families of children with cancer struggle with how to manage their concerns about maintaining a child's developing independence with closely monitoring symptoms that might be indicative of a cancer's return.Parents of children with cancer may be more likely to restrict their child's social involvement with peers because of concerns about infection, particularly when the child is undergoing treatment. The parents' overprotective stance is likely to lessen in intensity after the child's treatment is over.
- For parents of a child with a hereditary cancer, the "hovering" may continue long past the end of treatment, as anxious parents look for signs of a cancer recurrence with great intensity, given the known predisposition to multiple cancers.
- Struggles for independence by adolescent and young adult mutation carriers may, therefore, be more intense because of the ongoing concern of parents about their developing another cancer.
- When the adolescents or young adults assume responsibility for their own health care, parents may worry about their children's lack of vigilance for signs of recurrent or new cancers or failure to get recommended screening or immediately follow up with medical providers on symptoms of unclear significance.

Secondary Cancers (See Chapter 33, Pediatric Cancer Survivors).

- Having survived a cancer makes some young adults feel that even if they get another cancer, they will be able to "beat" it.
- Young adults who have a cancer syndrome need, however, to be watchful for early symptoms of associated cancers and may be advised to undergo regular screening. This runs counter to the wish to "put cancer behind me," and, as a result, some young adults avoid screening or regular follow-up.
- Those with increased hereditary predisposition would be well served to build a trusting relationship with a physician, such as an informed internist or oncologist, who can oversee any recommended screening and follow further studies.

Other Associated Conditions

- In addition to baldness and other growth- or cognitive-related side effects of treatment for childhood cancer, survivors who have a hereditary syndrome may experience other physical symptoms that can affect their social interaction and acceptance by peers.
- Beckwith-Wiedemann Syndrome (BWH), for example, is associated with macroglossia, or an enlarged tongue, may also cause craniofacial

(continued)

Box 9.3 (Continued)

abnormalities and an increased incidence of Wilm's tumor, adrenal carcinoma, and hepatoblastoma.

Dating, Marriage, and Childbearing

- Young adults who are members of hereditary cancer families worry about when to introduce this fact into conversations with those they date.
- They may fear that the familial syndrome might negatively influence or scare away a potential marriage partner out of concern for the health of future generations or worry about the health of the carrier or potential carrier.
- Some young adults in *BRCA1/2* families choose not to be tested in young adulthood before they meet a life partner so as not to have to discuss the test result with those they date.
- The next generation of mutation carriers face unprecedented decisions about whether, when, and how to have children and whether to utilize reproductive technologies that may greatly reduce the risk of having a child who is a mutation carrier.

Insurance

- Young adults are the age group with higher percentages of individuals without health insurance in the United States.
- Young adult survivors and especially those who carry hereditary predisposition to cancer should be encouraged to have continuous health-insurance coverage.
- In April 2009, a U.S. Federal law, often referred to as GINA (Genetic Information Nondiscrimination Act), went into effect. It provides protection against discrimination in health coverage and employment on the basis of genetic information. The employment protections are limited to companies with more than 15 employees. GINA does not provide protection against discrimination in life, disability or long-term-care insurance.[18] (https://www.genome.gov/Pages/PolicyEthics/GeneticDiscrimination/GINAInfoDoc.pdf)
- Getting disability and life insurance may not be problematic if individuals work for large companies with group insurance plans, but it may be more difficult or expensive if applied for individually.
- New insurance laws under the U.S. Affordable Care Act support coverage for many medical screening or other procedures related to prevention of disease, but the particulars should be carefully considered and checked with the individual's insurance company prior to undergoing screening.

Advice from Professionals Caring for Families of Children with Hereditary Cancers

Professionals can help parents and children in hereditary cancer families with the following common concerns:

Clarifications

- Passing on a mutated gene is part of the large complex of good and sometimes not-so-good genetic predispositions that parents give to their children without awareness of the implications of these characteristics.
- Hereditary cancers are not contagious, even though they may "run in families."
- Not everyone who inherits an altered gene, which increases the risk of cancer, develops cancer.
- Past family illness experiences will not necessarily be repeated in current or future generations. Much more is known and will be discovered about the hereditary causes for cancer. Also, improvements in cancer treatment will alter the experience of those in hereditary cancer families who do develop cancer.

Locating Genetic Counseling and/or Genetic Testing Services

- Providing an initial framework for understanding what genetic counseling and testing can and cannot offer.
- Helping families to evaluate timing of requests for counseling and/or testing.
- Helping them to understand family issues that could arise with gathering family history data or having more familial genetic information and possible resolutions for their family.
- Locating cancer genetic services through local providers or NCI database.

Family Communication

- Anticipation of how to talk with children, grandparents, adult siblings, and extended family before undertaking genetic counseling or testing can be helpful.
- Asking relatives what they would want to know before the information is available may reduce tension in subsequent sharing of results of genetic consultations or testing (see earlier).
- A letter from professionals explaining the genetic information presented can facilitate discussion with relatives.
- Urging by professionals to disseminate genetic information within the family is highly motivating.

References

1. Patenaude AF. *Genetic Testing for Cancer: Psychological Approaches to Helping Patients and Families*. Washington, DC: American Psychological Association; 2005.

2. Strahm B, Malkin D. Hereditary cancer predisposition in children: Genetic basis and clinical implications. *Int J Cancer.* 2006;119(9):2001–2006.
3. Schneider KA. *Counseling about Cancer: Strategies for Genetic Counseling.* 3rd ed. New York: Wiley-Liss; 2012.
4. Schiffman JD, Geller JI, Mundt E, Means A, Means L, Means V. Update on pediatric cancer predisposition syndromes. *Pediatr Blood Cancer.* 2013; 60:1247–1252.
5. Bennett R. *The Practical Guide to Genetic Family History.* New York: Wiley-Liss; 1999.
6. Howard HC, Avard D, Borry P. Are the kids really all right? Direct-to-consumer genetic testing in children: are company policies clashing with professional norms? *Eur J Hum Genet.* 2011;19:1122–1126.
7. Ross LF, Saal HM, David KL & Anderson RR and the American Academy of Pediatrics; American College of Medical Genetics and Genomics. Technical report: ethical and policy issues in genetic testing and screening of children. *Genet in Med.* 2013;15:234–245.
8. Bredenoord AL, deVries MC & van Delden JJM. Next-generation sequencing: Does the next generation still have the right to an open future? *Nature Rev Genet.* 2013;14: published online March 2013. doi:10.1038/nrgs3459
9. Clayton EW, McDullough LB, Biesecker LG, Joffe S, Ross LF, Wolf SM for the Clinical Sequencing Exploratory Research Cser Consortium Pediatrics Working Group. *Am J Bioeth.* 2014;14:3–9.
10. Douma KF, Aaronson NK, Vasen HG, et al. Psychological distress and use of psychosocial support in familial adenomatous polyposis. *Psycho-Oncol.* 2010;19:289–298.
11. Codori AM, Zawacki KL, Petersen GM, et al. Genetic testing for hereditary colorectal cancer in childhood: long-term psychological effects. *Am J of Med Genet.* 2003;116(2):117–128.
12. Van Dijk J, Imhof SM, Moll AC, et al. Quality of life of adult retinoblastoma survivors in the Netherlands. *Health Qual Life Outcomes.* 2007;5:30.
13. Smith KR, West JA, Croyle RT, Botkin JR. Familial context of genetic testing for cancer susceptibility: Moderating effects of siblings' test results on psychological distress one to two weeks after *BRCA1* mutation testing. *Cancer Epidemiol Biomarkers Prev.* 1999;8(4, Pt. 2):385–392.
14. Villani A, Tabori U, Schiffman J, et al. Biochemical and imaging surveillance in germline TP53 mutation carriers with Li-Fraumeni syndrome: a prospective observational study. *Lancet Oncol.* 2011;12:559–567.
15. Malkin D. Genetic testing: psychological impact on family members. Talk presented at Annual Meeting of the International Pediatric Oncology Society(SIOP), Hong Kong, China, September 27, 2013.
16. American Society of Clinical Oncology. American Society of Clinical Oncology policy statement update: genetic testing for cancer susceptibility. *J Clin Oncol.* 2003;21(12):2397–2406.
17. Brooks GA, Stopfer JE, Erlichman J, Davidson R, Nathanson KL, Domchek SM. Childhood cancer in families with and without BRCA1 or BRCA2 mutations ascertained at a high-risk breast cancer clinic. *Cancer Biol Ther.* 2006;5(9):1098–1102.
18. National Human Genome Research Institute, Genetic Information Nondiscrimination Act (GINA) of 2008, http://www.genome.gov/24519851

Section III

Specific Symptom Management

Chapter 10

Nausea, Vomiting, Anorexia, and Fatigue

Marilyn J. Hockenberry and Cheryl C. Rodgers

Distressing physical symptoms caused by childhood cancer and its treatment occurs frequently due to aggressive therapy regimens implemented to cure the disease. Common childhood cancer symptoms, such as nausea and vomiting, anorexia, and fatigue can disrupt a child's life when not relieved. Each symptom requires careful assessment and appropriate interventions to reduce the distress and improve daily life for children living with cancer and their families.

Nausea and Vomiting

Nausea and vomiting are two common symptoms associated with cancer treatment and can occur in up to 70% of pediatric patients.[1] These symptoms have distinct characteristics (Table 10.1). Either symptom can occur before the start of chemotherapy, referred to as anticipatory; during chemotherapy administration or within 24 hours after chemotherapy, referred to as acute; or more than 24 hours after completion of chemotherapy, referred to as delayed.

Pathophysiology

Major factors trigger and prolong nausea and vomiting following chemotherapy or radiation therapy. These factors include:

- Irritation or injury to certain cells within the stomach and digestive tract of the body.
- Neurotransmitters (serotonin, histamine) released from the stomach that signal the brain when a toxic substance is in the body.

Etiology

Many cancer chemotherapy agents are emetogenic (Table 10.2). Even when chemotherapy administration is preceded by antiemetic therapy, nausea and vomiting may still occur. Other factors that may affect the amount and severity of nausea and vomiting include:

- Prior experiences with motion sickness.
- Previous bad experience with nausea and vomiting.

Table 10.1 Nausea and Vomiting Characteristics

Nausea	Vomiting
• An unpleasant wavelike sensation in the stomach and back of throat that may lead to retching, vomiting, or both.	• Forcible voluntary or involuntary emptying of the stomach contents through the mouth.
• Can be accompanied by sweating, light-headedness, dizziness, increased salivation and weakness.	• Can be accompanied by nausea, rapid breathing, and abdominal cramping.
• Controlled by a part of the nervous system that controls the body's automatic functions, like breathing.	• Controlled by two areas of the brain: the vomiting center (in the area postrema located in the medulla) which has overall control of vomiting, and the nearby Chemoreceptor Trigger Zone (CTZ).

Table 10.2 Severity of Nausea and Vomiting Associated with Chemotherapy

High	Moderate	Low	Minimal
Actinomycin-D	Daunorubicin	Etoposide	Aparaginase
Carmustine	Doxorubicin	Teniposide	Vincristine
Cisplatin	Idarubicin	Paclitaxel	Bleomycin
Cyclophosphamide ($\geq$1.5 g/m^2)	Carboplatin	Topotecan	Busulfan
Dacarbazine	Cyclophosphamide (<1.5 g/m^2)	Methotrexate	Fludarabine
Mechlorethamine	Cytarabine (IV >1 gm/m^2)	Mitoxantrone	Rituximab
	Ifosfamide	Mitomycin	Vinblastine
		Cytarabine (<1 gm/m^2)	

- Fatigue.
- Emotional stress such as anxiety or fear.
- Sensitivity to odors.

Assessment

Patient assessment prior to chemotherapy administration can provide insight into strategies that can decrease nausea and vomiting. A pre-chemotherapy assessment should include the following:

- Type and dose of chemotherapy being administered.
- Previous history of nausea and vomiting.
- Determination of previous tolerance of chemotherapy treatment: what contributed to the symptoms.
- Previous effectiveness of antiemetic regimen.
- Effectiveness of supportive interventions: relaxation techniques, distraction, biofeedback, etc.

Nausea and vomiting can severely alter fluid and electrolyte balance in the pediatric patient. Although chemotherapy agents or intravenous hydration is infusing, assessment of intake and output must be monitored closely and any discrepancy may indicate dehydration or overhydration and should be reported promptly.

Preventing Nausea and Vomiting

- The goal is to prevent the child from ever experiencing nausea or vomiting to try to prevent the development of anticipatory symptoms (the conditioned response of developing nausea and vomiting before receiving the drug).
- Nonpharmacologic interventions (e.g., relaxation, distraction, cognitive behavioral therapy) can be useful in preventing and treating nausea and vomiting.
- Administration of an antineoplastic drug with a mild sedative at bedtime may be helpful for some children. Nighttime administration of drugs such as methotrexate and 6-mercaptopurine may be more effective than morning administration.

Additional strategies to decrease nausea and vomiting include:

- Eat foods served cold or at room temperature.
- Drink sips of liquids when nauseated.
- Eat smaller, frequent meals throughout the day.
- Eat easy-to-digest food such as gelatin, toast, rice, dry cereals, and crackers.
- Avoid foods that are fried, greasy, very sweet, spicy, hot, or strong flavored.
- Maintain good oral hygiene, and rinse mouth frequently.
- Use distraction such as music, television, games, or reading before, during, and after chemotherapy.
- Listen to relaxation tapes or use visual imagery before, during, and after chemotherapy.
- Exercise when possible.

Treatment

5-Hydroxytryptamine-3 (5-HT_3) receptor antagonists are the antiemetics of choice to manage nausea and vomiting in children caused by chemotherapy and radiotherapy. In addition to lack of sedation, the advantage of these agents over previously used medications is that they produce no extrapyramidal side effects, such as difficulty speaking or swallowing, shuffle walk, slow movements, trembling, stiffness of the arms and legs, or loss of balance. 5-HT_3 receptor antagonists, such as ondansetron, granisetron, and tropisetron, should be administered in children receiving high or moderate emetic chemotherapy but has not shown benefits for children receiving minimally emetic chemotherapy.[1] 5-HT_3 receptor antagonists given in combination with dexamethasone are more effective than 5-HT_3 receptor antagonists alone for chemotherapy induced nausea and vomiting.[2] NK-1 receptor antagonist (aprepitant) is an effective medication for nausea and vomiting associated with highly emetogenic chemotherapy, but it is currently restricted for use in children 12 years of age and older.[2]

Table 10.3 Common Medications for Nausea and Vomiting

Medication	Dose and Frequency	Routes	Side Effects
Front Line Antiemetics			
Ondansetron (Zofran®)	0.15 mg/kg if given as three doses, or 0.45 mg/kg as one dose	po, IV	Headache
Granisetron (Kytril®)	10 mg daily	po, IV	Headache
Tropisetron (Navoban®)	0.2 mg/kg daily	po, IV	Headache
Alternative Antiemetics			
Medication	Dose and Frequency	Routes	Side Effects
Metoclopramide (Reglan®)	1–2 mg/kg, q 2–4 hr	IV	EPS*, sedation
Prochlorperazine (Compazine®)	0.5 mg/kg, q 4–6 hr	po, IV	EPS, agitation
Promethazine (Phenergan®)	0.5 mg/kg, q 4 hr	po, IV	EPS, agitation
Adjuvant Medications			
Diphenhydramine (Benadryl®)	1 mg/kg, q 4–6 hr	po, IV	Sedation
Dexamethasone (Decadron®)	6 mg/m^2 as one dose or divided tid	po, IV	Facial flushing, hyperglycemia Electrolyte imbalance
Lorazepam (Ativan®)	0.025 mg/kg, q 6 hr	po, IV	Sedation

*EPS = extra pyramidal symptoms.

Alternative medications for the prevention and treatment of chemotherapy-induced nausea and vomiting include metoclopramide and phenothiazine medications. Promethazine (Phenergan®), chlorpromazine (Thorazine®), prochlorperazine (Compazine®) or trimethobenzamide (Tigan®) are effective phenothiazine agents. Metoclopramide (Reglan®) is a more effective antiemetic for severe vomiting. Unfortunately, the drug causes a number of side effects in children, particularly extrapyramidal reactions, such as muscle tremors or twitching, agitation, grimacing, dysarthria and oculogyric crisis (fixation of eyes in one position for minutes or hours). Metoclopramide (Reglan®) should be administered with dexamethasone (Decadron®) or diphenhydramine (Benadryl®).[3] Common medications to prevent nausea and vomiting during chemotherapy are found in Table 10.3.

Anorexia

Most chemotherapy causes some degree of anorexia, a decrease in or complete loss of appetite. Loss of appetite, as well as weight loss, may also result directly from effects of the cancer on the body's metabolism. Anorexia may be mild, or, if severe, it may lead to cachexia, a form of malnutrition with muscle wasting. Decreased appetite is generally temporary and returns when chemotherapy is finished. It may take a few weeks after chemotherapy is finished for the appetite to recover. Some chemotherapy may cause more severe loss of appetite.

There are many risk factors associated with an increased incidence of malnutrition in children with cancer.[3] These include:

- Advanced cancer (unfavorable histology Wilms' tumor, neuroblastoma, rhabdomyosarcoma, Ewing's sarcoma).
- Tumors of the head and neck.
- Poor prognosis leukemia, multiple relapse leukemia.
- High-grade brain tumors.
- Stem cell transplantation.

Some children gain weight during cancer treatment; however this may not be an indication of good nutrition. Steroids, inactivity, electrolyte imbalances, and fluid retention, are common causes of weight gain. A thorough nutritional assessment should be performed periodically during the child's cancer treatment.

Assessment

- Evaluate extent of appetite loss, vomiting, taste changes, diarrhea, and constipation.
- Evaluate nutritional intake, either through diet recall or food diary.
- Monitor weight closely: If <10th percentile or < 1 kg/year prepubertal or <1 kg/6 months pubertal, consult dietician and/or nutritionist.
- Monitor height closely. Loss of height acceleration could be a sign of poor nutrition.
- Monitor trends of laboratory values, such as albumin and prealbumin levels.

Intervention

Proper nutrition helps strengthen the body to fight disease and infection, and cope with cancer treatments. It is important to keep the child's body well-nourished during cancer treatment and include foods from all five basic food groups (Figure 10.1). However, maintaining good nutrition during cancer therapy may be difficult due to a variety of symptoms caused from the cancer treatment. Consulting a dietician/nutritionist can help the child and family learn ways to maintain an appropriate body weight. Table 10.4 lists a variety of interventions that can be performed to minimize symptoms and maximize nutritional well-being.

General Advice for Parents

- Don't push the child to eat.
- Try to get the foods they ask for.
- Explain reasons behind the need for good nutrition.

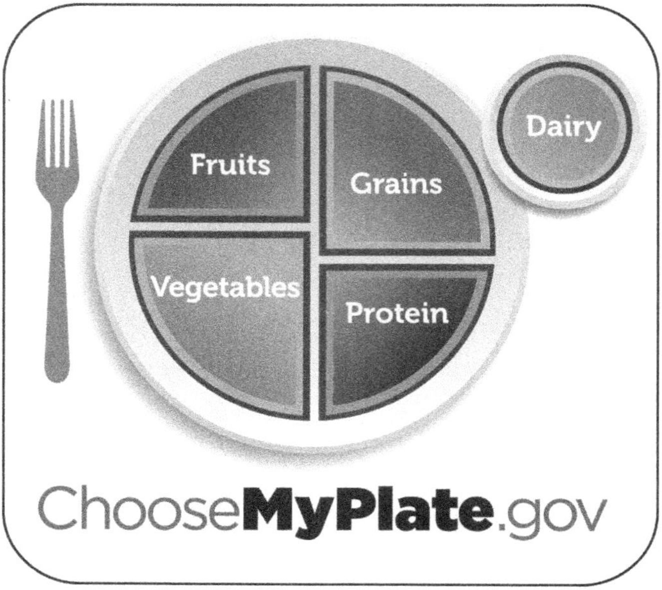

Figure 10.1 Choose My Plate. From: United States Department of Agriculture (USDA) Center for Nutrition Policy and Promotion. ChooseMyPlate. Alexandria, VA: USDA. http://www.choosemyplate.gov/. Accessed Aug 16, 2013.

Table 10.4 Maintaining Nutrition During Childhood Cancer Therapy[5]

Symptom	Intervention
Poor Appetite	• Smaller, more frequent meals and snacks • Let the child help with shopping and preparing meals • Offer high-calorie, high-protein meals and snacks • Avoid forcing a child to eat—this may make a child's appetite worse • Approach meal times as engaging, stimulating, pleasant times

Mouth Sores	• Use soft foods that are easy to chew
	• Avoid foods that may cause irritation to the mouth, including the following:
	  • citrus fruits or juices (i.e., orange, tangerine, grapefruit)
	  • spicy or salty foods
	  • rough, course, or dry foods (i.e., raw vegetables, crackers, toast)
	• Cut foods into small pieces
	• Serve foods cold or at room temperature—hot foods may irritate the mouth and throat
	• Use a blender to make foods softer and easier to chew

(continued)

Table 10.4 (Continued)

Symptom	Intervention
Dry Mouth	• Try sour foods in order to increase salivary production • Chew gum or eat hard candies • Offer small frequent sips of water while eating • Offer foods with liquid in them (i.e., soups) or sauce or gravy to dip the food into
Taste Changes	• Offer salty or seasoned foods • Use flavorful seasoning on foods • Marinate meats in fruit juice, teriyaki sauce, or Italian dressing • Try serving foods at different temperatures • Offer foods that look and smell good • Keep the child's mouth clean by rinsing and brushing • Use plastic utensils to avoid the metal taste
Nausea/Vomiting	• See previous section on nausea and vomiting

Diarrhea	• Try to avoid high-fiber foods including the following:
	  • nuts and seeds
	  • whole grains
	  • dried beans and peas
	  • raw fruits and vegetables
	• Try to limit greasy, fatty, gassy, or fried foods
	• Offer small, frequent meals and liquids throughout the day
	• Limit milk and milk products if lactose intolerance is a problem
	• Drink plenty of liquids throughout the day

Constipation	• Include high-fiber foods, including the following:
	  • whole grain breads and cereals
	  • raw fruits and vegetables
	  • raisins and prunes
	• Drink plenty of fluids; hot drinks are sometimes helpful
	• Keep the skin on vegetables when cooking them
	• Add bran or wheat germ to foods such as casseroles, cereals or homemade breads

Adapted from Cincinnati Children's Hospital Medical Center. Nutritional requirements for a child with cancer. Cincinnati, OH: CCHMC; 2011. http://www.cincinnatichildrens.org/health/info/cancer/home/nutritional-requirements.htm. Accessed Aug 16, 2013.

- Offer food multiple times throughout the day. Encourage the child to eat whenever hungry.
- "Power pack" the food so that each bite counts by adding extra margarine, cheese, gravy, or sauce to foods.
- Offer the high fat version of a food like fried chicken instead of baked, and whole milk instead of skim.

Fatigue

Fatigue is one of the most distressing and debilitating symptoms experienced during childhood cancer treatment.[6–8] Fatigue often develops

Table 10.5 Factors Related to Fatigue in Children with Cancer

Factors	Causes
Treatment-related	Chemotherapy, radiation therapy, surgery, biologic response modifiers, myelosuppression
Environmental	Long waits in the clinic and hospital, altered schedules or routines, hospital noise, sleep/rest interruptions in the hospital
Personal/ behavioral	Cognitive/developmental stage, emotions, moods, worry, boredom
Cultural/family	Parent cues, expectations of others (e.g., family, relatives or friends), being pushed too hard, lacking a schedule

during cancer treatment but can persist for years after treatment ends.[8] Survivors who report chronic fatigue have poorer physical, social, emotional, and school functioning than survivors who were not fatigued.[9] The fatigue a person with cancer feels is different from the fatigue of everyday life. It is unrelated to activity and may not be resolved with rest or sleep (Table 10.5).

Fatigue and depression symptoms are often associated with each other, although they have distinct features.[10] The following feelings are common with fatigue caused by chemotherapy:

- Weariness.
- Weakness.
- Lack of energy.
- Decreased ability for physical and mental work.
- Trouble thinking and concentrating.
- Forgetfulness.

In contrast, depression often causes feelings of sadness, irritability, or frustration, loss of interest in normal activities, and indecisiveness. Fatigued pediatric cancer survivors are 33 times more likely to be depressed than nonfatigued survivors and depressed pediatric cancer survivors have significantly higher rates of fatigue then survivors who are not depressed.[8] More research is needed to determine the exact relationship and causative factors among these two symptoms.

Assessment

Multidimensional questionnaires allow for assessment that captures the many characteristics of fatigue. In clinical practice, important questions to ask the child and parents during each clinic visit include:

- Are you feeling tired or weak? If yes, on a scale of 1–10 how bad is the feeling?
- Does feeling tired or weak prevent you from playing or doing your usual activities?

Several instruments have been tested and are recognized as valid and reliable measures of fatigue frequency and intensity.

Childhood Fatigue Scale (CFS)[11]—A 10-item questionnaire that asks children 7–12 years of age about their feelings of tiredness during the past week. The child is asked to rate each question on a four-point Likert scale. The CFS has three subscales that include Lack of Energy, Not Able to Function, and Altered Mood, and is available in English and Spanish.

Parent Fatigue Scale (PFS)[12]—Consists of 17 items that ask the parent their perceptions of the amount of fatigue experienced by their child in the past week. Four subscales of the PFS include Lack of Energy, Not Able to Function, Altered Sleep, and Altered Mood. The PFS is available in English and Spanish.

Fatigue Scale–Adolescent (FS-A)[13]—Created specifically to comprehensively measure cancer-related fatigue in adolescents 13–18 years of age. The FS-A consists of 13 questions designed to evaluate the intensity of fatigue experienced during the past week. Available in English.

Multidimensional Fatigue Scale[14]—An 18-item scale that has child and parent matching versions. Six of the items measure general fatigue, six measure sleep/rest fatigue and six items measure cognitive fatigue. Available in 22 languages.

Pediatric Functional Assessment of Chronic Illness Therapy—Fatigue (Peds FACIT-F)[15]—An 11-item scale for children with cancer that has stable measurement properties across age, sex, and cancer types. It is significantly correlated with the PedsQL Multidimensional Fatigue Scale and can be useful in clinical trials and other research. Available in English and Spanish.

Interventions to Decrease Fatigue during Childhood Cancer Treatment

Education

- Provide patient and family with knowledge of the impact cancer treatment can have on energy level and performance.
- Suggest keeping a diary to track energy level and changes in activity during treatment.
- Develop plan with patient and family to minimize energy expenditure.
- Provide discussion that is age and developmentally appropriate for the patient to understand.

Rest Patterns and Sleep

- Encourage patient and family to develop a specific bedtime and wake time.
- Emphasize importance of a schedule and routine prior to bedtime.
- Determine ways to prevent sleep interruptions during the nighttime.
- Encourage rest periods during the day but emphasize importance of keeping them short.

Exercise

- Discuss information on exercise as being beneficial in relieving fatigue.
- Encourage exercise that involves rhythmic or repetitive movement of large muscle groups (walking, cycling, swimming).
- Emphasize that the exercise program should be developmentally appropriate and initiated gradually and should occur several times a week.

Stress Management

- Teach patient and family stress reduction techniques such as relaxation therapy, guided imagery or distraction to facilitate rest.
- Nutrition.
- Discuss how regular exercise may improve appetite and increase nutritional intake and how improved nutrition can promote increased energy and less tiredness.

References

1. Jordan K, Roila F, Molassiotis A, Maranzano E, Clark-Snow R, Feyer P. Antiemetics in children receiving chemotherapy, MASCC/ESMO guideline update 2009. *Support Care Cancer.* 2011;19(Suppl1):S37–S42.
2. Dupuis LL, Boodham S, Holdsworth M, et al. Guideline for the prevention of acute nausea and vomiting due to antineoplastic medication in pediatric cancer patients. *Pediatr Blood Cancer.* 2013;60:1073–1082.
3. Berde CB, Billett AL, Collins JL. Symptom management in supportive care. In: PA Pizzo, DG Poplack, eds. *Principles and Practice of Pediatric Oncology.* 5th ed. Philadelphia, PA: Lippincott Williams & Wilkins; 2006:1348–1380.
4. United States Department of Agriculture (USDA) Center for Nutrition Policy and Promotion. ChooseMyPlate. Alexandria, VA: USDA. http://www.choosemyplate.gov/. Accessed Aug 16, 2013.
5. Cincinnati Children's Hospital Medical Center. Nutritional requirements for a child with cancer. Cincinnati, OH: CCHMC; 2011. http://www.cincinnatichildrens.org/health/info/cancer/home/nutritional-requirements.htm. Accessed Aug 16, 2013.
6. Chang CW, Mu PF, Jou ST, Wong TT, Chen YC. Systematic review and meta-analysis of nonpharmacological interventions for fatigue in children and adolescents with cancer. *Worldviews Evid Based Nurs.* 2013;10(4):208–217. doi: 10.1111/wvn.12007
7. Baggott C, Dodd M, Kennedy C, et al. Changes in children's reports of symptom occurrence and severity during a course of myelosuppressive chemotherapy. *J Pediatr Oncol Nurs.* 2010;27(6):307–315.
8. Meeske KA, Siegel SE, Globe DR, et al. Prevalence and correlates of fatigue in long-term survivors of childhood leukemia. *J Clinical Oncol.* 2005;23(24):5501–5510.
9. Meeske KA, Patel SK, Palmer SN, et al. Factors associated with health-related quality of life in pediatric cancer survivors. *Pediatr Blood Cancer.* 2007;49:298–305.
10. Whitsett SF, Gudmundsdottir M, Davies P, et al. Chemotherapy-related fatigue in childhood cancer: Correlates, consequences, and coping strategies. *J Pediatr Oncol Nurs.* 2008;25(2):76–96.
11. Hinds PS, Yang J, Gattuso JS, et al. Psychometric and clinical assessment of the 10-item reduced version of the Fatigue Scale-Child instrument. *J Pain Symptom Manage.* 2010;39(3):572–578.
12. Hockenberry MJ, Hinds PS, Barrera P, et al. (2003). Three instruments to assess fatigue in children with cancer: The child, parent and staff perspectives. *J Pain Symptom Manage.* 2003;25(4):319–328.

13. Mandrell BN, Yang J, Hooke MC, et al. Psychometric and clinical assessment of the 13-item reduced version of the fatigue scale-adolescent instrument. *J Pediatr Oncol Nurs.* 2011;28(5):287–294.

14. Varni JW, Burwinkle TM, Katz ER, Meeske K, Dickinson P. The PedsQL in pediatric cancer: Reliability and validity of the Pediatric Quality of Life Inventory Generic Core Scales, Multidimensional Fatigue Scale, and Cancer Module. *Cancer* 2002;94(7):2090–2106.

15. Lai JS, Cella D, Kupst MJ, et al. Measuring fatigue for children with cancer: Development and validation of the pediatric Functional Assessment of Chronic Illness Therapy-Fatigue (pedsFACIT-F). *J Pediatr Hematol/Oncol.* 2007;29(7):471–479.

Chapter 11

Pain

Lonnie Zeltzer and Elliot J. Krane

The treatment of pain is often divided into two broad categories: (a) non-pharmacologic methods, of which psychological/behavioral interventions, physical methods, and complementary and alternative medical (CAM) practices are the three most common examples, and (b) pharmacologic methods, which include drug therapy as well as interventional or invasive methods of analgesia.

Pain must be evaluated before therapy can ensue. In developing an effective therapeutic regimen, it is necessary to determine possible sources of the patient's pain, type of pain, and aggravating/alleviating factors, as well as developmental, psychological, and environmental contributions. The initial evaluation includes descriptors of the discomfort and pain location to help determine the type and sources of the pain, recognizing that multiple contributory sources may exist. Evaluation includes other factors that can enhance pain-related suffering and reduce the ability to tolerate discomfort such as sleep status (onset and maintenance), appetite, fatigue, dyspnea, nausea/vomiting, diarrhea/constipation, pruritus, mood, and emotional state. Assessment of comorbid anxiety, depression, posttraumatic stress syndrome, and a past history of negative and traumatic pain experiences are essential, because each of these might influence pain. If not addressed, these factors can create anticipatory anxiety, which enhances the pain experience and suffering. Table 11.1 provides some examples of different types of pain.

Table 11.2 provides some examples of both nonpharmacological and pharmacological treatments by type of pain. Examples of nonpharmacological interventions are not meant to indicate preference of some strategies over others not mentioned (e.g., cognitive-behavioral therapy versus biofeedback, etc.). Although interventional strategies are included for completeness, in practice they are less frequently used in the treatment of pediatric cancer pain and are reserved for specific indications when less invasive methods are not effective.

Table 11.1 Classification of Types of Pain

	Characteristics	Examples
Neuropathic	• Burning, shooting, electrical, stabbing • Allodynia (skin sensitivity)	• Phantom limb pain • Radiculopathy • Chemotherapy-induced neuropathy • Herpes zoster
Nociceptive	• Pressure, aching, throbbing, "just hurts" • Pain with palpation of affected organ	• Procedural pain • Mucositis • Pathologic fracture • Arthralgia and arthritis
Myofascial	• Aching pressure, external cramping • Pain with range of motion, activity, palpation • Muscle spasms	• Muscle strain • Myositis
Visceral	• Internal cramping pain • Nausea, vomiting • Radiologic pathology	• Pancreatitis • Small bowel obstruction • Bladder spasms • Capsular liver distension

Pain Scales

Several instruments have been tested and are recognized as valid and reliable measures of pain intensity.

The Numerical Rating Scale (11 point NRS)—This is a 0–10 verbal self-report numerical scale where 0 represents no pain and 10 represents severe/most pain possible.[1]

The Faces Pain Scale—Revised[2]—Self-report. This scale includes six, gender-neutral, line drawings of faces that are scored from 0–10. It has been shown to have adequate psychometric properties[3,4] and has been validated for use in children 4–16 years of age. The scale is available at http://painsourcebook.ca in 33 languages. Although there are many different "faces" scales for the measurement of pain intensity, this one has been validated in the most studies.

Color Analog Scale[5]—Self report. This scale is s a thermometer. As one moves up the page, the scale gradually gets wider and changes color from red (most pain) to white (no pain). At the bottom, it is 20 mm wide and white in color, whereas at the top it is 75 mm wide and red in color. The white color at the bottom indicates "no pain" and the red color at the top indicates "the most pain." The reverse side of the scale is numbered from 0 to 10 in 1-cm increments, allowing healthcare providers to quantify a child's response. This tool has been validated for general assessment of pain in children 3–17 years of age and for assessing pain severity, and for changes in pain severity in children 5–12 years of age. It is available in English and Spanish.

Table 11.2 Useful Pain Interventions by Classes of Pain

	Non-pharmacological	Pharmacological
Neuropathic	• Hypnosis • Biofeedback • Relaxation • Physical therapy • Desensitization • Hydrotherapy	• Conventional Analgesics • Opioids, nonsteroidal anti-inflammatory drugs (NSAIDs), coxibs • Unconventional Analgesics • Antiepileptic drugs, antidepressants, local anesthetics • Nerve Blocks • Sympathetic ganglion • Plexus and peripheral nerve • Subarachnoid and epidural • Neuroablation and neurolysis
Nociceptive	• Hypnosis • Biofeedback • Relaxation • Acupuncture/pressure • Distraction	• Conventional Analgesics • Opioids, NSAIDs, coxibs • Nerve Blocks • Sympathetic ganglion • Plexus and peripheral nerve • Subarachnoid and epidural • Neuroablation and neurolysis
Myofascial	• Hypnosis • Biofeedback • Relaxation • Acupuncture/pressure • Distraction • Massage • Cooling • Warming • Physical therapy • Iyengar yoga	• Conventional Analgesics • Opioids, NSAIDs, coxibs • Nerve Blocks • Local injection • Plexus and peripheral nerve • Subarachnoid and epidural
Visceral	• Hypnosis • Biofeedback • Relaxation • Acupuncture/pressure • Distraction	• Conventional Analgesics • Opioids, coxibs • Nerve Blocks • Subarachnoid, and epidural • Neuroablation and neurolysis

Visual Analog Scale[6]—Self report. This single item tool is s a 100-mm vertical pain thermometer. The bottom end point represents "no pain" and the top end point represents "as bad as it can be." The child indicates their current pain level by drawing a line on the thermometer corresponding to how much pain they are in. Validated in older children (9 years of age and up) and has been used in multiple studies that look at pain levels in children with chronic illnesses.

Pain Thermometer[7]—Self report. This single item assessment tool consists of a line drawing of a thermometer that has a bulb at the bottom and vertical lines. There are no corresponding descriptions of what the lines mean. The child is told that this "pain thermometer" works like an outside or oral thermometer, and if there is no pain, the mercury would not rise out of the bulb, but the more pain the child is experiencing the higher the mercury would rise. The child colors in the level of mercury to indicate the amount of pain he or she is experiencing.

McGill Pain Questionnaire (MPQ) (short version)[8,9]—Self report; 15-item tool; identifies the location, intensity, duration, and quality of a patients' pain. Following assessment, three pain scores are obtained: sensory, affective, and total pain score. MPQ has been validated in children ages 14 and older and has been used extensively in clinical settings. It is best used as a clinical tool to receive an immediate measure of pain. There is a longer version that also focuses on pain assessment, but not as simply as the short version. It inquires about the pain in fine detail. For example there are queries about associations with weather, time of day, etc., whereas the short form does not have those details. The short form is more appropriate for acute and surgical pain than is the long form. The long form takes about 10 minutes to complete, whereas the short form takes under five minutes. Another advantage of this measure is that it is available in several languages, including English, Spanish, French, Greek and even Norwegian.

Nonpharmacologic Treatment

Psychological/Behavioral/Physical Interventions

Children with significant pain virtually always experience some, often significant, adverse psychological effects of pain, including depression, social withdrawal, diminished self-esteem, anger, feelings of loss of control, and anxiety. These psychological associations with pain then feed back to enhance the perceptions and reports of pain, lower the pain threshold, and increase suffering.

- Although psychopharmacology is often useful in the management of anxiety and depression associated with pain, it is not a substitute for psychotherapeutic interventions, including psychotherapy; cognitive behavioral therapy (CBT); dialectic behavioral therapy (DBT); acceptance and commitment therapy (ACT); relaxation techniques; family therapy when needed; and a behavioral plan to enhance functioning, including school attendance when possible (see Table 11.3).[10,11]
- Parents, not knowing the best way to support their child, may inadvertently contribute to their child's pain by continually inquiring about pain, thereby focusing attention on it, arguing with each other or about the child causing feelings of fear, guilt, and other negative emotions in the child.
- If children stay home from school during aspects of treatment or because of disease- or treatment-related effects, they are removed from normal activities and may have fewer distractions and supports to divert attention away from pain.

Table 11.3 Psychological/Behavioral/Physical Therapies for Pain

Type of Therapy	Description
Cognitive-Behavioral Therapy (CBT)	• A structured format that combines strategies for altering negative thoughts, relaxation techniques, sometimes involving imagery, and behavioral strategies that enhance positive function
Psychotherapy • Insight-Oriented • Eclectic	• Helps child understand and express emotions related to feelings of anger, frustration, sadness or worry/fear; understand strengths • Helps child to develop strategies to cope and function, which in turn helps to improve feelings of control and mastery • Combinations of the above
Relaxation Techniques	• Breathing, with slow measured exhales • Progressive focus on parts of the body sequentially noticing feelings of warmth and relaxation in that body part with each breath • Sequential contraction and then relaxation of muscles as child progresses from one body part to the next, typically from feet to head
Distraction	• Helps keep the child's attention focused on interesting objects or activities, e.g., school, reading, stories, computer, videogames, TV, film, writing, music, friends, phone, etc.
Family Interventions and Therapies	• Education about strategies to help child cope and to use distraction techniques to help reduce anxiety • Help develop a structured behavioral incentive plan to enhance the child's functioning • Work with the family on communication about both positive and negative emotions; enhancing intra-family communication • Further support for couples in co-parenting and supporting one another in coping with their child's illness
Physical Therapy	• Development of a plan for graded appropriate exercise and movement; working with a therapist to reduce postural imbalance and enhance muscle circulation

- Children who are experiencing unrelieved pain may become more sedentary. This can create further pain through lack of exercise, and development of myofascial pain and contact pressure effects on the body, with reduced circulation to the affected body parts.

Medical procedures such as bone marrow aspirations/biopsies, intrathecal punctures for spinal fluid sampling or administration of medication, intravenous punctures, and intramuscular injections can cause acute pain and anxiety and lead to conditioned fear with increasing pain if pain and anxiety are not prevented or treated adequately. However, increasingly and appropriately more centers are using a short-acting intravenous

Table 11.4 Psychological/Behavioral/Physical Pain Reduction Methods for Medical Procedures (often mostly carried out by child-life specialists)

Type of Intervention	Description
Party Blowers Soap Bubbles Pop-Up Book Stories	• Good for younger children; facilitates focus of attention and deep breaths
Mutual Storytelling	• Engages child in participatory activity to focus attention and engage imagination
Hypnosis/Guided Imagery	• Engages child in focused attention on a set of images and imaginary experiences
Other Distractors	• Use of humor and jokes; magic tricks; singing and music; TV, videogames; counting, math games; telling or reading stories to the child; rhythmic breathing
Counter-Sensory Stimulation	• Having child squeeze parent's hand tightly, rubbing another part of the body, pressing a part of the body next to the procedural site

general anesthesia called propofol along with a local anesthetic as well as behavioral preparation and interventions for the more invasive procedures and topical local anesthetic and behavioral interventions for intravenous phlebotomies (see Table 11.4).

The following sections address a breadth of intervention approaches. Some will be more readily available than others. Referrals should always be made with consideration to the training, credentials, and expertise of the provider.

Complementary Therapies

See Chapter 21, Integrative Oncology. CAM incorporates the application of Eastern medical practices; spiritual practices; energy therapies; and other techniques, such as art, pet, music, and aroma therapies, to complement the use of conventional pharmacological and psychological Western medical practices. CAM is defined by the National Center for Complementary and Alternative Medicine (NCCAM) as a group of diverse medical and health-care systems, practices, and products that are not presently considered to be part of conventional medicine. NCCAM groups CAM therapies into five categories or domains: (a) biologically based therapies, (b) manipulative and body-based therapies, (c) energy therapies, (d) mind-body interventions, and (d) alternative medical systems. There are few well-studied CAM therapies for pain control in children with cancer other than hypnotherapy for medical procedure pain. Box 11.1 provides examples of CAM therapies that have been used with children, although as noted, strong evidence for the efficacy of many are lacking. See Zeltzer[12] for a review of state of the science on complementary therapies for pediatric pain.

Box 11.1 CAM Potential Treatment Approaches*

Hypnotherapy—Helping the child to imagine being somewhere else or dissociated from the current experience; this can involve induction strategies to help narrow the focus of child's attention, deepening strategies to enhance the narrowed focus, helping the child go to a "favorite place" where the child can feel safe and comfortable, and then enhancing the dissociation with a variety of strategies, including "pain switches," "magic glove," "central pain control station," etc. Posthypnotic suggestions can be given for enhanced entry into and maintenance of a hypnotic state as needed.

Acupuncture—The use of needles or pressure (acupressure) at key points along meridians or energy lines to enhance the flow of energy or "Qi" (pronounced "chee").

Massage/Craniosacral Therapy—Bodily tactile manipulation of soft tissues with differing degrees of pressure, depending upon the type of massage.

Meditation/Mindful Awareness—The focus on the present, often with the help of a focus on the breath as the mind wanders to other thoughts and feelings; loving kindness meditation involves feelings of connection and well-wishes for safety, health, happiness, and living in peace for self and others. A goal of meditation practice is to achieve loving kindness (metta), compassion (karuna), joy (mudita) and equanimity (upekka).

Iyengar Yoga—A form of yoga developed by BKS Iyengar in Puna, India, in which a selection of bodily poses (asanas) are held with the assistance of props, such as blocks, blankets, bolsters, and straps, to achieve bodily, emotional and spiritual balance. The training in this form of yoga is vigorous and studies have shown its benefits for people with chronic health conditions, especially chronic pain. Pranayama, or yogic breathing, comes later after learning and practicing specific poses in this form of yoga.

Art Therapy—The expression of emotions and thoughts through art, directed by a therapist with training in the psychodynamic understanding of human behavior and how to help children use the art medium for psychotherapeutic benefit. This forum of therapy is especially useful for children who are non-verbal or have difficulty with direct verbal communication.

Music Therapy—The same goal as art therapy but using music, usually in an interactive way with children. Group therapy through drumming circles is one example, and individual instruments or voice work with a trained music therapist is another.

Pet Therapy—The tactile sensation and connection made with specially trained animals with their trainers has been especially useful in the hospital setting and in situations where children are isolated.

Biofeedback—The use of computers or other forms of provision of feedback on biological systems, such as muscle tension, breathing, heart

(continued)

Box 11.1 (Continued)

rate, or skin temperature, with training in how to alter these systems to achieve a more relaxed state. Imagery and breathing techniques are often taught with the visual or other sensory feedback providing reinforcement of accomplishment.

Aroma Therapy—The use of different aromas to achieve a calming state, such as the use of lavender. For children who have developed conditioned anxiety to medical procedures or chemotherapy, pairing of calming interventions together with new aromas (e.g., oranges) can help such children to condition in a positive way to the new aroma.

Reiki Energy Therapy—The balancing of energy fields around and within the body by Reiki masters who are trained to assess and alter the flow of such energy.

*See ref. 12 for evidence base for each type of therapy.

Pharmacological Interventions

Drug Therapy

Although pain reduction is a goal of drug therapy, it is not the only goal, and indeed is not always the primary goal. Improvement of the patient's functional state should be the primary goal of drug therapy in all but the terminally ill patient. All too often, drug therapy reduces a child's report of pain but leads to sufficient drowsiness, nausea, dysphoria, or mood depression to diminish function. Therefore, in addition to the obvious goal of reducing the report of pain, the goals of drug therapy are improved sleep, reduced anxiety, improved mood, greater interaction with family and friends, and an improved ability to engage in the activities of daily living (ADLs) (see Table 11.5).

Appropriate selection of drugs depends upon the correct diagnosis of pain. It is particularly important to recognize the presence of or a contribution by neuropathic pain, because neuropathic pain is often refractory to the use of conventional analgesics, but amenable to the use of unconventional analgesics (see Tables 11.6 and 11.7).

Interventional Therapy

The selection of the most appropriate interventional technique is decided in consultation with an experienced interventional pain physician. These techniques are generally performed under anesthesia in children, using ultrasound and/or radiologic imaging to guide the operator.

The use of interventional regional anesthetic techniques usually provide the most profound analgesia, by blocking or destroying the nerves that provide sensation to the affected body part.

- Regional anesthetic techniques frequently allow children to wean and discontinue most or all of their conventional pain medications, reducing side effects and allowing the greatest degree of return to a functional state. Their greatest limitation is the inability of most techniques to provide relief over a period of greater than a few weeks, which may be

Table 11.5 Conventional Analgesics

Nonsteroidal Anti-inflammatory Drugs (NSAIDs)	Starting Dose	Maintenance Dose
Ibuprofen	10 mg/kg q6H	10 mg/kg q6H
Naproxen	3 mg/kg q8H	3 mg/kg q8H
Acetaminophen	10 mg/kg q6H	10 mg/kg q6H
Ketorolac (Toradol®)	0.25 mg/kg IV q6H	0.25 mg/kg IV q6H
Coxib NSAIDs	Starting Dose	Maintenance Dose
Celecoxib (Celebrex®)	1 mg/kg BID	2–3 mg/kg BID
Opioids (Intravenous)	Continuous Dose	Intermittent Dose
Morphine[a]	0.01–0.02 mg/kg/hr	0.05 mg/kg q4H
Hydromorphone[a]	0.002–0.004 mg/kg/hr	0.01 mg/kg q4H
Fentanyl[a]	0.5 mcg/kg/hr	Not used
Methadone[a]	Not used	0.1 mg/kg q12H
Weak Opioids (Oral)[b]	Starting Dose	Maintenance Dose
Tramadol (Ultram®)	1 mg/kg q6H	2 mg/kg q4H
Hydrocodone[a])	0.1 mg/kg q6H	0.15 mg/kg q4H
Strong Opioids (Oral)	Starting Dose	Maintenance Dose
Morphine[a]	0.1 mg/kg q4H	0.3 mg/kg q4H
Oxycodone[a]	0.1 mg/kg q6h	0.15 mg/kg q4H
Methadone[a]	0.05 mg/kg q12H	0.15 mg/kg q8H
Opioids by Alternative Routes	Starting and Maintenance Doses	
Transdermal fentanyl (Duragesic®)	Based upon established opioid requirement	
Transmucosal fentanyl (Actiq®, Fentora®)	Based upon established opioid requirement	
Rectal hydromorphone	Based upon established opioid requirement	

[a] Maintenance oral opioid doses listed are typical for the nontolerant patient. Some opioid-tolerant patients may require much higher doses. All opioids should be carefully titrated to effect as side effects allow.

[b] Codeine is a prodrug with weak if any primary analgesic effects. As many as 20% of individuals lack the hepatic microsomal enzyme to metabolize codeine to its active form, morphine; and dangerously, some patients are "supermetabolizers" who metabolize very rapidly, leading to rapid escalation of serum morphine levels and toxicity; therefore, codeine should not be routinely used as an oral opioid analgesic.

sufficient until either surgical healing occurs or tumor mass is palliated by radiation or chemotherapy.

- For longer durations of analgesia, particularly in the terminally ill child, catheters may be surgically implanted. The most significant risk and limitation in the insertion of nerve-block catheters is the risk of infection in immunocompromised children and the risk of bleeding in children who may have thrombocytopenia or prolonged clotting time.

Table 11.6 Common Oncological Causes of Neuropathic Pain

Neurotoxic drugs	Nerve invasion/infiltration/compression by tumor
• Vincristine • Vinblastine	• Neuroblastoma, Primary neuroectodermal tumor (PNET) • Sarcoma • Lymphoma • Spine metastases
• Nerve inflammation	• Surgical nerve injury
• Graft versus host disease • Herpes zoster	• Phantom limb pain following amputation • Concomitant surgical nerve injury during tumor resection

Table 11.7 Unconventional Analgesics Useful in Neuropathic Pain

Drug	Starting Dose	Maintenance Dose
Antiepileptic drugs (AEDs)		
Gabapentin (Neurontin®)	1.5 mg/kg PO TID	10 mg/kg PO TID
Pregabalin (Lyrica®)	0.5 mg/kg PO BID	3 mg/kg PO BID
Topiramate (Topamax®)	0.5 mg/kg PO BID	2.5 mg/kg PO BID
Levetiracetam (Keppra®)	10 mg/kg PO BID	30 mg/kg PO BID
Antidepressants		
Tricyclic Antidepressants		
Amitriptyline (Elavil®)	0.1–0.2 mg/kg PO HS	0.5–1 mg/kg PO HS
Nortriptyline (Pamelor®)	0.1–0.2 mg/kg PO HS	0.5–1 mg/kg PO HS
Desipramine (Norpramine®)	0.1–0.2 mg/kg PO HS	0.5–1 mg/kg PO HS
Selective Serotonin-Norepinephrine Reuptake Inhibitors (SSNRIs)		
Duloxetine (Cymbalta®)	0.1–0.2 mg/kg PO QD	1 mg/kg PO QD
Venlafaxine (Effexor®)	0.1–0.2 mg/kg PO QD	1 mg/kg PO QD
Anesthetics		
Intravenous lidocaine	15 mcg/kg/min IV	25 mcg/kg/min IV
Intravenous ketamine	50 mcg/kg/hr IV	300 mcg/kg/hr IV
Oral ketamine	0.25 mg/kg PO q4H	1 mg/kg PO q4H
Topical Agents		
Lidocaine (Lidoderm®)	5% Cream 12 hr/day	5% Cream 12 hr/day
Capsaicin Cream	1% Cream TID	1% Cream TID

Interventional techniques can be usefully divided into anesthetic techniques, in which the nerves are anesthetized for variable periods of time using single drug injection or catheter delivery techniques, and destructive techniques, in which the nerves are ablated (preserving the Schwann cell sheath and allowing axonal regrowth over time) or permanently destroyed using chemical lysis of the nerves.

- In children, neurolysis is generally reserved for terminally ill patients, since the long-term effects of nerve destruction in growing children expected to survive their malignancy is not known.

Table 11.8 Invasive Pain Techniques Useful in Cancer Pain

Clinical Condition	Recommended Invasive Technique
Short Term Interventions (≤4 weeks)	
Extremity Pain	
• Phantom Limb • Bone Pain • Neuropathic Pain	• Peripheral nerve or plexus block (e.g., brachial plexus, lumbar plexus, sciatic nerve) • Sympathetic nerve or ganglion block (stellate ganglion, lumbar sympathetic ganglion) • Epidural analgesia
Chest Pain	
• Surgical (Thoracotomy, Sternotomy) • Pain due to malignancy	• Thoracic epidural analgesia • Paravertebral nerve blocks and infusion (unilateral pain) • Intercostal nerve block
Abdominal Pain	
• Surgical • Pancreatitis • Hepatomegaly	• Epidural analgesia • Celiac plexus block
Long Term Interventions (>4 weeks)	
• Chest Pain • Abdominal Pain • Lower Extremity Pain	• Intrathecal catheter and implanted reservoir/pump • Spinal cord stimulation

- Occasionally, techniques known as neuromodulation are useful, in which nerve stimulators are surgically implanted in the epidural space or adjacent to peripheral nerves, to stimulate spinal nerves such that nociceptive input from the periphery is blocked at the point of stimulation (see Table 11.8).

Summary

The most successful pain treatment strategies for children with cancer depend upon a careful evaluation. Treatments for pain are most successful if a biopsychosocial approach is used. Psychological, behavioral, social/family, CAM, and physical strategies should be considered in conjunction with pharmacological management. Pharmacological analgesic consideration includes route of drug delivery, which depends upon the stage of disease, reason for the pain, and patient characteristics. This pharmacological approach includes interventional strategies as well as oral, transdermal, mucosal, intranasal, intravenous, per rectal, per G-tube and other drug delivery pathways as appropriate. Both pharmacological and behavioral trategies may be needed to treat pain-associated factors such as sleep, constipation, anxiety, and others as determined by history.

Typically, the combination of treatment strategies is more effective than any single approach alone. All pain treatments should include prevention of pain and anxiety associated with medical procedures to prevent conditioned procedure aversion. The latter can lead to anticipatory anxiety that will serve to enhance procedural pain with subsequent procedures. Children can be helped to cope with their cancer experience when expression of their thoughts and feelings is encouraged, and when eradication of their pain and suffering remains a primary goal.

References

1. von Baeyer C. Numerical rating scale for self-report of pain intensity in children and adolescents: recent progress and further questions. *Eur J Pain.* 2009;13(10):1005–1007.
2. Hicks C, et al. The faces pain scale—revised: Toward a common metric in pediatric pain measurement. *Pain.* 2001;93:173–183.
3. Chambers C, et al. A comparison of faces scales for the measurement of pediatric pain: children's and parents' ratings. *Pain.* 1999;83(1):25–35.
4. Chambers C. Johnston C. Developmental differences in children's use of rating scales. *J Pediatr Psychol.* 2002;27(1):27–36.
5. McConahay T, Bryson M, Bulloch B. Clinically significant changes in acute pain in a pediatric ED using the Color Analog Scale. *Am J Emerg Med.* 2007; 25(7):739–742.
6. Schanberg L, et al. Pain coping and the pain experience in children with juvenile chronic arthritis. *Pain.* 1997;73(2):181–189.
7. Williamson G, Walters A, Shaffer D. Caregiver models of self and others, coping and depression: predictors of depression in children with chronic pain. *Health Psychol*, 2002;21(4):405–410.
8. Melzack R. The McGill Pain Questionnaire: major properties and scoring methods. *Pain.* 1975;1(3):277–299.
9. Melzack R. The short-form McGill Pain Questionnaire. *Pain.* 1987;30(2):191–197.
10. Palermo TM. *Cognitive-Behavioral Therapy for Chronic Pain in Children and Adolescents.* New York, NY: Oxford University Press; 2012.
11. Eccleston C, et al., Psychological therapies for the management of chronic and recurrent pain in children and adolescents. *Cochrane Database Syst Rev.* 2012;12:CD003968.
12. Zeltzer LK. Complementary therapy in paediatric pain In: *Oxford Textbook of Paediatric Pain*, Patrick BJS, McGrath J, Walker SM, Zempsky WT, ed. New York, NY: Oxford University Press; 2012: 623–632.

Further Reading

1. Casillas J, Zeltzer LK. Cancer Pain in Children. In: *Bonica's Management of Pain, 4ed*, Ballantyne JC, Fishman SM, Rathmell JP, eds. Hagerstown, MD: Lippincott Williams & Wilkins; 2009: 669–680.
2. Krane EJ, Casillas J, Zeltzer LK. Pain and Symptom Management. In: *Principles and Practice of Pediatric Oncology, 6th* ed, Pizzo PA, Poplack DG, eds. Philadelphia: Lippincott Williams & Wilkins; 2010: 1256–1287.
3. Collins JJ, Grier HE, Kinney HC, Berde CB. Control of severe pain in children with terminal malignancy. *J Pediatr.* 1995;126(4):653–657.

4. Dworkin RH, O'Connor AB, Backonja M, et al. Pharmacologic management of neuropathic pain: Evidence-based recommendations. *Pain.* 2007;132(3):237–251.
5. Solomon MZ, Browning D. Pediatric palliative care: Relationships matter and so does pain control. *J Clin Oncol.* 2005;23(36):9055–9057.
6. Spagrud LJ, Piira T, von Baeyer CL. Children's self-report of pain intensity: The Faces Pain Scale—Revised. *Am J Nurs.* 2003;103(12):62–64.
7. Stanford EA, Chambers CT, Craig KD. A normative analysis of the development of pain-related vocabulary in children. *Pain.* 2005;114(1-2):278–284.
8. Stinson JN, Kavanagh T, Yamada J, Gill N, Stevens B. Systematic review of the psychometric properties, interpretability and feasibility of self-report pain intensity measures for use in clinical trials in children and adolescents. *Pain.* 2006;125(1-2):143–157.
9. Zernikow B, Meyerhoff U, Michel E, et al. Pain in pediatric oncology—children's and parents' perspectives. *Eur J Pain.* 2005;9(4):395–406.

Chapter 12

Anxiety and Depression

Maryland Pao and Anne E. Kazak

Anxiety in Pediatric Oncology Patients

Anxiety in Childhood Cancer

- Uneasiness and apprehension are the hallmarks of anxiety, ranging from transient mild discomfort to persistent, escalating, and/or paralyzing fear. Anxiety has psychological symptoms such as dread, anticipation of negative outcomes, and difficulty sleeping as well as physical symptoms such as feeling tense, palpitations, and chest tightness (see additional symptoms that follow).
- Anxiety is a normal reaction to life stressors and uncertainties, but is thought to be problematic when its intensity and duration begin to impact functioning and quality of life even in the context of childhood cancer.
  - Providers need to distinguish between anxiety symptoms and anxiety disorders (continuum from normal response to variant to impairment).
  - Anxiety may be acute or chronic; important to identify the underlying etiology.
  - It may exist as a primary disorder, psychological reaction to illness, a secondary disorder, or any combination of the three (Table 12.1).
  - It may be comorbid with other psychiatric disorders (e.g., depression).
  - Akathisia (motor restlessness) may be misdiagnosed as anxiety.

Why Is Diagnosis and Treatment of Anxiety Important in a Pediatric Oncology Setting?

- Different types of anxiety are seen in pediatric oncology and may vary at different points in the course of cancer treatment.
- The diagnosis of a life-threatening illness, such as cancer, and the subsequent aggressive treatment may be disruptive, frightening, and potentially traumatic for children and their families.
- Patients feel anxious during and immediately after diagnosis and treatment, as well as during survivorship, treatment for relapses, and palliative care.

Table 12.1 Anxiety Disorders in the Child with Cancer[a]

Primary anxiety disorder	Anxiety disorder secondary to organic etiology
• Generalized anxiety disorder • Panic disorder • Simple phobia • Separation anxiety	• Anxiety disorder due to another medical condition • Substance/medication-induced anxiety disorder
Obsessive compulsive and related disorders	Trauma- and stressor-related disorders • Acute stress disorder • Posttraumatic stress disorder Adjustment disorder with anxiety

[a] May exist independently or in combination.

- Anxiety may affect symptom management, treatment adherence, medical outcome or the ability of the patient to cope with the illness.
- Anxiety related to the anticipation or performance of medical procedures can impede treatment.
- Anxiety can worsen preexisting physical conditions, such as asthma, irritable bowel syndrome (IBS), or movement disorders.
- Anxiety is common in parents, which can make it more difficult for parents to hear and understand complex treatment related information. In general, presenting information in shorter conversations, asking parents questions to assure understanding, and encouraging questions is helpful for all parents, but especially those who are particularly anxious.
- Parental anxiety can exacerbate the child's anxiety. Understanding family history of anxiety may be helpful in understanding the extent to which anxiety may be characteristic of the family.
- Pediatric medical traumatic stress is a set of psychological and physiological responses of children and their families to pain, injury, serious illness, medical procedures, and invasive or frightening treatment experiences.
  - Traumatic stress responses are more related to one's subjective experience of the medical event than its objective severity.
  - Traumatic stress responses include symptoms of arousal, re-experiencing and avoidance, or a constellation of these symptoms consistent with Posttraumatic Stress Disorder (PTSD) or Acute Stress Disorder (ASD).
  - Traumatic stress responses are sometimes seen in children and adolescents but are very common in parents across the course of treatment and into survivorship. These responses can emerge at any time in the course of treatment, and even years after treatment has ended.

Signs and Symptoms of Anxiety

General symptoms of anxiety may be psychological and/or physical. Symptoms may be intermittent or persistent throughout the day. Table 12.2 provides further classification of specific *DSM-5* anxiety disorders.

Table 12.2 Considerations for Classifying Anxiety Disorders in Medically Ill Children; All Include Functional Impairment[1]	
Classification	**Key Symptoms/Considerations**
Generalized Anxiety Disorder	Excessive worry >6 months, with associated restlessness, fatigue, difficulty concentrating, irritability, muscle tension, sleep disturbance
Panic Disorder	Severe palpitations, diaphoresis, and nausea; feeling of "impending doom;" resulting panic attacks lasting at least several minutes and result in persistent worry of future attacks or lead to avoidance
Phobias	Specific fear of blood/needle phobia, claustrophobia, agoraphobia, "white coat syndrome"; may lead to difficulty with MRI scans, confinement in isolation, treatment nonadherence etc.
Separation Anxiety Disorder	Inappropriate/excessive worry about separation from home/family; repeated complaints of physical symptoms when separations occur, common in children younger than age 6, resurgence around age 12
Obsessive-Compulsive Disorder	Obsessive preoccupation or fears about physical illness; compulsive, repetitive behaviors to avoid dread or decrease anxiety
Anxiety Disorder Due to General Medical Condition	Should be considered if history is not consistent with symptoms of primary anxiety disorder/is resistant to treatment; more likely if physical symptoms (shortness of breath, tachycardia, tremor) are pronounced
Substance-Induced Anxiety Disorder	May result from direct effect of substance or withdrawal. Be particularly aware of medication history, start of new medication, change in dosage
Acute Stress/Posttraumatic Stress Disorder (PTSD)	Numbness, intrusiveness, avoidance, and hyperarousal; diagnosis depends on duration greater than one month; can occur as a reaction to hearing diagnosis, aspects of medical treatment, or memories of treatment; common in chronic physical illness. PTSD for 6 years or younger show negative emotional and behavioral changes, avoidance, play reenactment

Adapted and reprinted with permission from the Diagnostic and Statistical Manual of Mental Disorders Fifth Edition (DSM-5). © 2013, American Psychiatric Association.[1]

Psychological symptoms

- Feeling worry, fear, and sadness, possibly without being able to identify a source of symptoms.
- Crying spells.
- Inability to "turn off" one's thoughts.

Physical symptoms

- Tachycardia, tachypnea, nausea, insomnia, anorexia, diaphoresis, and tremor.

Table 12.3 Psychological Reactions to Illness[2]	
Diagnosis and Prognosis of Illness	Acute stress reactions of family members being affected by the cancer, parental reactions to diagnosis; uncertainty of medical outcome, recurrence, family history of disease, concerns of emotional impact of death on family
Physical Concerns	Fears concerning the physical effects of illness (e.g., amputation, scarring, pain), cosmetic outcomes (e.g., hair loss during chemotherapy treatment), social stigma
Hospital Anxiety	Separation from caretakers, particularly younger than age 5, association of hospital staff with distress of illness, conditioned responses to chemotherapy treatments
Impact of Illness	Concerns about missing school, separation from friends, feeling different, needing more attention and assistance from family members, financial worries
Adapted and reprinted with permission from the Clinical Manual of Pediatric Psychosomatic Medicine. © 2006, American Psychiatric Association.[2]	

Etiology/Evaluation of Anxiety

Developing anxiety may involve a variety of factors, including a preexisting vulnerability, psychological reactions, and life experiences. Some children are more genetically predisposed to anxiety or have a prior history of an anxiety disorder. Psychological reactions and symptoms may be "triggered" by a serious illness (Table 12.3). Children with no prior history of anxiety who suddenly present with striking anxiety symptoms during serious medical illness should receive a comprehensive evaluation. Certain medical conditions may precipitate symptoms of anxiety (Tables 12.4 and 12.5).

Assessment Measures for Anxiety

Clinicians may choose to administer an anxiety-rating scale to patients in addition to using clinical judgment, evaluation of laboratory tests, and review of medical/psychiatric history. These scales are often also utilized in outcomes research. They include:

State-Trait Anxiety Inventory for Children (STAIC)[3]—Age range 9–12 years; 44-item self-report measure of subjective feelings of anxiety at a particular moment in time and relatively stable levels of anxiety for an individual; administration time 10 minutes; use STAI for ages 13 and older. Available in 17 languages.

Multidimensional Anxiety Scale for Children (MASC)[4]—Age range 8–19 years; 39-item self-report measure; examines anxiety across four domains of physical symptoms, social anxiety, harm avoidance and separation/panic; administration time 10 minutes. Available in 18 languages.

Revised Children's Manifest Anxiety Scale (RCMAS)[5]—Age range 6–19 years; 37-item self-report measure; examines four domains: physiological anxiety, worry/over-sensitivity, social concerns/concentration and a lie scale; administration time 10–15 minutes. Available in 6 languages.

Table 12.4 Possible Medical Conditions Precipitating Anxiety in Oncology Patients[2]

Metabolic	Neurologic	Cardiovascular
• Electrolyte disturbances • Uremia • Vitamin B12/folate deficiency	• Encephalopathy • Mass-lesion • Poststroke • Postconcussion • Seizure • Vertigo	• Ischemic heart disease • Arrhythmias • Congestive heart failure • Hematologic (e.g., anemia)
Pulmonary	Endocrinologic	Neoplasms
• Hypoxia • Pneumothorax • Pulmonary edema/ embolism • Asthma • Anaphylaxis	• Cushing syndrome • Adrenal insufficiency • Hypopituitarism • Pheochromocytoma • Thyroid dysfunction	• Brain Tumors • Insulinoma
		Other
		• Transplantation • Pain (uncontrolled) • Caffeine • Substance abuse or withdrawal

Adapted and reprinted with permission from the Clinical Manual of Pediatric Psychosomatic Medicine. © 2006, American Psychiatric Association.[2]

Child PTSD Symptom Scale (CPSS)[6]—Age range 8–18 years; 24 item self-report measure that assesses symptoms of posttraumatic stress and PTSD diagnosis; administration time 10 minutes. Available in 7 languages.

Interventions for Anxiety

Behavioral and Cognitive Behavioral Interventions for Procedural Distress

- Behavioral and cognitive behavioral approaches for reducing procedural distress are well established.[7] These should be tailored developmentally and include distraction, guided imagery, and relaxation. Parents and staff members can be trained in the use of these approaches.

Other Treatments for Anxiety

- In general, individual psychotherapy, cognitive behavioral therapy, and family-therapy approaches are important in reducing anxiety and in providing patients and families with adaptive strategies to use in coping with the illness and its treatment. Play therapy may be useful in treating younger cancer patients.

Pharmacological (See Table 12.10 for medications used in children and adolescents with anxiety.)

- Considerations before prescribing anxiolytic agents:
  - Body weight, Tanner staging, clinical status, and drug-drug interactions should be factored into medication and dose selection.
  - Benzodiazepines can cause sedation, confusion, and behavioral disinhibition especially in children.

Table 12.5 Considerations in the Assessment of Anxiety in a Pediatric Setting[2]

Medical history • Current subjective symptoms • Possible medical conditions precipitating anxiety (Table 10.3) • Use of prescribed medication • Pain evaluation Psychiatric history • Particular attention to anxiety disorders • Family history of psychiatric disorders especially anxiety or mood disorders Psychosocial sources of anxiety • Diagnosis of illness • Hospital anxiety, fear of needles, procedures • Anticipatory anxiety (chemotherapy) • Separation from home and/or other familiar settings/people • Impact on family members • Isolation, loss of control and privacy • Physical effects of illness, concerns about disfigurement • Uncertainty of prognosis • Worries of death • Academic and social impact • Financial burden of illness	Use of drugs or alcohol • Alcohol, Amphetamine, Barbiturates, Benzodiazepines, Caffeine and other stimulants, Cocaine Review of vital signs and laboratory tests/procedures • Heart rate • Complete blood count • Glucose • Electrolytes • Blood urea nitrogen, Creatinine • Liver enzymes • Thyroid function tests • Urinalysis with toxicology screening • Chest imaging if indicated/Arterial blood gas/oxygen saturation measurements (to rule out respiratory causes) • Central nervous system scans

Adapted and reprinted with permission from the Clinical Manual of Pediatric Psychosomatic Medicine. © 2006, American Psychiatric Association.[2]

- Antihistamines are not helpful for persistent anxiety, and their anticholinergic properties can precipitate or worsen delirium.
- Combining brief pharmacological (e.g., midazolam (Versed®) and psychological interventions is also effective.
- The needs for intervention may continue after the end of cancer treatment. For adolescent survivors of childhood cancer and their families, participation in a combined cognitive behavioral therapy (CBT)/Family therapy intervention reduced symptoms of traumatic stress across members of the family.[8]
- Resources for multidisciplinary members of pediatric teams, including a toolbox for providing trauma informed practice can be found at the Center for Pediatric Traumatic Stress website (www.healthcaretoolbox.org), part of the National Child Traumatic Stress Network (www.nctsn.org).

Depression in Pediatric Oncology Patients

Childhood Depression in Pediatric Cancer

- Depression ranges from a transient low mood change to impairment in overall functioning and may present with both psychological and physical symptoms. In general, the most prominent symptoms of depression are sadness (dysphoria) and lack of pleasure (anhedonia).
  - Depression may exist as a primary disorder, psychological reaction to illness, secondary disorder to organic etiology, or any combination of these three (Table 12.6).
  - Depression may be comorbid with other psychiatric disorders (e.g., anxiety).
  - Even if patients do not meet diagnostic criteria for a depressive disorder, they should still receive appropriate follow-up and continued monitoring from healthcare professionals.
- Childhood depression can differ from adult depression, largely linked to the importance of developmental factors.
  - Childhood depression may be expressed in symptoms of anxiety, somatic complaints, social withdrawal, nonadherence and behavior problems.
  - Adolescents who are depressed may have sleep and eating problems.
  - Depression affects school performance and peer relationships and can be associated with substance use and suicidality.
- There are important challenges to assessing depression in pediatric cancer. Consideration must be given to the following:
  - Medical symptoms and/or side effects of cancer treatments can be confused with, or co-exist with, symptoms of depression.
  - Depressive responses may be a "normal" response to the diagnosis and treatment of cancer and to medical events that occur during the course of treatment.
  - Physicians and nurses are less accurate at assessment of depression than of physical distress. They should seek consultation from mental health professionals who can help determine if the depression is part of adaptation to the child's diagnosis or is more severe or urgent in nature. Mental health professionals can help patients, parents and siblings cope with "normal." reactive depression.

How Common Is Depression?

- Estimates of depression in medically ill samples vary. Meta-analysis estimates a relatively low rate—a 9% prevalence of depression in chronically ill children and some studies show a lower than normal rate of depression in pediatric cancer. Generally, studies using clinical interview methodologies (rather than self-report) tend to report higher levels than self-report.
- Depression in a pediatric hospital setting is one of the most frequent reasons for a psychiatric consult especially within one year of diagnosis of cancer.

Table 12.6 Mood Disorders in Children with Cancer[a]

Depressive Disorders • Major depressive disorder • Unspecified depressive disorder • Persistent depressive disorder (Dysthymia) Bipolar disorders (I, II, cyclothymia, unspecified) Mood disorder secondary to organic etiology • Mood disorder due to another medical condition • Substance/medication-induced mood (depressed or bipolar) disorder	Mood disorder as psychological reaction to physical illness • Adjustment disorder with depressed mood • Regression • Bereavement

[a] May exist independently or in combination.

- Antidepressants are commonly prescribed by pediatric oncologists.
  - A multi-institute survey of 151 pediatric oncologists found that many oncologists (71%) prescribed SSRIs but do not follow FDA guidelines. They should seek consultation from mental health professionals on best prescribing and monitoring practices for SSRIs in youth.[9]

Why Is Diagnosis and Treatment of Depression Important in a Pediatric Oncology Setting?

- Depression affects children and adolescents' quality of life and psychological well-being.
  - Depression is associated with future adverse behaviors such as: impaired school performance and social relationships, drug/tobacco abuse, and suicidal behavior.
- In the medically ill, depression may affect symptom management, treatment adherence, and medical outcome.
  - Depression is associated with higher morbidity, increased length of hospital stay, and increased complaint of somatic symptoms.
  - Depression is a risk factor for nonadherence with medical care.
- Patients may feel depressed at multiple stages: during and immediately after diagnosis and treatment, as well as during survivorship, treatment for relapses, and palliative care. For example:
  - Diagnosis of a serious illness such as cancer and the subsequent aggressive treatment may trigger feelings of helplessness and result in depression.
  - Depression can emerge throughout the course of treatment and often after the immediate crisis of diagnosis has passed. It is helpful to keep this in mind and re-assess for depression, as needed.
  - At terminal stages of cancer, oncologists, nurses, and mental health professionals can help the child and family work through feelings of loss and should recognize symptoms of depression as part of the grieving process.

Signs and Symptoms of Depression

Children and adolescents are more likely than adults to present with irritability, guilt, and somatic complaints. Physical symptoms include joint pain, limb pain, back pain, abdominal pain, headaches, gastrointestinal problems, fatigue, weakness, and change in appetite. Table 12.7 provides further classification of specific *DSM-5* mood disorders.

Etiology/Evaluation of Depression

A detailed patient history is needed to determine the etiology of psychological/physical symptoms consistent with depression. Symptoms of depression can be difficult for clinicians to differentiate from medical and treatment side effects of cancer, which often include fatigue, decreased appetite, and sleep disturbances. Careful attention is needed to discern whether physical symptoms can be attributed to the physical illness process/treatment or a depressive disorder. Often, the diagnosis of depression is based on cognitive symptoms (anhedonia, feelings of worthlessness, etc.).

Determining whether depressive symptoms are related to an expected course of grief or a clinical depression is another important consideration, particularly in terminally ill patients. Consideration must be given to the patient's past psychiatric history and family psychiatric history, which may reveal genetic vulnerability for mood disorders. Evaluation for depression includes the assessment of the following: symptom severity, duration and impact on quality of life. The patient and primary caregivers should be interviewed to most comprehensively obtain information (Tables 12.8 and 12.9).

Assessment Measures for Depression

Clinicians may choose to administer a screening scale for mood disorders in addition to relying upon their clinical judgment, evaluation of laboratory tests, and review of medical/psychiatric history. These scales include the following.

Children's Depression Inventory (CDI)[11,12]—Age range 7–17 years; 27-item self-report measure that assesses a range of depressive symptoms including disturbed mood, anhedonia, and interpersonal behavior in the past 2 weeks; high specificity and accurate predictor of depression in medically ill pediatric population with cut-off score of 11 or 12. Available in 22 languages. Also a short 10-item version available.

Children's Depression Rating Scale (CDRS)[13,14]—Age range 6–12 years; 17-item clinician's interview that assesses severity of depression; 14 items are based on subject's responses and 3 items are based on clinician's evaluation of child's nonverbal behavior. Available in English. CDRS-Revised also in Hebrew and German.

Memorial Symptom Assessment Scale (MSAS)[15,16]—Reliable and valid for ages 7–12 years; assesses symptoms of medically ill children: tiredness, pain, insomnia, change in appetite, worry, sadness, nausea. Available in 3 languages.[17]

Treating Depression in Pediatric Oncology

Accurate and effective assessment and treatment of depression in pediatric cancer is best accomplished in collaboration with a mental health

Table 12.7 Considerations for Classifying Mood Disorders in Medically Ill Children; all include functional impairment[1]

Classification	Key Symptoms/Considerations
Major Depressive Disorder	Primary mood disorder most often associated with previous psychiatric history. Must exhibit at least 5 symptoms of: persistent depressed mood, anhedonia, irritability, change of weight, change of appetite, sleep disturbance, fatigue, feelings of worthlessness/guilt, diminished ability to concentrate, recurrent thoughts of death for at least 2 weeks.
Dysthymia	Chronically depressed or irritable mood for at least 1 year that is less disabling than MDD. At least 2 symptoms of: sleep disturbance; fatigue; diminished ability to concentrate; feelings of hopelessness.
Adjustment Disorder (e.g., the adjustment to diagnosis, course and treatment of cancer)	Depressed mood in reaction to medical illness; the most common mood disorder in cancer patients. Symptoms of depression do not meet criteria for major depression but are associated with mildly impaired functioning or shorter duration.
Mood Disorder Due to Other Medical Condition	Depressed mood, elevated mood, or irritability due to underlying medical condition; may be one of the first symptoms of medical illness. Relationship to significant physical examination and study findings; particular attention to any CNS lesions in frontal, limbic and temporal lobes as possible cause.
Substance/ Medication-Induced Mood Disorder	Depression induced by medication, drugs or alcohol. Usually resolves within 2 weeks of abstinence. Important to note the course of depression in initiation/dosage of a medicine (e.g., high dose Interferon-alpha).
Primary or secondary mania	Manic symptoms as a primary disorder, secondary to medical condition, induced by medication (e.g., corticosteroids) or toxicity. Symptoms include the following: abnormally elevated, expansive, or irritable mood, rapid speech. Patients with brain atrophy or sleep deprivation are more prone.
Behavioral considerations	Regression: When stress of illness leads to behavioral regression and manifests as clinginess, social withdrawal, tearfulness, depressed mood. Very common in children and adolescents. Generally resolves after illness/hospitalization.
Bereavement	Fleeting thoughts of sadness or suicide that are part of the normal mourning process. Complicated Bereavement with prolonged and more persistent symptoms of mourning needs to be distinguished from depression.

Adapted and reprinted with permission from the Diagnostic and Statistical Manual of Mental Disorders, Fifth Edition (DSM-5). © 2013, American Psychiatric Association.[1]

Table 12.8 Additional Considerations for Etiology of Mood Disorder in Oncology Patients[10]

Medications • Corticosteroids (may cause depressive or mania symptoms) • Opioid analgesics • Benzodiazepines • Barbiturates • Narcotics • Interferon-alpha • Interleukin-2 (IL-2) • Chemotherapy agents (e.g., prednisone, vincristine, vinblastin, procarbazine, L-asparaginase)	Metabolic abnormalities • Electrolytes • Calcium • B-12 • Folic acid • Parathyroid function • Thyroid function
Stroke Tumor • Primary brain tumors • Central nervous system lymphomas or metastases • Carcinoma of pancreas	Pain • Severe, uncontrolled pain • Fear of unrelieved pain

Adapted and reprinted with permission from the *Bethesda Handbook of Clinical Oncology*.

professional. Clinical social workers, psychologists, and/or child psychiatrists familiar with children with serious illness should be consulted in this process.

There are few reports of interventions for depression that are specific and exclusive to pediatric cancer. Fortunately, literature in this area is growing and the results of other, more general literatures are relevant. For example, individual psychotherapy for depression (especially cognitive behavioral therapy) is effective for youth in general, both alone and in combination with medication. In small studies, both citalopram (Celexa®) and fluvoxamine (Luvox®) have been shown to be well-tolerated in pediatric oncology patients.[18,19] Similarly, there is evidence for family interventions in childhood disorders, including depression.[20] Prescribing information for anxiolytics and antidepressants in children is provided in Table 12.10.

Management for Suicide in Children and Adolescents

Completed suicide is rare in children in general and in children and adolescents with cancer and cancer survivors, but suicidal ideation should be screened in survivors particularly if they have persistent health problems or pain conditions.[21] However, suicide risk increases with age and through adolescence, so assessing risk specific to suicide is important as patients grow older. When assessing any child or adolescent's depression, clinicians should inquire about current suicidal ideation and history of previous

Table 12.9 Considerations in the Assessment of Depression in a Pediatric Hospital Setting[2]

Medical history • Current subjective symptoms consistent with depression (e.g., anhedonia) • Possible medical conditions precipitating depression (cf. Table 10.3) • Use of prescribed medication • Pain evaluation • Extent of hospitalizations and separations from family and home community • Treatment intensity (although not generally associated with psychological outcomes, treatment factors may precipitate depressive reactions) • Uncertainty of prognosis	History and response to diagnosis/treatment • Psychiatric history, with attention to mood disorders, past suicide attempts • Family history of psychiatric disorders • History or current use of drugs or alcohol • Psychosocial risk factors in the child/family (e.g., social support, family functioning, pre-illness functioning of child and family members; prior school attendance and achievement; other problems including conflict, separations, etc.) • Prior losses (serious illness and/or death of family members, loss of pet, disappointments in school or social relationships)
Mental status examination • Focus on mood, cognition and psychotic symptoms (for mania) • Comorbid anxiety symptoms are common	Review of vital signs and laboratory tests/procedures • Heart rate • Complete blood count • Electrolytes • Renal/hepatic function tests • Thyroid function tests • Central nervous system scans • EEG

Adapted and reprinted with permission from the Clinical Manual of Pediatric Psychosomatic Medicine. © 2006, American Psychiatric Association.[2]

Table 12.10 Preparations and Dosages of Anxiolytics and Antidepressants in Children

Medication	Prescribing Information	FDA approval in children?
Benzodiazepines		
Clonazepam (Klonopin®)	0.25–3 mg/day 0.01 mg/kg/24 hr ÷ q8 hr po	Yes, up to 10 yr or 30 kg for epilepsy
Diazepam (Valium®)	2–10 mg/day 0.04–0.25 mg/kg	No
Lorazepam (Ativan®)	0.5–6 mg/day 0.05 mg/kg	Yes, ≥12 yr for insomnia, premed anesthesia
Midazolam (Versed®)	0.025–0.05 mg/kv iv Max 0.4 mg/kg 0.25–1 mg/kg po Max 20 mg	No

(continued)

Table 12.10 (Continued)

Medication	Prescribing Information	FDA approval in children?
SSRIs		
Citalopram (Celexa®)	5–40 mg/day	No
Escitalopram (Lexapro®)	5–20 mg/day	Yes, ≥ 12 yr for depression
Fluoxetine (Prozac®)	5–60 mg/day	Yes, 7–17 yr for depression/OCD
Fluvoxamine (Luvox®)	25–200 mg/day Max 300 mg	Yes, 7–17 yr for OCD
Paroxetine (Paxil®)	5–20 mg/day	No
Sertraline (Zoloft®)	12.5–150 mg/day Max 200 mg	Yes, 6–17 yr for OCD
TCAs		
Amitriptyline (Elavil®)	5–50 mg/day Max 300 mg	Yes, ≥12 yr for depression
Desipramine (Norpramin®)	10 mg/day Max 300 mg	No
Nortriptyline (Pamelor®)	10 mg/day Max 150 mg	No
Other antidepressants		
Bupropion (Wellbutrin®)	37.5–300 mg/day	No
Venlafaxine (Effexor®)	18.75–300 mg/day	No
Duloxetine (Cymbalta®)	20–60 mg/day	No
Alternative anxiolytic		
Buspirone (Buspar®)	15–60 mg/day	No

suicide attempts/ideation in order to provide a comprehensive evaluation. (See Chapter 14, Psychiatric Emergencies.)

References

1. American Psychiatric Association: *Diagnostic and Statistical Manual of Mental Disorders*. 5th ed. Arlington, VA: Author; 2013.
2. Shaw RJ, DeMaso DR. *Clinical Manual of Pediatric Psychosomatic Medicine*. Washington, DC: American Psychiatric Publishing; 2006.
3. Spielberger CD, et al. Measuring the psychological vital signs of anxiety, anger, depression, and curiosity in treatment planning and outcomes assessment. In: Maruish ME, ed. *The Use of Psychological Testing for Treatment Planning and Outcomes Assessment*. Mahwah, NJ: Erlbaum; 2004: 421–447.
4. March JS, Parker JD, Sullivan K, Stallings P, Conners CK. The Multidimensional Anxiety Scale for Children (MASC): factor structure, reliability, and validity. *J Am Acad Child Adolesc Psychiatr*. 1997;36(4):554–565.

5. Perrin S, Last CG. Do childhood anxiety measures measure anxiety? *J Abnorm Child Psychol.* 1992;20(6):567–578.
6. Foa E, Johnson K, Feeny N, Treadwell K. The child PTSD Symptom Scale: A preliminary examination of its psychometric properties. *J Clin Child Psychol.* 2001;30(3):376–384.
7. Spirito A, Kazak A. *Effective and Emerging Treatments in Pediatric Psychology.* New York, NY: Oxford University Press; 2006.
8. Kazak A, Alderfer M, Streisand R, et al. Treatment of posttraumatic stress symptoms in adolescent survivors of childhood cancer and their families: A randomized clinical trial. *J Fam Psychol.* 2004;18(3):493–504.
9. Phipps S, Buckholdt KE, Fernandez L, et al. Pediatric oncologists' practices of prescribing selective serotonin reuptake inhibitors (SSRIs) for children and adolescents with cancer: A multi-site study. *Pediatr Blood Cancer.* 2012;58:210–215.
10. Rosenstein DL, Pao M, Fleisch SB, Elswick DE. Psychopharmacologic management in oncology. In: Abraham J, Allegra CJ, Gulley J, eds. Bethesda Handbook of Clinical Oncology. Philadelphia, PA: Lippincott, Williams, & Wilkins; 2014: 480–489.
11. Sitarenios G, Stein S. Use of the Children's Depression Inventory. In: Maruish M, ed. *The Use of Psychological Testing for Treatment Planning and Outcomes Assessment: vol. 2: Instruments for Children and Adolescents.* 3d ed. Oxford, UK: Taylor & Francis; 2004: 4.
12. Knight D, Hensley VR, Waters B. Validation of the Children's Depression Scale and the Children's Depression Inventory in a prepubertal sample. *J Child Psychol Psychiat.* 1988;29(6):853–863.
13. Poznanski EO, Cook SC, Carroll BJ. A depression rating scale for children. *Pediatrics.* 1979;64(4):442–50.
14. Poznanski EO, Grossman JA, Buchsbaum Y, Banegas M, Freeman L, Gibbons R. Preliminary studies of the reliability and validity of the children's depression rating scale. *J Am Acad Child Psychiatry.* 1984;23(2):191–197.
15. Portenoy RK, Thaler HT, Kornblith AB, et al. The Memorial Symptom Assessment Scale: An instrument for the evaluation of symptom prevalence, characteristics and distress. *Eur J Cancer.* 1994;30A(9):1326–36.
16. Collins JJ, Devine TD, Dick GS, et al. The measurement of symptoms in young children with cancer: The validation of the Memorial Symptom Assessment Scale in children aged 7–12. *J Pain Symptom Manage.* 2002;23(1):10–16.
17. Lam WW, Law CC, Fu YT, Wong KH, Chang VT, Fielding R. New insights in symptom assessment: the Chinese Versions of the Memorial Symptom Assessment Scale Short Form (MSAS-SF) and the Condensed MSAS (CMSAS). *J Pain Symptom Manage.* 2008;36(6):584–95.
18. DeJong M. Fombonne E. Citalopram to treat depression in pediatric oncology. *J Child Adolesc Psychopharmacol.* 2007;17(3):371–377.
19. Gothelf D, Rubinstein M, Shemesh E, et al. Pilot study: Fluvoxamine treatment for depression and anxiety disorders in children and adolescents with cancer. *J Am Acad Child Adolesc Psychiatry.* 2005;44(12):1258–1262.
20. Diamond G, Josephson A. Family-based treatment research: A 10-year update. *J Am Acad Child Adolesc Psychiatry.* 2005;44(9):872–887.
21. Recklitis CJ, Diller LR, Li XC, Najita J, Robison LL, Zeltzer L. Suicide ideation in adult cancer survivors: A report from the childhood cancer survivor study. *J Clin Oncol.* 2009;28:655–661.

Chapter 13

Fertility and Sexuality

Jennifer M. Levine, Kevin C. Oeffinger, Jennifer S. Ford, and Charles A. Sklar

From the perspective of the adolescent and young adult survivor, alterations in gonadal function and the loss of fertility (or even the fear of impaired fertility) are perhaps the most life altering sequelae of childhood cancer influencing a survivor's developing body image, sexuality, dating relationships, marriage patterns, and sense of well-being.

Fertility is one of the most difficult outcomes to study in survivors, as the primary endpoint is pregnancy, which is influenced by many physical and societal factors beyond the direct effect of the cancer therapy on the reproductive organs.

- Many men are not willing to have a semen analysis, and self-reporting a successful impregnation is subject to both over-and under-reporting biases.
- The investigation of fertility in both genders is hampered by the often overlapping effects of different cancer therapies on the reproductive system, and the sometimes late recovery of function.
- Pregnancies may occur when survivors are no longer in contact with treating physicians or long-term follow-up clinics, thereby limiting accurate assessment of this outcome.

A survivor's (and a parent's) understanding of fertility and sexuality and how it is impacted by cancer and cancer therapy evolves through the stages of survivorship. During the stress-laden period of diagnosis, when therapeutic decisions are made and as a parent faces the possibility of losing a child, details regarding the potential for infertility and gonadal dysfunction are often not understood or remembered by families, and sometimes they are not adequately provided by the cancer treating team. Later, as the cancer is cured and the patient matures into adulthood, issues of fertility and sexuality become more immediate and prevalent. This chapter presents an overview of fertility (including therapies associated with gonadal dysfunction and methods of fertility preservation) and sexuality. See Tables 13.1–13.5. Further reading on the effects of cancer treatment on ovarian and uterine function and reproductive potential in women and testicular function in men is available.[1,2]

Table 13.1 Acute Ovarian Failure and Premature Menopause in Female Survivors of Childhood Cancer

Acute Ovarian Failure

- Definition: loss of ovarian function during or shortly following completion of therapy
- Occurs in 5–7% of females treated in childhood or adolescence[3]
  - High risk groups:
    - Stem cell transplant recipients
    - Total body irradiation (TBI)—nearly all women treated with TBI after age 10 years; about 50% of those treated prior to 10 years of age
  - High dose myeloablative therapy (e.g., busulfan, cytoxan, melphalan, thiotepa)
- Ovarian (pelvic or abdominal) irradiation >1000 cGy
- Ovarian irradiation <1000 cGy with concomitant alkylating agents (e.g., cyclophosphamide) or older age at exposure

Nonsurgical Premature Menopause

- Female survivors who do not develop acute ovarian failure are potentially at risk of developing premature menopause[4]
- Definition: menopause prior to age 40 years
- High risk groups:
  - older attained age
  - increasing dose of radiation to the ovaries
  - increasing dose of alkylating agents
  - diagnosis of Hodgkin lymphoma
  - cranial radiation doses >3000 cGy to the hypothalamic-pituitary axis may lead to gonadotropin deficiency affecting fertility
- For women treated with an alkylating agent plus abdominopelvic radiation, the cumulative incidence of nonsurgical menopause approaches 30% by 40 years of age

Evaluation for Ovarian Dysfunction

- Detailed history of menstrual cycle:
  - age at menarche
  - for women with cancer prior to menarche—precocious or delayed puberty
  - for women with cancer following menarche—change in menstrual history during and following cancer therapy
  - frequency, duration, intensity of menstruation
  - use of estrogen replacement
- Symptoms of hypoestrogen state
  - hot flashes
  - night sweats
  - vaginal dryness
  - variable sexual interest
  - altered, depressed or irritable mood
- Laboratory evaluation of ovarian potential and reserve:
  - Difficult to predict premature menopause by biochemical testing
  - Affected by use of oral contraceptives.
  - Follicle stimulating hormone (FSH) and estradiol levels
    - If menstruating, obtain on day 3 of cycle
    - FSH will be elevated and estradiol level low in menopause
    - FSH levels often fluctuate and may need repeating
  - Anti-Mullerian hormone (AMH) is a newer method that may provide additional information regarding ovarian reserve
  - Further testing should be conducted by a reproductive specialist and may include a pelvic or transvaginal ultrasound to assess ovarian volume and antral follicle count

Table 13.2 Infertility and Androgen Deficiency in Male Survivors of Childhood Cancer

<table>
<tr><td>Infertility
• Germinal epithelium of the testis is sensitive to radiation.
• Germinal epithelium of the testis is also sensitive to chemotherapeutic drugs, including alkylating agents (e.g., cyclophosphamide and ifosfamide), procarbazine and cisplatin. Outcomes are agent specific and dose-dependent.
• High-risk groups:
• Radiation doses (to the testes) above 200 cGy invariably cause oligospermia or azoospermia.
  • TBI—fractionated dose of 1200 to 1500 cGy often results in infertility.
  • Males with ALL who are treated with irradiation of the testis
  • Though the testes are shielded with modern techniques, scatter radiation from high dose radiation can result in oligospermia or azoospermia. Examples include pelvic, inguinal or spinal radiation.</td><td>• Chemotherapy
• Moderate to high dose cyclophosphamide or ifosfamide often results in azoospermia. The combination of these two agents, used in the treatment of patients with Ewing sarcoma, causes infertility in virtually all males.
• Combination of cisplatin with either ifosfamide or cyclophosphamide, used in the contemporary treatment of osteosarcoma, results in oligospermia or azoospermia in a majority of males.
• High-dose melphalan or busulfan used in preconditioning regimens prior to a stem cell transplant causes impaired spermatogenesis in the majority of males.
• Radiation to the hypothalamic-pituitary axis with doses >3000 cGy (e.g., cranial radiotherapy for a brain tumor) may result in a gonadotropin deficiency, thus indirectly affecting spermatogenesis and reproductive potential.</td></tr>
<tr><td colspan="2">Evaluation for Infertility in Males
• Pubertal staging—reduced testicular volume (<12 ml), measured by Prader orchidometer, is strongly suggestive of impaired spermatogenesis
• An elevated FSH suggests impaired spermatogenesis but is insufficient to determine fertility potential.[5]
• Semen analysis is the gold standard to evaluate sperm count, motility, mobility, and volume.</td></tr>
<tr><td>Androgen Deficiency
• In comparison with the germinal epithelium, the Leydig cells are less affected by chemotherapy and radiotherapy.
• Testicular irradiation with doses of greater than 2000 and 3000 cGy are associated with Leydig cell dysfunction in prepubertal and sexually mature males, respectively.</td><td>• Even with high-dose cyclophosphamide, frankly subnormal levels of testosterone are rare, though Leydig cell dysfunction may be evidenced by an elevated luteinizing hormone (LH) level. Regardless of whether there are frankly subnormal levels of testosterone, mild Leydig cell dysfunction will lead to premature androgen deficiency as this population ages is not known.
• Androgen deficiency can also result from hypogonadotropic hypogonadism following cranial radiotherapy.</td></tr>
<tr><td colspan="2">Evaluation of Androgen Deficiency
• In postpubertal males, elevated LH and decreased testosterone levels indicate Leydig cell dysfunction.</td></tr>
</table>

Table 13.3 Fertility Preservation Options
The American Society of Clinical Oncology (ASCO) recommends that oncologists discuss fertility preservation options as appropriate and refer interested patients and their families to reproductive specialists.[6] In a survey of pediatric oncology practitioners, 75% of respondents indicated that they offer sperm banking to postpubertal male patients ≥50% of the time, whereas 12% of practitioners responded that they referred postpubertal female patients to a fertility specialist ≥50% of the time.[7]
Females • When radiation fields include the pelvis, the ovaries can be surgically transposed to a more protected location. However, even after transposition of the ovaries, some women will develop premature menopause secondary to their chemotherapy. • Radical trachelectomy, in which the cervix but not the entire uterus is surgically removed, may preserve fertility in patients with early stage cervical cancer. • There is insufficient evidence to support the use of gonadotropin releasing hormone (GnRH) analogues in protecting the ovaries during cancer directed treatment. • Oocyte cryopreservation is now considered a nonexperimental intervention. This process requires hormonal hyperstimulation for approximately 10–12 days with subsequent oocyte retrieval under anesthesia. Unfertilized oocytes are then cryopreserved and can be thawed and fertilized utilizing assisted reproductive techniques in the future. The cost is not usually covered by insurance. • Ovarian tissue cryopreservation is an investigational method of fertility preservation that has the advantage of requiring neither a sperm donor nor ovarian stimulation.
Males • Sperm cryopreservation is an effective method of fertility preservation in *postpubertal* males. Spermarche does not occur until about 13 to 14 years of age, thus limiting sperm banking to adolescents. • Anterograde ejaculation is the most common method for obtaining sperm. In individuals who cannot ejaculate via masturbation, alternative methods of obtaining sperm for cryopreservation include vibrostimulatory ejaculation and testicular sperm extraction (TESE). TESE is a surgical procedure performed under anesthesia. • Methods to preserve fertility in younger males, including testicular tissue cryopreservation, have had little success to date.

Practical Applications

- A majority of patients and parents do not recall receiving information on fertility, despite having been informed.
- Many patients are unaware of their fertility status.
- Patients want their treatment team to tell them the facts about cancer-related infertility and sperm banking, directly and openly. Patients (older adolescents and young adults) want to make their own choice of whether to bank sperm.
- It is important to discuss fertility and fertility concerns several times throughout treatment and posttreatment, because they may become more relevant as the patient gets older and further out from treatment.

Table 13.4 Body Image

- Definition: Mental perception of one's physical body and its function. It forms an important part of one's entire self-image.
- Develops gradually, from positive experiences of satisfaction in early childhood.
- In adolescence, the altered, sexually mature body and images of it are integrated into an individual's identity. This integration and development can be influenced by experience of physical illness.
- Body image has been found to be inferior in survivors of childhood leukemia as compared to peers.[8]
- Most disturbing physical changes for adolescents includes hair loss, presence of a central venous catheter, weight changes, scars from surgery, amputation, acne (typically medication-induced), slowed linear growth and delay in development of secondary sexual characteristics.
- Body image concerns persist and may even appear for the first time after treatment, even when many of the physical changes are no longer apparent.
- Body-altering side effect of cancer treatments (both in the short- and long-term) are reported by adolescents and young adults to be one of the worst aspects of the diseases.
- Physical changes are distressing for children and adolescents with cancer of all ages. Self-consciousness about appearance can lead to social withdrawal[9] and can affect both the formation of romantic relationships and the development of physical and emotional intimacy within those relationships.[10]
- High-risk groups:
  - Those who report physical late-effects that interfere substantially with daily activities.
  - Older age at diagnosis (especially adolescence and young adulthood).
  - Those undergoing active treatment.
  - Those undergoing cranial irradiation.
  - Those undergoing treatment that limits growth or is associated with infertility.

Also, diagnosis and treatment planning create tremendous anxiety for patients and their families. It is difficult for patients and families to remember all the new medical information they receive. Guidelines exist for the assessment and management of female and male reproductive health in survivors.[17,18]

- Since most sexual information processed by adolescents and young adults is either learned at school or from peers, missing educational and social experiences because of treatment may affect sexual-identity formation. If this is the case, sexual-health education, similar to the information being provided in school, should be offered to the patient.
- It is important to take into account the patient's developmental stage when deciding whether to discuss certain aspects of the treatment effects (sexual health and body image issues such as scaring). Involving parents may be beneficial for younger adolescents, whereas it may hinder self-esteem and growth in older ones.
- Teenagers interviewed about sperm banking preferred to hear about sperm banking privately, without having their parents present.

Table 13.5 Sexuality

- Definition: The development of one's sexuality and sexual identity is a process that occurs during adolescence and leads to an understanding and appreciation of oneself as a sexual being.
- WHO Definition of sexual health: state of physical, emotional, mental, and social well-being related to sexuality...which requires a positive and respectful approach to sexuality and sexual relationships as well as the possibility of having pleasurable and safe sexual experiences.[11]
- Sexuality is positively associated with body image and self-esteem and inversely associated with depressed mood.[12] An association also exists between sexual function and health status. Survivors of childhood cancer often have persistent health concerns.[13]
- Establishing positive sexual identity depends on obtaining sexual health knowledge, developing interpersonal relationships and dealing with body image concerns. All of these are challenged by the cancer experience.
  - Survivors may have relatively limited sexual knowledge which may impair the development of a healthy sexual identity.
  - Barriers to interpersonal relationships include: feelings of being unattractive or different, possible impairments in social skills, fears felt by potential partners about the cancer diagnosis, isolation from peers and treatment-related cognitive impairments.
  - Positive body image is an integral element of sexual health.
- Hormonal, interpersonal. or psychological problems can affect sexuality.
- Recent studies have identified some degree of difficulty in sexual functioning in 41–43% of young adult survivors of childhood cancer survivors, with women experiencing a greater degree of dysfunction.[14,15]
- High-risk groups:
  - Those who have had high-dose chemotherapy and bone marrow transplantation.
  - Those with impaired fertility.
  - Those with body image disturbance.
  - Those with delayed puberty.
- Sexual dysfunction (problems with libido, arousal, orgasm, resolution) can occur as a result of treatment (radiation/surgery in the pelvic area), physical symptoms (fatigue, pain, nausea), psychological factors (anxiety, depression, guilt), and social and interpersonal factors. It is important that adolescent and young adult cancer patients are given permission to talk about sexuality, as well as concerns about fertility with knowledgeable providers. (Cf. corresponding handbook for adults).[16]

(See MMQL-AF measurement of health-related quality of life in Appendix, Health-Related Quality of Life in Pediatric Oncology)

Tips and Suggestions

- Acknowledge the sensitivity of the topic in terms of emotions and values.
- Separate sexuality and fertility.
- Provide information on contraception and sexually transmitted infections.
- Tips on making the discussion easier:
  - Try to find a place for the discussion where you have privacy and will not be overheard. Plan ahead for privacy as much as possible.
  - Make sure to set aside enough time for discussion.

    - Make eye contact with your patient.
    - If the patient and/or family get upset, be supportive. You cannot take away the pain and loss of potential infertility but you can let them know you empathize.
    - Avoid minimizing or negating the importance of infertility.
    - This topic can bring up a lot of emotions. Ask patients if they would like to discuss their feelings with a social worker, psychologist, or with clergy.
- Have information readily available about regionally appropriate referrals to sperm banks or reproductive specialists.
- Have information readily available about multiple pathways and options regarding family building.
- Have information readily available for local therapists and/or counselors with a specialty in body-image dysfunction and/or sexual dysfunction.
- Provide links to relevant websites for information and financial assistance, e.g., http://www.fertilehope.org/index.cfm

Summary

Infertility and premature gonadal dysfunction are common outcomes following therapy for childhood cancer and influence a survivor's quality of life, body image, and sexuality. It is imperative that clinicians address the fears and concerns of survivors in a sensitive manner. Moreover, recognizing the complexity of this topic and the evolving options for fertility preservation, a multidisciplinary team that includes a reproductive specialist and a mental health provider who is familiar with the issues of cancer survivors (or ready availability by referral) is preferred.

Oncology teams can facilitate the development of positive self-esteem and development of sexual health in several ways: facilitating personal control and individuation, offer opportunities for sexual health education, connect the patient/survivor with other teens diagnosed with cancer. Evaluate sexual development to ensure puberty is proceeding normally. Those with late effects that alter sexual functioning, physical appearance, or fertility should be referred to heath-care providers who specialize in these issues.

Any patient or survivor with sexual problems that result from treatment for childhood cancer needs both medical and psychological follow-up. A team approach that provides rehabilitation and psychological assistance to address concerns about body image, fertility, and sexuality is crucial.

References

1. Levine J. Gonadotoxicity of cancer therapies in pediatric and reproductive-age females. In: Gracia C, ed.,*Oncofertility Medical Practice*. New York, NY: Springer; 2012: 3–14.
2. Ginsberg JP, Gonadotoxicity of cancer therapies in pediatric and reproductive-age males. In: Gracia C, ed. *Oncofertility Medical Practice* 2012, New York, NY: Springer; 2012: 15–23.

3. Chemaitilly W, Mertens A., Mitby P., et al., Acute ovarian failure in the childhood cancer survivor study. *J Clin Endocrinol Metab.* 2006;91(5):1723–1728.
4. Sklar CA, et al. Premature menopause in survivors of childhood cancer: a report from the childhood cancer survivor study. *J Natl Cancer Inst.* 2006;98(13):890–896.
5. Green DM, Zhu L. Zhang N. et al. Lack of specificity of plasma concentrations of inhibin B and follicle-stimulating hormone for identification of azoospermic survivors of childhood cancer: a report from the St Jude lifetime cohort study. *J Clin Oncol.* 2013;31(10):1324–1328.
6. Loren AW, Mangu P. Beck. et al. Fertility preservation for patients with cancer: American Society of Clinical Oncology clinical practice guideline update. *J Clin Oncol.* 2013;31(19):2500–2510.
7. Kohler TS, Kondapalli T. Shah A. Chan S. Woodruff T. Brannigan R. et al. Results from the survey for preservation of adolescent reproduction (SPARE) study: gender disparity in delivery of fertility preservation message to adolescents with cancer. *J Assist Reprod Genet.* 2011;28(3):269–277.
8. Puukko LR, Sammallahti P. Aalberg V. et al. Childhood leukemia and body image: interview reveals impairment not found with a questionnaire. *J Clin Psychol.* 1997;53(2):133–137.
9. Evan EE, Kaufman M. Cook A. Zeltzer L. et al. Sexual health and self-esteem in adolescents and young adults with cancer. *Cancer.* 2006; 107(7 Suppl):1672–1679.
10. Thompson, AL, Long KA, Marsland AL. Impact of childhood cancer on emerging adult survivors' romantic relationships: a qualitative account. *J Sex Med.* 2013;(10 Suppl 1):65–73.
11. Available from: http://www.who.int/reproductivehealth/topics/sexual_health/sh_definitions/en/index.html
12. Pendley JS, Dahlquist LM, Dreyer Z. *J Pediatr Psychol.* 1997;22(1):29–43.
13. Jacobs LA, Pucci DA. Adult survivors of childhood cancer: the medical and psychosocial late effects of cancer treatment and the impact on sexual and reproductive health. *J Sex Med.* 2013;(10 Suppl 1):120–126.
14. Zebrack BJ, et al. *Sexual functioning in young adult survivors of childhood cancer.* Psychooncol. 2010;19(8):814–822.
15. van Dijk EM, van Dulmen-den Broeder E. Kaspers G. Van Dam E. Braam K. Huisman J. et al. Psychosexual functioning of childhood cancer survivors. *Psychooncol.* 2008;17(5):506–511.
16. Hughes M. Physical symptom management: Sexual dysfunction. In: *Quick Reference for Oncology Clinicians: The Psychiatric and Psychological Dimensions of Cancer Symptom Management.* Charlottesville, VA: IPOS Press; 2006: 90–96.
17. Metzger ML, Meacham L. Patterson B. et al. Female reproductive health after childhood, adolescent, and young adult cancers: guidelines for the assessment and management of female reproductive complications. *J Clin Oncol.* 2013;31(9):1239–1247.
18. Kenney LB, Cohen L. Shnorhavorian M. et al., Male reproductive health after childhood, adolescent, and young adult cancers: a report from the Children's Oncology Group. *J Clin Oncol.* 2012;30(27):3408–3416.

Chapter 14

Psychiatric Emergencies

Travis Mickelson, D. Richard Martini, and Maryland Pao

This chapter addresses three problems that require urgent psychiatric intervention in the medical setting: (1) patients who are suicidal or self-harming, (2) patients who are delirious, and (3) patients who are aggressive and potentially dangerous to others. In general, these are rare occurrences in children and adolescents with cancer but are highly distressing and urgent for families and staff alike when they occur. Research shows that asking adolescents directly about suicide reveals important clinical information.[1] Iatrogenic risk of inquiring about suicidal thoughts has been refuted.[2] Mental health providers should be involved at the earliest signs of suicidal behavior, delirium, or aggressive behaviors.

Management of the Suicidal/Self-Harming Pediatric Patient

Basic Questions in the Evaluation of the Suicidal Patient

- Always ask adolescents about suicide in a direct manner.[1]
- Screening and assessment instruments[3] to guide evaluation include:
  - Ask Suicide-Screening Questions (ASQ),[1] Behavioral Health Screen (BHS),[4] Columbia Suicide Severity Rating Scale (CSSRS),[5] and others.[6]
- Distinguish between active (with plan) and passive (without plan) suicidal ideation. Is there any intent?
- Suicide attempts (definition): potentially self-injurious act with at least some wish to die as a result of this act.
- Has the patient ever made an attempt, had an interrupted attempt, an aborted attempt, or made preparations for suicide?
- How potentially lethal was the attempt?
- Is the patient considered to be at high risk for a successful suicide attempt?
- Will the patient follow through on a referral for necessary treatment?

Epidemiology of Suicidal Behavior in the General Pediatric Population

Suicide Behavior and Oncology Patients

Suicidal behavior and attempts in children and adolescents undergoing treatment for cancer are not well described. Suicidal symptoms have been reported in adult survivors of childhood cancer.[7]

General Patient Characteristics

- Suicide rates increase with age through childhood and adolescence.
- 60 to 90% of adolescent suicides are associated with psychiatric disorders (although the rate is as low as 60% for adolescent completers under 16), including major depressive disorder.[8,9] This raises questions about whether these adolescents received psychiatric services prior to their suicide.

Behavioral Characteristics

- According to the CDC,[10] of high school students in the U.S. in 2011:
  - 15.8% seriously considered attempting suicide.
  - 12.8% developed a suicide plan.
  - 7.8% made a suicide attempt.
  - 2.4% injured themselves to a degree that required medical attention.

"Cluster phenomena," wherein patients display increased suicidality after being exposed to suicidal behavior has been described. Typically, this lasts no more than one to two weeks and affects 1–5% of all adolescent suicides.

Risk factors for Suicidality in Adolescents [Adapted from Ash (2006)[11]]

Patient

- Stated intent of suicide with or without plan (active/passive).
- Previous suicide attempt.
  - Preparatory acts.
  - Aborted attempts.
  - Interrupted attempts.
  - Actual attempts.
- Females are more likely to consider, plan, attempt, and require treatment for a suicide attempt.[12]
- Males are more likely to complete a suicide attempt.[13]
- Co-morbidity/history of psychiatric disorder.
- Symptoms of helplessness, hopelessness, impulsivity.
- Social isolation.
  - Peer relationships.
- Uncontrolled pain.
- Advanced medical disease.
- Recent stressors.
- History of abuse or violence.

- Access to means such as firearms, weapons, or toxins.
- Drug/alcohol abuse.
- School/academic problems.

Family

- Lack of parental awareness and connectedness to family.
- Family history of suicidal behavior/suicide.
- Family history of psychopathology.

Assessment of Suicidal Behavior in Pediatrics

Patient Examination

- Evidence of hematological, neurological, endocrine, gastrointestinal, autoimmune, and infectious diseases.
- Evidence of medication side effects.
- Evidence of previous suicide attempts.
- Evidence of self-injury.
- Indicators of physical and sexual abuse.
- Toxicology screen and a drug and alcohol screen.
- Pregnancy test for adolescent girls.
- Access to means (e.g., firearms, weapons, medications in the home, etc.)
- Evidence of a psychiatric disorder such as a mood or anxiety disorder.

Assessment of Lethality

- Not necessarily related to the intent of the patient.
- Overdose is the most common method of attempt.
- Pediatric patients tend to over- or underestimate drug toxicity.

Assessment of Intent

- Evaluate method chosen.
- Evaluate expectations from the attempt (e.g., stated intent to die).
- Reversibility of the attempt.
- Ambivalence about living.
- Evidence of premeditation (e.g., telling others, suicide note).

Precipitants

- Problematic relationships with peers and family.
- Desire to escape from a situation perceived as hopeless.
- Depressive or perfectionistic tendencies.
- School problems.
- Bullying.

Current Risk Factors

- Presence of suicidal ideation with a plan.
- Lack of available strong social supports.

- Access to means such as a gun and/or potentially lethal doses of medications.
- Unsuccessful treatment of a recurrent psychiatric disorder.
- Use of alcohol or drugs.
- Family history of suicide.

Cognitive Functioning Considerations

- Patients with developmental delay or intellectual disabilities require assessments that are consistent with their level of functioning, because these patients may also be at risk for suicide and suicidal behavior.[14]

Management Considerations for Suicidal Children and Adolescents[6]

Patient Protection:

- Environmental restrictions (e.g., secure bullets or other weapons, and medications; firearms removal from home).
- Appropriate support, observation, and monitoring at home or in the hospital (e.g., constant monitoring by a responsible person [1:1]).
- Available care providers to be contacted in emergency.

Ongoing Assessment of Suicide Risk by Trained Mental Health Provider:

- Beginning at first report of suicide ideation.
- After signs of change in mental status.
- During worsening of illness-related symptoms/pain.
- At times of management transition (e.g., change of healthcare provider).

Treatment of Underlying Psychopathology:

- May include psychopharmacology and/or psychotherapy (including cognitive behavioral therapy).
- Important to address any disease-related factors, such as pain, contributing to mood disorder, or anxiety.

Management of the Delirious Pediatric Patient[15]

Definition of Delirium

Disturbance of cognition and level of consciousness.
Acute presentation.
Waxing and waning course.
Etiology from a medical condition.

Epidemiology of Delirium in Patients

- Often diagnosis and treatment of delirium is neglected in pediatric patients
- Occurs in 30% of critically ill children[16]

Typical causes of Delirium in Pediatric Patients

- Critical illness (e.g. trauma, infection, respiratory failure, metabolic disturbance, CNS disease) or its treatment (e.g., anticholinergic agents, sedatives, analgesics).
- Substance use or withdrawal.
- Toxin exposure.
- Sleep–wake cycle disturbance.
- Inadequate or excessive pain management.

Risk Factors for Delirium in Children

- Few studies in pediatric populations.
- Genetic predisposition.
- Chronic neurologic illness.
- Pre-existing psychiatric disorder.
- Pre-existing cognitive deficits.
- Severity of medical illness.
- Infection (especially with CNS involvement).
- Auto-immune disorders (e.g., lupus).
- Postorgan or bone marrow transplant.

Symptom Presentations of Delirium in Pediatric Patients[17]

Most Common

- Disorientation.
- Irritability.
- Inattention.
- Memory loss.
- Diffuse cognitive deficits.
- Clouded consciousness.
- Disturbances in sleep-wake cycle.

Less Common

- Disorganized thinking.
- Language abnormalities.
- Inconsolability.
- Autonomic dysregulation.

Infrequent

- Delusions.
- Visual or auditory hallucinations.
- Illusions.
- Affective lability.

Diagnosing Delirium in Pediatric Patients

Pediatric patients are more vulnerable to acute mental status change than adults. Assessment is directed at identifying delirium and its medical causes in order to treat the underlying disorder(s) and to simplify medication regimens whenever possible. Clinicians may misidentify symptoms of delirium as indicators of inadequate pain management and add opiates to the treatment regimen. Although this may immediately sedate the patient and appear calming, the long-term effect is to exacerbate the deterioration in mental status if the cause of delirium is not corrected as well.

Hyperactive Delirium

- Irritability.
- Agitation.
- Restlessness.
- Disorientation.
- Abnormalities of thought and perception.
- Presents as oppositional behavior and management problems.
- Greatest risk for self-inflicted harm.

Hypoactive Delirium

- Quietly confused.
- Anxious and tentative.
- Apathetic.
- Withdrawn.
- Unrecognized and poorly understood, misdiagnosed as depression or as compliance.

Mixed States

- Fluctuate between hypoactive and hyperactive delirium.
- Most commonly observed.

Subclinical Delirium

- Decreased awareness.
- Restlessness.
- Inconsolability.
- Purposeless actions.
- Poor autonomic regulation.

Assessment

- Monitor fluctuating levels of severity with lucid intervals followed by periods of confusion; requires serial evaluations.
- Use modified structured interviews that are developmentally appropriate—the Delirium Rating Scale (DRS) or the Pediatric Confusion Assessment Method for the Intensive Care Unit (PCAM-ICU) is applicable to pediatric patients.[18,19]
- Obtain information from parents, nurses and the medical team on behavioral change.
- Provide explanation of the symptoms to the patient and family as a consequence of the medical illness and/or treatment.
- Identify the organic cause(s), which may be multifactorial.

Psychiatric Differential Diagnosis

- Acute stress disorder.

- Acute anxiety state.
- Adjustment disorder.
- Dissociative disorder.
- Childhood-onset psychosis.
- Mania.

Treatment for Delirium in Pediatric Patients

Environmental interventions and psychopharmacologic interventions may provide symptomatic relief while the underlying medical causes of delirium are identified and corrected.

Environmental Interventions

- Frequent orientation by consistent caregivers in the family and on the clinical staff.
- Establish a calm and reassuring environment that neither over nor under stimulates the patient.
- Establish a day/night routine with periods of uninterrupted rest.
- Encourage participation in daily routines (hygiene, exercise).
- Assess the need for tubes, lines, and restraints.
- Continually calm and inform the patient and family of the relationship between medical course and mental status.

Psychopharmacology

- Recommended when symptoms are persistent and severe and affect the child's medical outcome.
- Recommend child and adolescent psychiatry consultation to discuss off label use of these medications.
- Haloperidol (Haldol®)
  - Check vital signs and obtain an EKG.
  - IV or PO.
  - Available in low doses (0.25–1 mg titrated up by 0.25 mg to 0.5 mg increments every 30 to 45 minutes).
  - Parental doses are twice as potent.
  - Particularly effective for hyperactive delirium.
- Atypical antipsychotic medications.
  - Recommended in the adult literature because of the lower risk of extrapyramidal and cardiac side effects.
  - Risperidone (Risperdal®) available as a liquid or orally disintegrating tablet.
  - Olanzapine (Zyprexa®, Zydis®) available IM, as a pill, and as a disintegrating tablet.
  - Ziprasidone (Geodon) available PO.
  - May be preferred for hypoactive delirium.
- Benzodiazepines [alprazolam (Xanax®), diazepam (Valium®), lorazepam (Ativan®)].
  - Rarely effective alone and may complicate and exacerbate symptoms.
  - Lorazepam (Ativan®) available IV or PO.

- Given in combination with antipsychotic medications in adults but no studies are available in children.
- Dexmedetomidine (Precedex) may sedate without a risk for delirium.

Management of the Aggressive/Disruptive Pediatric Patient

In the pediatric oncology setting, these extreme behaviors are uncommon but may be seen in the following conditions.

Differential Diagnosis

- Delirium.
- Uncontrolled pain.
- Difficulty modulating emotions.
- Poor impulse control/impulsivity.
- Intoxication with opiates or benzodiazepines.
- Alcohol or benzodiazepine withdrawal.
- Drug intoxication.
- Acute grief reactions.
- Medication side effects.
- Brain metastases.
- Organic mood disorder on steroids.
- History of physical or sexual abuse.
- Psychiatric diagnosis.
  - Depression.
  - Bipolar Disorder.
  - Psychotic Disorder.
  - Intermittent Explosive Disorder.
  - Separation Anxiety Disorder.
  - Generalized Anxiety Disorder.
  - Posttraumatic Stress Disorder.
  - Pervasive Developmental Disorder.
  - Oppositional Defiant Disorder.

Steps to Follow in the Initial Evaluation

1. Approach the patient in a calm and solicitous manner that avoids confrontation.
2. The primary medical care team should set aside sufficient time to identify the circumstances that triggered the patient's loss of control.
3. Inform the patient of the impact of his or her behaviors on others including the medical staff and the interviewer; denying the impact may be perceived as provocative and escalate the aggression.
4. Enlist help from family, friends or staff member with whom the patient has established relationships.
5. Attempt to meet the patient's immediate needs including voluntary medications to calm the agitation.

6. Alert hospital security if the patient does not respond to verbal reassurance and work with security personnel to plan an approach that will offer safety and support to all involved.
7. Intervene physically only when the patient's behaviors are an obvious danger to himself or others. This may require the administration of medication or the application of physical restraints and/or seclusion.
8. Be prepared to initiate direct interventions when the patient rapidly escalates.
9. Leave the patient in the company of a family member, caregiver or staff member at all times in order to decrease the risk of escalating anxiety and agitation.

Restraint and Seclusion

Under extreme circumstances, such as the need to provide life-threatening treatment to a combative or confused child, it may be necessary to restrain a child using physical force. Restraint, seclusion or continuation of such procedures can only be ordered by qualified and trained individuals authorized by the hospital or treatment facility. Additional care must be taken if restraint is needed in cancer patients due to frailty, blood clotting impairments and fragile bones. Guidelines for Restraint and Seclusion have been published by Brown et al.[20] It is important to be familiar with and to follow one's own hospital policies regarding restraint and seclusion.

Purpose

- Prevention of harm to patient and others.

Physical Restraint

- Centers for Medicare and Medicaid Services define the use of restraints as follows:

  "Managing behavioral emergencies is allowed only when all less restrictive measures have failed and unanticipated severely aggressive or destructive behavior places the patient or others in imminent danger."

Seclusion

- Seclusion is only very rarely necessary for pediatric oncology patients and should be considered only under extreme circumstances, when it is considered the only reasonable method to calm the patient. It should be undertaken with very careful monitoring if allowed by hospital rules, taking into consideration the patient's emotional and physical status.

Ordering Seclusion or Restraint

- Trained staff members can initiate procedures before an order is obtained

- Licensed independent practitioner (LIP) provides a verbal or written order within **one hour** of the initiation of restraint or seclusion and reviews the patient's condition
- Must perform an in-person evaluation within **2 hours** of the initial intervention (ages 17 and younger).
  - Within **1 hour** for Medicare/Medicaid-funded program (CHA guidelines).
- If the patient is no longer in seclusion or restraint when the order expires, the LIP must evaluate the patient within 24 hours if the initial intervention.
- Verbal and written orders are time limited.
  - 4 hours if 18 years and older.
  - 2 hours if between 9 and 17 years.
  - 1 hour if under 9 years.
- Continuation can be ordered by a qualified trained individual authorized by the hospital.
- LIP must perform an in-person reevaluation every 4 hours when 17 years or younger, 8 hours when 18 years and older.
- Does not apply for holds of 30 minutes or less.

Medical Immobilization

- Necessary restrictive procedures that facilitate healing.
- Support a level of compliance that is beyond the developmental capabilities of the young patient.

Chemical Restraint

- Use of medications to control the patient's behaviors including agitation or violence.
- Difficult to consistently identify when used in a medical setting.
- Inadequate documentation frequently accompanies it use.
- Concept is particularly challenging in emergent situations.
- Not chemical restraint if the medication is part of a plan of care for a diagnosable condition.
  - Implies that the patient is appropriately assessed and the medication prescribed is consistent with the diagnosis.
  - Considered treatment and not simply a means of controlling the patient.

Use of Chemical Restraint

- The patient is struggling violently while in physical restraints.
- Physical restraints are not preferred.
- Exercise caution to not oversedate the patient and limit effective assessment.
- Intervention is included in a Plan of Care.

References

1. Horowitz, LM, Bridge, JA, Teach, SJ. Ask suicide-screening questions (ASQ). *Arch Pediatr Adolesc Med.* 2012;166:1170–1176.

2. Gould, MS, Marrocco, FA, Kleinman, M, et al. Evaluating iatrogenic risk of youth suicide screening programs. *JAMA*. 2005;293:1635–1643.
3. Oquendo M. A., Halberstam B. & Mann J. J. Risk factors for suicidal behavior: utility and limitations of research instruments. In First MB, ed., *Standardized Evaluation in Clinical Practice*. 2003: 103–130.
4. Diamond G, Levy S, Bevans KN, et al. Development, validation and utility of internet-based, behavioral health screen for adolescents. *Pediatrics*. 2010;126:163–170.
5. Posner K, Brown GK, Stanley B, et al. The Columbia-Suicide Severity Rating Scale: initial validity and internal consistency finding from three multisite studies with adolescents and adults. *Am J Psychiatry*. 2011;168(12): 1266–1277.
6. Berman AL, Jobes DA, Silverman MM. Adolescent Suicide: Assessment and Intervention. 2nd ed. Washington, DC: American Psychological Association; 2006.
7. Recklitis CJ, Lockwood RA, Rothwell MA, Diller LR. Suicidal ideation and attempts in adult survivors of childhood cancer. *J Clin Oncol*. 2006;24(24):3852–3857.
8. Bridge JA, Goldstein TR, Brent DA. Adolescent suicide and suicidal behavior. *J Child Psychol Psychiat*. 2006;47:372–394.
9. Shaffer D, Gould MS, Fisher P, et al. Psychiatric diagnosis in child and adolescent suicide. *Arch Gen Psychiat*. 1996;53(4):339–348.
10. 3. Centers for Disease Control. Youth risk behavior surveillance—United States, 2011. http://www.cdc.gov/mmwr/pdf/ss/ss6104.pdf
11. Ash P. Children and adolescents. In: RI Simon, RE Hale, eds. Textbook of Suicide Assessment and Management. Washington, DC: American Psychiatric Publishing; 2006:35–55.
12. Centers for Disease Control. Youth risk behavior surveillance system: selected 2011 national health risk behaviors and health outcomes by sex. 2011. http://www.cdc.gov/healthyyouth/yrbs/pdf/us_disparitysex_yrbs.pdf
13. Centers for Disease Control. Suicide: Facts at a glance. http://www.cdc.gov/violenceprevention/pdf/suicide_datasheet_2012-a.pdf
14. Ludi E, Ballard E, Greenbaum R, et al. Suicide risk in youth with intellectual disabilities: The challenges of screening. *J Dev Behav Pediatr*. 2012;33:431–440.
15. Schieveld JN, Leroy PL, van Os J, Nicolai J, Vos GD & Leentjens AF. Pediatric delirium in critical illness: Phenomenology, clinical correlates and treatment response in 40 cases in the pediatric intensive care unit. *Intensive Care Med*. 2007;33(6):1033–1040.
16. Silver G, Traube C, Kearney J. Detecting pediatric delirium: development of a rapid observational assessment tool. *Intensive Care Med*. 2012;38:1025–1031.
17. Turkel SB, Tavaré CJ. Delirium in children and adolescents. *J Neuropsychiatry Clin Neurosci*. 2003;15(4):431–435.
18. Turkel SB, Braslow K, Tavare CJ, Trzepacz PT. The delirium rating scale in children and adolescents. *Psychosomatics*. 2003;44(2):126–129.
19. Smith HA, Boyd J, Fuchs DC. Diagnosing delirium in critically ill children: validity and reliability of the pediatric confusion assessment method for the intensive care unit. *Crit Care Med*. 2011;39:150–157.

20. Brown RL, Genel M, Riggs JA. Use of seclusion and restraint in children and adolescents. Council on Scientific Affairs, American Medical Association. *Arch Pediatr Adolesc Med*. 2000;154(7):653–656.

References—General

American Psychiatric Association. Practice guideline for the treatment of patients with delirium. *Am J Psychiatry*. 1999;156(Suppl. 5):1–20.

Gould MS, Greenberg T, Velting DM, Shaffer D. Youth suicide risk and preventive interventions: A review of the past 10 years. *J Am Acad Child Adolesc Psychiatry*. 2003;42(4):386–405.

Hem E, Loge JH, Haldorsen T, Ekeberg Ø. Suicide risk in cancer patients from 1960 to 1999. *J Clin Oncol*. 2004;22(20):4209–4216.

Joint Commission on Accreditation of Healthcare Organizations. Provision of care, treatment, and services. In: *2006 Comprehensive Accreditation Manual for Hospitals (CAMH): The Official Handbook*. [Standard PC.12.90, EP4, Restraint and Seclusion, Rev. Sep 2, 2007]. Oak Brook, IL: Joint Commission Resources; 2006.

Spinetta JJ, Masera G, Eden T, et al. Refusal, non-compliance, and abandonment of treatment in children and adolescents with cancer: A report of the SIOP Working Committee on Psychosocial Issues in Pediatric Oncology. *Med Pediatr Oncol*. 2002;38(2):114–117.

Section IV

Treatment Issues and Interventions

Chapter 15

Medical Aspects of Transplantation

Allistair Abraham and Terry J. Fry

Transplantation

Blood and marrow transplantation (BMT) is curative for a number of malignant and nonmalignant conditions (Tables 15.1–15.3). For patients with inadequate or ineffective blood cell production, *allogeneic* transplant ("*allo-*" = genetically different) BMT from a donor provides replacement with normally functioning bone marrow. In refractory cancer, the use of additional chemotherapy and/or radiation therapy is often limited by significant negative side effects, including myelosuppression. The role of transplantation in these patients is to rescue blood cell production.[1] An *autologous* ("*auto-*" = self) transplant refers to the case in which the patient's own blood-producing cells (hematopoietic stem cells, or HSCs) are collected ahead of time and re-infused following cytotoxic therapy. When an allogeneic BMT is performed for cancer (as in the case of leukemia) the donor immune cells can also attack residual cancer cells contributing to the therapeutic potential of the procedure. This phenomenon is often referred to as the graft-versus-tumor (GVT) or graft-versus-leukemia (GVL) effect.

Although successful BMT can result in life-long cure of a major illness, it is not without risks including short-and long-term toxicities.[2,3] One major potential sequela of allogeneic BMT is a condition known as graft-versus-host disease, or GVHD. This occurs when the transferred immune cells attack the recipient's nonmalignant tissues. GVHD has two general classifications. Acute GVHD is inflammatory in nature and has a predilection for the skin, gut, and liver. Conversely, the chronic version more resembles autoimmune and rheumatologic diseases of the skin, lungs, liver, gut, eyes, connective tissues, and genitalia. Determining what drives transplanted immune cells to attack the tumor (GVT, GVL) versus the patient's normal tissue (GVHD) is the focus of ongoing research efforts.[4–7] In addition to GVHD, BMT also carries the risk of several complications (Table 15.4). The psychosocial aspects of BMT are particularly important, and should be an essential part of the comprehensive care of these patients (Table 15.5). BMT can be burdensome to family members, who find themselves caring for a child with a severely deficient immune system. The logistical burdens of taking medications multiple times per day

Table 15.1 Indications for Autologous Transplant Malignancy

Diagnosis	Therapeutic Considerations
Neuroblastoma	• High-risk patients • Done in addition to standard chemotherapy, surgery, radiation, and antibody therapy • Single or double transplants associated with high-dose chemotherapy or radioactive agent (e.g., MIBG) administration
Hodgkin lymphoma	• Relapse after standard therapy
Non-Hodgkin lymphoma	• Relapse after standard therapy
Retinoblastoma	• Relapse after standard therapy • Refractory or metastatic disease
Acute promyelocytic leukemia (APL)	• Relapse after standard therapy
Brain tumors	Facilitates high-dose chemotherapy for certain brain tumors including • Medulloblastoma • Atypical teratoid/rhabdoid tumor • Pineoblastoma • Germ cell tumor (high risk)
Ewing sarcoma	• Investigational for relapsed/refractory disease
Germ cell (extracranial)	• Investigational for relapsed/refractory disease
Wilms tumor	• Investigational for relapsed/refractory disease
Rhabdomyosarcoma	• Investigational for relapsed/refractory disease

Table 15.2 Indications for Allogeneic Transplant Malignancy

Diagnosis	Therapeutic Considerations
Acute lymphoblastic leukemia (ALL)	• Relapse after standard therapy • Transplant usually involves high-dose chemotherapy and total-body irradiation
Acute myeloid leukemia (AML)	• High-risk disease in remission • Relapse after standard therapy • Considered consolidation if matched sibling available
Chronic myeloid leukemia (CML)	• High-risk disease • Disease not controlled with tyrosine kinase inhibitors
Juvenile myelomonocytic leukemia (JMML)	• Transplant considered first line
Myelodysplastic syndrome (MDS)	• Considered for higher-risk disease
Hodgkin lymphoma	• Relapse after autologous transplant
Non-Hodgkin lymphoma	• Relapse after autologous transplant

Table 15.3 Indications for Allogeneic Transplant Nonmalignant disease

Diagnosis	Therapeutic Considerations
Hemoglobinopathy • Sickle cell disease • Thalassemia major	• Matched sibling donor considered for symptomatic patients • Unrelated donors considered experimental • Stable mixed chimerism sufficient for disease symptom resolution • Increased risk of rejection
Bone marrow failure • Fanconi anemia • Dyskeratosis Congenita • Shwachman- Diamond • Severe Aplastic anemia	• Increased transplant related toxicity associated with hereditary bone marrow failure syndromes • Increased risk of rejection in severe aplastic anemia
Immunodeficiency • Severe combined immunodeficiency (SCID) • Wiskott Aldrich • Chronic granulomatous disease • Hemophagocytic syndromes	• Minimal to no preparative regimen needed for most severe SCID • Stable mixed lymphocyte chimerism can be curative
Metabolic disease • Hurler syndrome • Adrenoleukodystrophy • Gaucher disease • Krabbe disease	• Transplanted cells serve as factories to produce missing enzyme from primary disease • Best outcomes with transplants done prior to development of disease symptoms
Osteopetrosis	• Best outcomes with transplants done early in disease course

and attending clinic visits frequently for many months can also take their toll on caregivers.

Current and Future Directions of BMT

- Transplant is reserved for the patients who have life-threatening diseases that can be most optimally treated using hematopoeitic stem cells. However, modern era indications for BMT continue to be refined, as the toxicity of BMT has improved over the last decade with better supportive care and the use of less intense chemotherapy and radiation regimens prior to transplantation.[8]
- More sensitive methods are used to ensure a high level of matching and compatibility between transplant donors and recipients at the DNA level (referred to as HLA matching). This has contributed to the expansion of donor pools with increasing use of HLA mismatched family members and unrelated donors when HLA matched siblings are unavailable.

Table 15.4 Common Acute and Late Effects of Transplantation

Organ system/Complication	Evaluations and Interventions
Immune mediated • Rejection • Graft-versus-host disease	• Monitor chimerism (contribution of donor blood cell production) • Immunosuppression • Tissue biopsy
Infectious risk	• Blood counts • Immune recovery blood testing • Surveillance for infection • Routine antiviral and antifungal prophylactic medications • Isolation from others • Revaccination
Cardiac • Cardiomyopathy • Hypertension	• Electrocardiogram • Echocardiogram • Hypertension screening • Cardiologist referral
Pulmonary • Bronchiolitis obliterans organizing pneumonia (BOOP) • Idiopathic pneumonia syndrome	• Oxygen saturation • Pulmonary function tests • Imaging studies (high resolution CT scan) • Bronchoscopy • Pulmonologist referral
Endocrine • Growth delay • Infertility • Metabolic syndrome	• Growth velocity, bone age • Sexual development and fertility assessment • Hormone levels • Lipid profile, body mass index—diet and exercise counseling, lipid lower medications • Endocrinologist referral
Transfusion requirements • Iron overload	• Blood counts • Surveillance for bleeding • Phlebotomy or iron chelation
Liver • Veno-occlusive disease	• Liver function test monitoring • Liver biopsy
Gastrointestinal • Mucositis • Nausea/vomiting • Poor nutrition • Diarrhea	• Pain medication • Tube feeds • Total Parenteral nutrition (TPN) • Biofeedback

(continued)

Table 15.4 (Continued)	
Organ system/Complication	**Evaluations and Interventions**
CNS • CNS hemorrhage • Seizure/Posterior reversible encephalopathy syndrome (PRES) • Developmental/cognitive delay[9] • Neuropathies (medication-induced)	• Cognitive and neuropsychological assessments (See Chapter 18 on Cognitive Sequelae of Cancer Treatment) • Neuropathic pain medications • Imaging • Blood pressure control • Neurologist referral
Ophthalmologic: • Cataracts • Visual impairment • Eye dryness	• Visual acuity • Ophthalmologic examination • Artificial tears
Skeletal • Osteopenia • Osteonecrosis	• Bone mineral density imaging • MRI • Vitamin D • Calcium • Weight-bearing exercises
Secondary malignancy	• Complete blood count • Imaging studies • High risk behavior counseling

Table 15.5 Common Psychosocial Effects of Transplantation	
Effect	**Possible Interventions to Consider**
Psychosocial • Anxiety, depression • Adjustment (school, work, relationships) • Social isolation • Problems with adherence	• Referral to social worker/psychologist • Individual and group therapy • Cognitive-behavioral therapy • School counselor support • Support groups • Spiritual support • Discussion with psychosocial team to consider whether referral to psychiatry is indicated
School absenteeism	• Home and hospital teaching • School re-entry program • Distance learning/video-conferencing with school to facilitate class participation (social and academic) • Online classes for college students/vocational training

(continued)

Table 15.5 (Continued)

Effect	Possible Interventions to Consider
Financial concerns • Healthcare expenses • Parental loss of work	• Social work support • National marrow donor program financial assistance program • Referral to other local and national resources
Complex ongoing care • Frequent medical follow-up during first year posttransplant • Multiple ongoing health concerns posttransplant • Inadequate insurance • Maintaining an environment free of infectious risks	• Social work to provide emotional support, assist with job, transportation, and financial needs, and to reduce barriers to care • Coordination and scheduling of clinic appointments for families • Multidisciplinary long term follow-up clinic if available to better coordinate care • Temporary medical housing

- There has been increasing use of alternative graft sources, such as umbilical cord blood grafts and peripheral blood, in addition to traditional bone marrow. Collectively, these changes have made transplant an option for more patients but have increased the complexity of the process of donor selection.

Summary

Bone marrow transplant increases our ability to effectively cure some high-risk cancers, hemoglobinopathies, immunodeficiencies, and other nonmalignant disorders. Traditionally, the high doses of chemotherapy and radiation used in transplant medicine posed several risks to patients. Current efforts and research aim to reduce toxicity by using lower doses of better-tolerated chemotherapy and radiation. Transplant has become available to more patients with the increase in donors and types of transplant grafts being used. Post-transplantation monitoring for long-term side effects is necessary to ensure the best outcomes, which highlights the need for sound long-term follow-up in a multidisciplinary setting. Additionally, the transplant process can be physically, mentally, and emotionally long and complicated for the patient and family, and, therefore, necessitates a well-structured psychosocial assessment and support system. The past two decades have seen major advancements in the treatment and supportive care of the patient undergoing BMT, resulting in more widespread applicability of curative transplant techniques to treat chronic debilitating diseases such as sickle cell disease. Investigation into engineered cellular therapies targeted to treat cancers more precisely and effectively may make the toxicities of chemotherapy and radiation things of the past.

References

1. Thomas ED, Buckner CD, Banaji M, et al. One hundred patients with acute leukemia treated by chemotherapy, total body irradiation, and allogeneic marrow transplantation. *Blood.* 1977;49(4):511–533.
2. Oliansky DM, Camitta B, Gaynon P, et al. Role of cytotoxic therapy with hematopoietic stem cell transplantation in the treatment of pediatric acute lymphoblastic leukemia: update of the 2005 evidence-based review. *Biol Blood Marrow Transplant.* 2012;18(4):505–522.
3. Oliansky DM, Rizzo JD, Aplan PD, et al. The role of cytotoxic therapy with hematopoietic stem cell transplantation in the therapy of acute myeloid leukemia in children: an evidence-based review. *Biol Blood Marrow Transplant.* 2007;13(1):1–25.
4. Shindo T, Kim TK, Benjamin CL, Wieder ED, Levy RB, Komanduri KV. MEK inhibitors selectively suppress alloreactivity and graft-versus-host disease in a memory stage-dependent manner. *Blood.* 2013;121(23):4617–4626.
5. Spierings E, Kim YH, Hendriks M, et al. Multicenter analyses demonstrate significant clinical effects of minor histocompatibility antigens on GvHD and GvL after HLA-matched related and unrelated hematopoietic stem cell transplantation. *Biol Blood Marrow Transplant.* 2013;19(8):1244–1253.
6. Haarberg KM, Li J, Heinrichs J, et al. Pharmacologic inhibition of PKCalpha and PKCtheta prevents GVHD while preserving GVL activity in mice. *Blood.* 2013;122(14):2500–2511.
7. Meyer EH, Hsu AR, Liliental J, et al. A distinct evolution of the T-cell repertoire categorizes treatment refractory gastrointestinal acute graft-versus-host disease. *Blood.* 2013;121(24):4955–4962.
8. Mateos MK, O'Brien TA, Oswald C, et al. Transplant-related mortality following allogeneic hematopoeitic stem cell transplantation for pediatric acute lymphoblastic leukemia: 25-year retrospective review. *Pediatr Blood Cancer.* 2013;60(9):1520–1527.
9. Smedler AC, Winiarski J. Neuropsychological outcome in very young hematopoietic SCT recipients in relation to pretransplant conditioning. *Bone Marrow Transplant.* 2008;42(8):515–522.

Chapter 16

Psychosocial Issues for Transplant Patients and Donors

Sean Phipps

Stem cell or bone marrow transplant (SCT) has evolved over the past three decades from a heroic, experimental therapy of last resort, to a standard therapy for many high-risk malignancies.[1] At the same time, advances in supportive care have led to improved survival outcomes, and thus to a rapidly growing number of long-term survivors of SCT. Despite these advances, SCT remains a high risk medical procedure involving a prolonged and physically demanding treatment regimen that can challenge the coping capacities of patients and their families. Research indicates that SCT is a stressful experience that can negatively impact on the social functioning, self-esteem, and general emotional well-being of survivors.[2–5] The literature also points to the overall positive adjustment of the great majority of transplant survivors.[6] A number of studies have also focused on parental response to SCT, suggesting that parents may be at greater risk of psychosocial distress than their children, and that parental distress in turn may impact child adaptation to SCT.[2,7–11]

Much of the literature to date focuses on long-term outcomes in survivors, particularly neurocognitive and academic outcomes, and a smaller number of studies have addressed the short- and intermediate-term outcomes, such as the general adjustment of patients and parents, and measures of distress. The transplant process is conceptualized in four phases, labeled the pretransplant phase, the acute phase, the transition phase, and the long-term follow-up phase. Each phase is associated with unique stresses and psychological issues as outlined in Box 16.1.

Pretransplant Phase

Given the risks associated with the SCT process, the decision to undergo the procedure can be very stressful, as can be the consent process, where the myriad potential adverse outcomes must be presented. Pretransplant psychosocial evaluations are recommended as a means of identifying potential problems and identifying the optimal approaches for supporting the patient and family through the procedure see Table 16.2.

Box 16.1 Stresses and Psychological Issues Associated with the Transplant Process

- Pretransplant Phase:
  - Decision to undergo procedure.
  - Search for a donor.
  - Consent process.
  - Psychosocial evaluation of patient, family, donor.
- Acute Phase:
  - Admission, conditioning, transplant, early engraftment.
  - Prolonged hospitalization/isolation.
  - Physical demands/somatic distress.
  - Disruption in family processes.
- Transition Phase:
  - Discharge, return home.
  - Less contact with the medical team and hospital.
  - School and social reintegration.
  - Return to "normal."
- Long-term Follow-up Phase:
  - Surveillance for late effects.
  - Neurocognitive and psychoeducational outcomes.
  - Social and vocational outcomes.

Acute Phase of Transplant Hospitalization

First line interventions are typically medical and pharmacological, including anti-emetics for nausea, including serotonin receptor antagonists such as ondansetron, and opioid analgesics for mucositis. Very little data is available regarding behaviorally oriented interventions, with only a few small trials involving cognitive-behavioral approaches, and some mind-body or complementary therapies.[12] Much of what is recommended is based on clinical experience, anecdote, or case studies.

Issues During Acute Phase of Transplant Hospitalization

- Somatic distress associated with conditioning: nausea, vomiting, mouth sores.
- Sleep disturbance, disruption in diurnal rhythm.
- Appetite disturbance, requirement of TPN (may be prolonged).
- Compliance issues: mouth care, oral medications, exercise, daily routine.
- Mood disturbance: anxiety, depression.
- Polypharmacy: multiple psychotropic or sedating agents.

Strategies to Reduce Acute Phase Distress, Maintain Compliance

- Facilitate maintenance of daily routine, wake up time, bedtime.
- Keep maximally active, using physical therapy, occupational therapy, child life services where possible.

Box 16.2 Pretransplant Psychosocial Assessment

- Patient
  - Past medical history.
    - Tolerance for prior chemotherapy, invasive procedures (if applicable).
    - Tolerance for prolonged hospitalizations (if applicable).
    - Past adjustment history.
      - Behavioral issues, mood.
      - Coping styles, preference for information.
    - Current cognitive functioning.
      - Developmental status, school history.
    - Understanding the transplant procedure.
    - Concerns/worries about the procedure.
      - Dispel misconceptions.
      - Coping with uncertainty and fluctuations in daily status of the patient.
      - Anticipate logistics of extended hospitalization.
- Parent/Family
  - Child adjustment history.
    - Specific parental concerns regarding patients' coping.
  - Family adjustment history.
    - Mental health history in the family.
    - Family adjustment to patient's illness.
    - Sibling adjustment (see Chapter 24, the Impact of Cancer on Family and Siblings).
  - Family logistical plans for transplant procedure.
    - Which parent will be present.
    - Availability of other caregivers.
    - Special concerns for other family members.

- Routine monitoring of pain, discomfort; early, aggressive pharmacological therapy, use of patient controlled analgesia (PCA's) where possible.
- Encourage p.o. intake, but avoid struggles.
- Developmentally appropriate distraction techniques; e.g., video games.
- Encourage contact with peers via social media.
- Teach pill swallowing (preferably prior to admission).
- Operant reinforcement plans to reward compliance, reduce stalling.
- Provide opportunity of emotional expression, and ongoing support.

Transition Phase

In the period following discharge from initial transplant hospitalization, patients and families remain at risk for a number of behavioral or psychosocial difficulties, and ongoing monitoring during this phase is important. Patients are no longer readily available as they were when they were inpatient, and their functioning is perhaps now less transparent to the medical team. The patient generally requires close outpatient medical monitoring, and psychosocial caregivers are encouraged to participate in this, with intermittent monitoring over the course of the first year posttransplant. It may be as long as a full year before the allogeneic transplant patient is ready to return to school and a full range of social activities. These re-integration activities may be particularly problematic for some patients. A subset of patients that may be at particular risk are those experiencing chronic graft-vs-host-disease (GVHD).[1,13] This can cause complications in multiple organ systems requiring aggressive medical management, often involving multiple medications with problematic side-effect profiles, including prolonged steroid use leading to changes in physical appearance. Given the potential effects of GVHD on patient quality of life, these patients require particularly close monitoring.[13]

Monitoring During the Transition Phase

- Assess for disturbance in mood, sleep, appetite, symptoms of posttraumatic stress (avoidant behaviors, intrusive thoughts about any part of the cancer experience).
  - Monitor same in parents who may be at greater risk.
    - Intervene or refer for local mental health services as needed.
- Monitor social functioning and degree of social reintegration.
- Anticipate return to school.
  - Discussion with school personnel.
    - Review of psychoeducational assessment results where applicable.
    - School visit depending on age of child, feasibility.
- Monitor patient energy level and resumption of normal activities.
- Patients experiencing GVHD require particularly close monitoring.

Long-Term Follow-up: Neurocognitive Late Effects

An issue of great concern in regard to psychological outcomes in transplant survivors relates to potential neurocognitive changes. Survivors of pediatric SCT are thought to be at risk for late neurocognitive deficits as a result of their exposure to a number of potentially neurotoxic agents.[14–17] Among the agents used in pretransplant conditioning, total body irradiation (TBI) has been a primary focus, but other cytotoxic conditioning agents are potentially neurotoxic as well. CNS toxicities also are associated with agents commonly used for the prophylaxis and/or treatment of graft-versus-host- disease (GVHD). More speculative is the possibility of direct effects of GVHD on the CNS.

Studies of neurocognitive outcomes have been hindered by small sample sizes, retrospective designs, or limited prospective follow-up.[14] The findings reported have been contradictory, with a few studies indicating declines in cognitive function following SCT, but a larger number of studies reporting normal neurodevelopment, with no evidence of decline.[4,14–17] Discrepancies between studies appear to relate largely to age effects, with younger children appearing to be at higher risk. A consensus in the literature is beginning to emerge, indicating that SCT, even with TBI, poses low to minimal risk for late cognitive and academic deficits in patients who are at least 6 years old at the time of transplant. For younger patients, the risk of cognitive impairment may be increased.

In most cases, appropriate surveillance of neurocognitive functioning for SCT survivors requires only an interval assessment of the child's school performance, perhaps supplemented by parental questionnaire data. Exceptions might be made for children who were younger ≤5 years at the time of transplant, particularly if they received TBI, and those for whom cognitive problems have already been identified, where more extensive, performance-based assessment, supplemented by possible teacher input, may be indicated.

Suggested Approach for Handling Neurocognitive/Psychoeducational Issues

- Pretransplant:
  - Review developmental, school history.
  - Provide anticipatory guidance for parents:
    - Explain that risks for cognitive problems are generally low.
    - Risks may be increased slightly for younger children.
- First Year Posttransplant:
  - Interview regarding developmental, school progress.
    - Parental questionnaire data that assesses the child's quality of life and psychosocial functioning.
    - Comparable self-reports for older children and adolescents.
    - Developmental screening/psychometric assessment for youngest patients and those for whom problems are suspected.
- Ongoing Surveillance:
  - Inquire regarding school progress.
    - Brief parental/self-report questionnaires.
    - Psychometric assessment for those with identified or suspected difficulties.

Long-Term Effects

More recently, there has been growing attention toward the very long term effects of SCT as survivors reach adulthood (see Chapter 13, Fertility and Sexuality, and Chapter 33, Pediatric Cancer Survivors).[14,18,19] The available data thus far indicate that most long-term survivors are functioning well as adults, and lead productive, normal lives, although a small subset experience difficulties. This subset of survivors evidence poorer health-related quality of life (in the physical but not the mental health domains), higher perceived cognitive problems (problems with memory and concentration), and have higher rates of unemployment and financial difficulties.[18,19] This information can be used in providing anticipatory guidance to survivors as they transition from pediatric to adult care and in planning for long-term follow-up.

Donor Issues

In the early period of SCT, the majority of pediatric transplants utilized sibling donors. Since most of these donors were minors, considerable attention was paid to the ethical and legal aspects of this process, with comprehensive psychosocial assessments of the parents and potential donors, and in some cases, appointment of a guardian *ad litem* through the juvenile court system to ensure protection of the donors' rights.[4,20] As SCT has become more routine, such scrutiny has relaxed considerably, and court involvement is rarely invoked. Moreover, matched sibling transplants now represent a minority of cases, with use of unrelated donors or cord blood samples through donor registries, or parental haplotype donors.[1] Very little empiric data is available regarding the impact of marrow donation on the sibling.[2,21] Recommended practices, based largely on anecdotal evidence and clinical experience, include a pretransplant evaluation process, with a separate interview with the prospective donor beginning at age 5 or 6.

Suggested Procedures for Donor Assessment/Follow-up

- Pretransplant
  - Parental interview (may be done by social work, psychology)
    - Parental perceptions of donation process for family.
      - Level of discussion that has occurred with donor, recipient.
    - Donor reaction, whether there are concerns about the donor's ability to cope with being a match, the donation, or the uncertain transplant outcome.
    - Donor Interview (may be done by child life team, social worker, psychologist, or child psychiatrist)
    - Assess donor's age-appropriate understanding of the process.
      - Dispel any misconceptions.
      - Ensure the absence of coercion, confirm perception of "voluntary choice."
    - Anticipatory guidance regarding process.
- Posttransplant
  - Assess donor's perception of the process in the period immediately following procedure.
    - Obtain additional parental report 1–3 months postdonation.
      - Assess any disturbance in donor's mood, sleep, appetite, symptoms of posttraumatic stress.
    - If transplant is unsuccessful/patient dies, additional follow-up with sibling donor by face-to-face visit or phone is important.

Conclusion

There have been many medical and technological advances in stem cell transplantation, along with improvements in supportive care, that have led to increased usage, and decreased morbidity and mortality associated with the procedure. Nevertheless, it remains a very demanding and stressful process for both the patient and his/her family. Although research suggests that most patients adjust reasonably well to this challenge, ongoing psychosocial monitoring is an essential aspect of care, beginning in the pretransplant period, during transplant hospitalization, and throughout long-term follow-up. Mental health professionals comprise an important part of the care team, to aid in monitoring, and when indicated, to provide empirically supported interventions (see Chapter 19, Psychotherapeutic Interventions).

References

1. Bollard CE, Krance RA, Heslop HE. Hematopoetic stem cell transplantation in pediatric oncology. In Pizzo PA, Poplack DG, eds., *Principles and Practice of Pediatric Oncology*, 6th ed. (Ch. 16). Philadelphia, PA: Lippincott, Williams & Wilkins, 201.
2. Packman W, Weber S, Wallace J, Bugescu N. Psychological effects of hematopoietic SCT on pediatric patients, siblings and parents: a review. *Bone Marrow Transplant.* 2010; 45:1134–1146.
3. Barrera M, Atenafu E, Pinto J. Behavioral, social, and educational outcomes after pediatric stem cell transplantation and related factors. *Cancer.* 2009;115:880–889.
4. Phipps, S: Psychosocial and behavioral issues in stem cell transplantation. In Brown RT, ed., Comprehensive handbook of childhood cancer and sickle cell disease: A biopsychosocial approach. New York, NY: Oxford University Press, 2006: 75–99.
5. Tremolada M, Bonichini S, Pillon M, Messina C, Carli M. Quality of life and psychosocial sequelae in children undergoing hematopoietic stem cell transplantation: A review. *Pediatric Transplantation.* 2009;13:955–970.
6. Phipps S, Peasant C, Barrera M, Alderfer MA, Huang Q, Vannatta K. Resilience in children undergoing stem cell transplantation: results of a complementary intervention trial. *Pediatrics.* 2012;129:e762–e770.
7. Barrera M, Atenafu E, Doyle J, Berlin-Romalis D, Hancock K. Differences in mothers; and fathers' psychological distress after pediatric SCT: a longitudinal study. *Bone Marrow Transplant.* 2012;47:934–939.
8. Manne S, DuHamel K, Ostroff J, et al. Coping and the course of mother's depressive symptoms during and after pediatric bone marrow transplantation. *J Am Acad Child & Adolesc Psychiat.* 2003;42:1055–1068.
9. Phipps S, Dunavant M, Lensing S, Rai SN. Patterns of distress in parents of children undergoing stem cell transplantation. *Pediatric Blood & Cancer.* 2004;43:267–274.
10. Streisand R, Rodrigue JR, Houck C, Graham-Pole J, Berlant N. Parents of children undergoing bone marrow transplantation: documenting stress and piloting a psychological intervention program. *J Pediatr Psychol.* 2000;25:331–338.
11. Jobe-Shields L, Alderfer MA, Barrera M, Vannatta K, Currier JM, Phipps S. Parental depression and family environment predict distress in children before stem cell transplantation. *J Development & Behavioral Pediatr.* 2009;30:249–256.
12. Phipps S, Barrera M, Vannatta K, Xiong X, Doyle JJ, Alderfer MA. Complementary therapies for children undergoing stem cell transplantation: report of a multisite trial. *Cancer.* 2010;116:3924–3933.

13. Bevans MF, Mitchell SA, Barrett AJ, et al. Function, adjustment, quality of life and symptoms (FAQS) in allogeneic hematopoietic stem cell transplantation (HSCT) survivors: a study protocol. *Health Qual Life Outcomes*. 2011;9:24.

14. Parsons SK, Phipps S, Sung L, Baker KS, Pulsipher MA, Ness KK. NCI, NHLBI/PBMTC First international conference on late effects after pediatric hematopoietic stem cell transplantation: health-related quality of life, functional, and neurocognitive outcomes. *Biol Blood & Marrow Transplant*. 2012;18:162–171.

15. Simms S, Kazak AE, Golumb V, Goldwein J Bunin N. Cognitive, behavioral, and social outcome of childhood stem cell transplantation. *J Pediatric Hematology/Oncology*. 2000; 24:115–120.

16. Kupst MJ, Penatic B, Debban B. Cognitive and psychosocial functioning of pediatric hematopoietic stem cell transplant patients: A prospective longitudinal study. *Bone Marrow Transplant*. 2002;30:600–617.

17. Phipps S, Rai SN, Lensing S, Leung W, Dunavant M. Cognitive and academic consequences of stem cell transplantation in children. *J Clin Oncol*. 2008 Apr 20;26(12):2027–2033.

18. Sanders JE, Hoffmeister PA, Storer BE, Appelbaum FR, Storb, RF, Syrjala KL. The quality of life of adult survivors of childhood hematopoietic cell transplant. *Bone Marrow Transplant*. 2010;45:746–754.

19. Lof CM, Winiarski J, Ljungman P, Forinder U. The socioeconomic and psychosocial circumstances of adult long-term survivors of hematopoietic stem cell transplantation in childhood. *Pediatric Transplant*. 2011;15:691–698.

20. Patenaude AF, Rappeport JM, Smith BR. The physician's influence on informed consent for bone marrow transplantation. *Theor Med*. 1986;7:165–179.

21. Wiener LS, Steffen-Smith E, Battles HB, Wayne AS, Love CP, Fry T. Sibling stem cell donor experiences at a single institution. *Psychooncol*. 2008;17:304–307.

Chapter 17

Medication Adherence

Ahna L. H. Pai and Dennis Drotar

Medical treatments for pediatric cancer vary widely in the degree to which the patient and their family are responsible for managing the treatment regimen and these expectations change over time. For instance, during induction for ALL there is typically close monitoring by the medical and nursing team, but in maintenance therapy, complex and prolonged oral medication regimens are largely managed by the patient and his/her parents.

Nonadherence represents a significant, though often unrecognized clinical issue for pediatric patients with cancer and their families, especially among adolescents.[1–4] Rates of nonadherence with prednisone and 6-Mercaptopurine (6MP) have been found to range from 10% to 42%[5] with up to 53% of adolescents with bioassay results consistent with nonadherence to treatment.[6] It has been estimated that 6MP an adherence rate of less than 95% is associated with an increased risk of relapse in ALL.[1] The potential clinical consequences of nonadherence can be significant, including lower survival rates and increased mortality due to relapse.[1,7–9] Anticipating, assessing, monitoring and, when necessary, treating adherence to the medical regimen are critical components of comprehensive clinical care.[10]

Anticipatory Guidance for Adherence

Prevention is the most effective approach to adherence. Anticipatory guidance should be provided to the patient (age dependent) and family (see Tables 17.1 and 17.2):

- Immediately prior to assuming self-management responsibilities.
- Whenever there is a change in a treatment regimen.

Ongoing Assessment and Monitoring of Adherence

Difficulties with maintaining adequate adherence to pediatric cancer treatment are very common and a particular patient's adherence behaviors will most likely change over time. Therefore, it is recommended that adherence assessment and monitoring occurs during every clinic visit for all patients and families who have the primary responsibility for managing cancer treatment (see Table 17.3). To most effectively monitor adherence, the patient,

Table 17.1 Anticipatory Guidance to Provide to All Patients and their Families

Goal	Key Points to Cover
General education about medication and treatment	• Provide general education about each medication or treatment procedure including what the medication/treatment is for, how it works and why it is important. • Provide information in verbal and written format if possible.

Discuss previous experiences taking medication	• Assess the patient's history of adherence behaviors. Ask:
	  • "Have you had to take medications regularly in the past? If so, what was that like?"
	  • "Did anything make taking the medication difficult/easy?"

Education concerning the importance and prevalence of adherence problems	• Introduce the idea that many patients (up to half) may have some problems adhering to their treatment regimens. • Note that adherence is necessary to get adequate medication exposure. • Discuss the potential consequences of inadequate exposure to a medication. • Highlight that adherence is difficult, there are many barriers to adherence, and the barriers change over time. • Tell the family that the team is available to help manage these barriers.

Promotion of adherence as a collaborative effort	• Create a collaborative working relationship by:
	  • Telling the families that you want to hear about adherence challenges, problems and successes at the beginning and throughout treatment.
	  • Encourage the family to talk about adherence difficulties.
	  • Emphasize that adherence issues may change throughout treatment. Therefore, the family and the team will need to work together over time to manage adherence.

Highlight the impact of the patient's developmental stage on adherence	• Encourage the family to talk about changes in adherence. • Emphasize that adherence can be influenced by the developmental stage of the patient (e.g., adolescence).

Develop a plan to monitor adherence that includes patient, parent and physician	• Monitoring adherence is necessary regardless of the age of the child.
	• Decide who will monitor each aspect of a treatment regimen. Identify a role for patient, parent and physician.
	• Examples of monitoring roles for each individual:
	  • Patient: Watching parent dispense medication, asking if a medication is correct, if it looks unfamiliar or incorrect.
	  • Parent: Watching the child taking their medication, asking if the child took their medication, counting pills.
	  • Physician: Confirming that there is a strategy in place to facilitate adherence, discussing adherence issues at every appointment, and documenting adherence management plans.

(continued)

Table 17.1 (Continued)

Goal	Key Points to Cover
Encourage basic skills for promoting adherence	• Encourage the family to make adherence plans at the beginning of a treatment. Plans should include details about how they will successfully accomplish a particular regimen task. • Encourage the family to develop a routine for taking medication (e.g., tie medication schedule with other regularly scheduled activities in the home such as meal time). • Tell family to explicitly discuss who will be responsible for each aspect of the treatment regimen (e.g., who will fill the prescriptions, who will remind the child to take their medication, who will confirm that medication has been taken).

Encourage basic skills for promoting adherence (continued)	• Advocate the use of reminder tools:
	  • Set reminder alarms.
	  • Send reminders to patient via text message, e-mail, or phone.
	• Teach organizational tools:
	  • Use pill boxes and/or pill calendars.
	  • Place medication in a visible location.
	• Encourage the development of backup plans:
	  • Carry extra doses of medication at all times.
	  • Keep doses of medication at houses of family members.
	  • Have pharmacy and physician numbers available at all times.

Emphasize importance of social support	• Educate the family that everybody needs help to successfully adhere to a long-term treatment plan. • Educate the family on the importance of involving friends and family in their plan for adherence as appropriate. • Emphasize the importance of general support (not necessarily focused on adherence) from family and friends in facilitating adherence.

and work collaboratively to monitor and facilitate adherence behaviors. Use of open-ended questions as much as possible when assessing adherence or factors that may impact adherence.

Ongoing Management and Intervention Strategies

Interventions to promote adherence may be indicated at several points throughout a treatment course due to changes in developmental level, lifestyle, and the treatment itself. The majority of interventions must be delivered often. Interventions are best administered using a team approach in which the patient and family, clinical care team and anyone closely involved

Table 17.2 General Risk Factors Associated with Nonadherence	
The frequency and pattern of risk factors provides critical information to allow tailoring of interventions to treat adherence issues. Factors are:	
• Child age (adolescents have poorer adherence than younger children) • Low socioeconomic status • History of psychological or psychiatric problems	• Limited cognitive functioning in child or parent • High family conflict and poor communication • Presence of other significant family stressors (employment problems, medical challenges, etc.) • Further out from diagnosis/longer time since diagnosis

Table 17.3 Routine Adherence Assessment and Monitoring
Medication confirmation • Have patient bring their medications to each appointment. • Review medications with patient and/or their family at each appointment. Note discrepancies between patient report and the chart. • "What medications are you currently prescribed? What dose? How often do you take [medication]? What is [medication] for?"
Access to Medication • "How do you obtain your medication from the pharmacy?" • "When you are away from the house, how do get your medication?"
General Monitoring • "Take me through a typical day and tell me about how you and your family manage your medication." • For each aspect of the treatment ask, "Who is responsible for [aspect]?" • "What has taking this medication been like for you and your family? What is the most difficult part? What is the easiest part?" • "What has helped you to take the medication?" • "How do you remind yourself to take your medication?" • "Has anything made you decide to stop taking your medication?" • What role does each of you play in managing the treatment regimen?
Parental Involvement • How do you know whether your son/daughter has taken their medications? • How do you support your son/daughter's adherence?

Side Effects
• Ask whether the patient is experiencing specific side effects:
  • What is it like to swallow the medication? Does [medication] have a bad taste or is it difficult to swallow?
  • "What side effects have you noticed from taking the medication?"
  • "What changes do you notice from taking the medication, either physically or emotionally?"
  • "Has [side effect] changed since your last visit? Is it better or worse?"
  • "How does [reported side effect] influence your decision to take your medicine day to day?"

(continued)

Table 17.3 (Continued)
Frequency of Non-adherence • "About how many doses of [medication] did you miss in the last 7 days?" • "When was the last time you missed [medication]?" • "Are there certain times when you forget your medication more than others?" • "How many times did you take your medication late? If, the patient took the medication late one or more times ask, "How late did you take your doses?"
Psychological Factors Influencing Adherence • "Has taking the medication been what you expected?" • "What does it mean to you to take this medication?" or "What do you think about when you are taking your medication?" • "How do you take your medications when you are out in public or with friends? What is that like?" • "What will happen if you decide not to take your medication?" • "Has taking your medication interfered with your daily life or the things you like to do? If yes, how so?"
Blood assays • Run labs to determine blood assay levels of medication metabolites and other serum indicators (e.g., ANC) of poor adherence (e.g., protocol AALL0331).[11] • Provide feedback to patient when appropriate.

Table 17.4 Management of Adherence in the Context of Ongoing Treatment

Adjust treatment to minimize interference with lifestyle or normative developmental events
• Simplify medication regimen
  • Dose
  • Timing of administration
  • Frequency of administration
  • Method of administration

Directly Address Side Effects • If possible, adjust medication (i.e., type, dose, timing) to minimize side effects or provide medications/interventions to counteract side effects if they directly hinder adherence. • Acknowledge that although side effects are very burdensome, they indicate that the treatment is effective. • Discuss costs and benefits of taking medication with patient.
Increase Monitoring • Increase frequency of appointments. • Increase practice of monitoring techniques listed in Table 17.3.
Behavioral Intervention Strategies • Reinforce adherence (or approximations to adherence). • Reinforce the family's use of strategies to improve adherence. • Reinforce discussion of adherence issues.

(continued)

Table 17.4 (Continued)

Indications for Assessment/Treatment by a Psychologist or Other Behavioral Specialist
• At the beginning of treatment, patient presents with multiple risk factors for non-\adherence (e.g., high family conflict, history of psychological difficulties) or has a history of non-\adherence with previous illnesses. • If routine adherence assessments identify potential adherence difficulties, then a more detailed assessment of adherence barriers is clinically indicated. • If patient or parent expresses concerns about their ability to follow the treatment regimen prior to starting or during treatment. • If patient or parent report difficulties following the regimen. • Interventions by the medical team have not improved adherence.
Interventions for Extreme and/or Dangerous Nonadherence
• In extreme cases, consider hospitalization for stabilization, education, and developing a treatment plan to increase adherence. • Involvement of child protective services for the assessment of and intervention for medical neglect.

in the child's care have clearly defined roles. Pediatric psychologists, among others, are team members who may consult in the implementation of adherence interventions. See Table 17.4 for a list of ongoing management and intervention strategies. Given the complexity of the treatment regimens and the multidisciplinary nature of adherence management and intervention, documentation of adherence management and intervention strategies is critical for effective communication between the patient, the patient's family, and medical team members.

References

1. Bhatia S, Landier W, Shangguan M, et al. Nonadherence to oral mercaptopurine and risk of relapse in hispanic and non-hispanic white children with acute lymphoblastic leukemia: a report from the children's oncology group. *J Clin Oncol.* 2012;30, 2094–2101.
2. Partridge AH, Avorn J, Wang PS, Winer EP. Adherence to therapy with oral antineoplastic agents. *J Natl Cancer Inst.* 2002;94(9):652–661.
3. Spinetta JJ, Masera G, Eden T, et al. Refusal, non-compliance, and abandonment of treatment in children and adolescents with cancer. A report of the SIOP Working Committee on psychosocial issues in pediatric oncology. *Med Pediatr Oncol.* 2002;38(2):114–117.
4. Kennard BD, Stewart SM, Olvera R, et al. Nonadherence in adolescent oncology patients: Preliminary data on psychological risk factors and relationships to outcome. *J Clin Psychol Med Settings.* 2004;11(1):31–39.
5. Davies HA, Lilleyman JA. Compliance with oral chemotherapy in childhood lymphoblastic leukaemia. *Cancer Treat Rev.* 1995;21(2):93–103.
6. Pai ALH, Drotar D, Kodish E. Correspondence between objective and subjective reports of adherence among adolescents with acute lymphoblastic leukemia. *Children's Health Care.* 2008;37(3):225–235.

7. Koren G, Ferrazini G, Sulh H, et al. Systematic exposure to 6-mercaptopurine as a prognostic factor in acute lymphoblastic leukaemia in children. *N Engl J Med*. 1990;323:17–21.
8. Lilleyman JS, Lennard L. Mercaptopurine metabolism and risk of relapse in childhood lymphoblastic leukemia. *Lancet*. 1994;343(8907):1188–1190.
9. Relling MV, Hancock ML, Boyett JM, Pui C-H, Evans WE. Prognostic importance of 6-Mercaptopurine dose intensity in acute lymphoblastic leukemia. *Blood*. 1999;93:2817–2823.
10. Drotar D. *Psychological Interventions in Childhood Chronic Illnesses*. Washington, DC: American Psychological Association; 2006.
11. National Cancer Institute. COG-AALL0331: *Phase III Randomized Study of Different Combination Chemotherapy Regimens in Pediatric Patients With Newly Diagnosed Standard-Risk B-Precursor Acute Lymphoblastic Leukemia*. Washington, DC: NCI; 2008. http://www.cancer.gov/clinicaltrials/COG-AALL0331. Accessed Sep 12, 2008.

Chapter 18

Cognitive Sequelae of Cancer Treatment

Brian P. Daly and Ronald T. Brown

Childhood cancers are chronic conditions that impact development across a number of domains, including cognitive function. Pathophysiology and adverse effects resulting from standard treatment modalities impact higher-order cognitive skills and academic achievement, thereby compromising daily functioning including school and play activities, and overall quality of life.

- Cognitive problems resulting from the disease and/or treatment may affect multiple aspects of a child's functioning associated with various cognitive domains and are frequently encountered during the late-effects period (typically defined as one-year following the cessation of treatment).
- Children and adolescents surviving leukemia, lymphoma, and brain tumors are at greatest risk for these cognitive toxicities.
- Assessment of cognitive toxicities are best accomplished by a comprehensive neurocognitive assessment that targets both broad domains and specific functions conducted by psychologists trained in neuropsychological assessment of children with chronic illness as well as behavioral ratings scales completed by parents and teachers.
- Since cognitive late effects vary in time of when they may (or may not) appear, monitoring is important. Patients at high risk for neurocognitive effects should work with their physician, a hospital- or community-based psychologist, and an appropriate contact within the school setting (i.e., school psychologist) to make a plan regarding the frequency and type of monitoring necessary to detect concerns early. In general, it is recommended that youth surviving leukemia, lymphoma, and brain tumors receive annual screening for academic functioning, and more comprehensive cognitive assessments on a biennial basis.[1] Parents and school personnel are often the first to notice changes in the child's functioning, which then warrant further evaluation by a qualified psychologist that focuses on areas of concern.
- Therapies most commonly employed to treat cancer (e.g., chemotherapy, radiation) often result in adverse long-term CNS related toxicities, commonly referred to as *neurocognitive late effects*. Neurocognitive late

effects may manifest months or years after completion of cancer treatment and are generally believed to progress and persist for years.

Neurocognitive Dysfunction

- The prevalence rates of neurocognitive dysfunction in long-term survivors of acute lymphoblastic leukemia (ALL) or central nervous system (CNS) tumors range widely, from 20% to 80%, due to differences in patient samples and cognitive processes studied, assessment measures, and definitions of impairment.[2–4]
- A recent meta-analysis of neurocognitive sequelae in survivors of brain tumors found pervasive and substantial impairments across a range of broad and specific neurocognitive domains.[5]
  - Children treated for brain tumors exhibited deficits in overall cognitive functioning, academic achievement, attention, psychomotor and visual-spatial skills, verbal memory, and language.
  - These delays were consistent with performance approximately a full standard deviation below expected levels based on normative data.[5]
- Several meta-analyses that examined the neurocognitive sequelae of treatment for childhood acute lymphoblastic or ALL suggest similar declines in both global and specific areas of neurocognitive functioning.[6,7]
- There is a growing literature indicating that declining white matter in the brain is directly associated with decrements in intellectual functioning.[8,9]

Prevention Interventions

- Prevention and intervention efforts that target cognitive sequelae and have demonstrated promise include academic prevention approaches,[10] parent directed approaches,[11] clinic based cognitive remediation/rehabilitation programs,[12] computer-based cognitive training,[13] and psychopharmacological treatment.[14]
- Although each of these strategies has demonstrated improvement on select areas of neurocognitive functioning (e.g., attention, working memory), outcome data on broad domains or other specific functions have been less compelling.
- More research efforts are needed before endorsing these approaches as both safe and effective.

Neurocognitive Late Effects Resulting from Radiation or Chemotherapy Treatment[2–4]

- Declines in intellectual functioning.
- Deficits in memory, attention/concentration, executive function, and processing speed.
- Delays in academic achievement.

- Diminished school performance relative to their healthy peers.
- Impaired nonverbal intelligence and reasoning, arithmetic academic achievement, visual-motor integration, visual-perceptual ability, sequencing, verbal fluency, perceptual localization, and nondominant hand motor skills. (Tables 18.1–18.3).

Table 18.1 Cognitive Sequelae: Impairment by Cognitive Domain

Intellectual Functioning	Processing Speed
Nonverbal intelligence (Performance)	Information-processing speed (rate and efficiency)
Nonverbal reasoning	Memory
Verbal intelligence	Visual and verbal short term
Verbal fluency	Working memory
Academic Achievement	Visual-Spatial and Visual-Motor
Arithmetic (computational)	Visual-motor control
Reading (comprehension)	Visual construction and integration
Spelling	Perceptual localization
Executive function	Nondominant hand motor skills
Planning	Perceptual motor skills
Insight	Judgment of long duration
Initiative	Interval judgment
Organizational skills	Motor timing
Attention/Concentration	Fine motor control
Attention flexibility and control	
Focused or divided attention	
Sustained attention	
Selective attention	

Table 18.2 Cancers That Place Children at Greatest Risk of Developing Treatment-Related Neurocognitive Effects

	Leukemia and Lymphoma	Brain Tumors
Mechanisms for impairment	Chemotherapy or radiation administered intrathecally to prevent proliferation of cancer cells into the CNS	Presence of tumors in the central nervous system (CNS), and specifically the brain

Table 18.3 Treatments Associated with Neurocognitive Late Effects[15]

• Surgical intervention in the brain	• Chemotherapy
• Cranial radiation therapy (CRT)	• Methotrexate
• Bone marrow transplantation	• Cytarabine
	• Corticosteroids

Table 18.4 Greatest Risk Factors for Neurocognitive Late Effects and Academic Problems[2–4]

• Gender (Females are at greater risk) • Age (Children treated under the age of 5 are at greatest risk) • Tumor location (Brain tumors, particularly tumors located in the supratentorial region) • Neurological severity • Receiving CNS radiation • Magnitude of radiation dose (there is an established dose-response relationship with those getting higher-dose cranial radiation therapy experiencing more neurocognitive late effects)	• Time since treatment (Greater time since treatment is predictive of more permanent cognitive impairment. Cognitive late effects can occur anywhere from several months to years following the end of treatment; however, it is unlikely that cognitive late effects will initially appear after 4 years posttreatment). • Those who experience relapse • Numerous or prolonged school absences • A history of learning problems that is premorbid to the diagnosis of cancer • Cancer treatment that affects hearing or vision • Cancer treatment that results in physical challenges

Multiple important risk factors are associated with neurocognitive late effects and academic problems. A thorough assessment of risk and protective factors for the individual patient is important in determining follow-up care recommendations and referrals (Table 18.4).

Testing Batteries

Cognitive assessment, including neurocognitive or neuropsychological assessment, utilizes objective measures to detect impairment in one or more cognitive domains. Scores from the assessment regimen are evaluated in relation to established norms of the general population. Brief neurocognitive evaluations frequently include global measures of intellectual functioning (e.g., WISC-IV) and measures of academic achievement. These evaluations usually last between two to four hours and result in a short report (1–5 pages). More comprehensive neuropsychological batteries also include: global measures of intellectual functioning and measures of academic achievement, with a particular focus on writing, math calculation, and reading comprehension skills. In addition, these evaluations frequently assess neurocognitive measures of processing speed; attention and concentration; executive functions and memory; motor/visual-motor skills; visual-perceptual skills and language; and parent, teacher, and self-report measures of adaptive, socio-emotional, and behavioral functioning.[5] These comprehensive batteries last anywhere from 4 to 12 hours, and may be scheduled over multiple days. Detailed reports from these evaluations can range from 5 to 25 pages. Regardless of whether the battery is short or long, tests should be selected based on the specific questions raised for the child referred for evaluation.

Table 18.5 details a novel assessment battery employed primarily for research purpose by the Children's Oncology Group (COG), a consortium

Table 18.5 Children's Oncology Group Standardized Neuropsychological and Behavioral Battery[16]

Test	Child's Age (Years: Months)					
	<2:0	2:0 ↓ 4:11	5:0 ↓ 5:11	6:0 ↓ 16:11	17:0 ↓ 17:11	≥18:0[b]
Children						
Intelligence						
WPPSI-III (Vocabulary, Block Design) *(15 min)*		X[a] (2:6 to 5:11)				
WISC-IV (Vocabulary, Block Design) *(15 min)*				X		
WAIS-IV (Vocabulary, Block Design) *(15 min)*					X	X
Processing Speed/Attention						
WPPSI-III (Symbol Search, Coding) *(10 min)*		X (4:0 to <6:0)				
WISC-IV (Symbol Search, Coding) *(10 min)*				X		
WAIS-IV(Symbol Search, Coding) *(10 min)*					X	X
Memory						
CMS (Story Memory, Faces, Dot Location) *(15 min)*			X	X		
CVLT-C *(15 min)*			X	X		
WISC-IV (Digit Span) *(5 min)*				X		
WAIS-IV (Digit Span) *(5 min)*					X	X
WMS-III (Logical Memory, Faces, Spatial Span) *(15 min)*					X	X
CVLT-II *(15 min)*					X	X
Parents						
COG Language Preference Questionnaire		X	X	X	X	
Attention and Behavior/Social/Emotional Function						
BASC-2 *(20 min)*		X	X	X	X	X[b]
Executive Function						
BRIEF-P *(5 min)*		X	X			
BRIEF*(5 min)*				X	X	
BRIEF-A *(5 min)*						X[b]
Adaptive Function						
ABAS-II *(15 min)*	X	X	X	X	X	X[b]
Quality of Life						
PedsQL 4.0 (Generic Version, NOT Cancer Module)		X	X	X	X	X[b]

(continued)

Table 18.5 (Continued)	
Index of Test Abbreviations	
WPPSI-III	Wechsler Preschool and Primary Scale of Intelligence—3rd Edition
WISC-IV	Wechsler Intelligence Scales for Children—4th Edition
WAIS-IV	Wechsler Adult Intelligence Scales—4th Edition
CMS	Children's Memory Scale
CVLT-C	California Verbal Learning Test—Children's Version
CVLT-II	California Verbal Learning Test—2nd Edition
WMS-III	Wechsler Memory Scale—3rd Edition
BASC-2	Behavior Assessment System for Children—2nd Edition
BRIEF-P	Behavior Rating Inventory of Executive Function—Preschool Version
BRIEF	Behavior Rating Inventory of Executive Function Scales
ABAS-II	Adaptive Behavior Assessment System—2nd Edition
PedsQL 4.0	Pediatric Quality of Life Inventory Version 4.0 (Generic Version, NOT Cancer Module)

[a] For patients < 4:0: administer Receptive Vocabulary, for patients ≥ 4:0: administer Vocabulary.

[b] Patients ≥ 18 years of age will complete a self-report form. No parent report will be used for patients 18 and older.

of cancer centers across North America, Australia, New Zealand, and Europe sponsored by the National Cancer Institute.[16] This standardized, brief battery evaluates cognitive, social, emotional, and behavioral functioning and was designed to collect psychometrically sound neurocognitive data across many premiere pediatric cancer institutions.[16]

Suggested guidelines for the role of general pediatricians in assisting survivors of childhood cancer who are evidencing possible neurocognitive problems include the following: (a) awareness of the potential for neurocognitive late effects; (b) identifying and then referring the family to qualified professionals in the community who can conduct neurocognitive or neuropsychological evaluations; (c) educating and providing the family with information about patients' rights; and, (d) providing relevant summaries of the child's medical and cancer history that can be used as supporting documentation for school placement and accommodations see Table 18.6.[17]

Prevention and Intervention

Although researchers have made significant strides in identifying the mechanisms of disease and its treatment, and cognitive toxicities that give rise to neurocognitive late effects, empirically supported interventions that remediate these learning impairments have yet to be firmly established. Several promising techniques are listed in Tables 18.7 and 18.8.

Table 18.6 Proposed Guidelines for the Assisting Survivors of Childhood Cancers [1,15,18, *]

1.0 Awareness of the potential for neurocognitive late effects	Evaluate disease and treatment factors.
1.1 Young age as a pervasive risk factor	Young age at time of treatment is one of the greatest risk factors for cognitive late effects.
1.2 Gender	Females also are especially at risk for cognitive late effects.
1.3 Chemotherapy	Assess for acute and subacute adverse side effects of chemotherapy treatments: Methotrexate (MTX), Cisplatinum, Vincristine.
1.4 Cranial radiation therapy (CRT)	Evaluate potential adverse impact of magnitude of total dose, fraction per dose, volume of brain treated and time elapsed since completion of treatment.
2.5 Neurosurgical procedures (brain tumors)	Assess for neurological deficits following neurosurgical procedure. Evaluate potential impact of tumor location, volume, invasiveness, acute and chronic central nervous system complications, shunts.
2.0 Identify and refer family to qualified professionals in the community	Refer patient to a psychologist for a neurocognitive or comprehensive neuropsychological evaluation.
2.1 Neurocognitive domains	Identify concerns in the following areas: intellect and achievement; social adjustment; dexterity and visual motor skills; attention and processing speed; learning and memory; visual perceptual skills.
2.2 Serial	Academic functioning should be screened annually.
2.3 Comprehensive	Comprehensive cognitive assessments may be conducted biennially.
3.0 Educate and provide the family with information about patients' rights	Children with mental or physical disabilities are entitled to school and community services and accommodations.
3.1 Educate	Educate families about local, state, and federal laws that protect the rights of children with disabilities: Individuals with Disabilities Education Act (IDEA); Section 504 of the American with Disabilities Act (ADA); Individualized Education Program (IEP).
3.2 Consultation	Pediatric neuropsychologists can provide the family with more detailed information about the potential impact of cognitive late effects.

(continued)

Table 18.6 (Continued)

3.3 Resources	Refer family to additional information from sources such as the Children's Oncology Group, the National Childhood Cancer Foundation collaborative, and the National Cancer Institute.
4.0 Provide summaries of the child's medical and cancer history	This information can be used as supporting documentation for school placement and accommodations.
1.1 Prenatal	Summarize any prenatal complications.
1.2 Developmental	Summarize any developmental delays or concerns.
1.3 Medical History	Summarize type of cancer and any medical complications (e.g., deficits in vision or hearing; deficits in attention or concentration; occurrence of chronic fatigue, seizures, headaches).
1.4 Treatment History	Summarize history of treatment for cancer and medical complications.
1.5 Current Treatment	Indicate which medications are currently being prescribed, if any.
1.6 Previous interventions	Summarize any previous school or community interventions.

* See Chapter 28, School and Academic Planning.

Table 18.7 Cognitive Sequelae Prevention and Intervention Strategies

1. Education of family, child, and school
2. Specific-skills training Training in specific skills such as study skills, organization skills and social skills
3. Compensatory strategies Teaches children how to compensate for deficits in a specific function. Strategies include classroom accommodations and assistive technology for functional deficits that are not likely to be remediated by traditional rehabilitative approaches.
4. Psychopharmacological interventions There is some preliminary support for the efficacy and safety of stimulant medication for survivors of acute lymphoblastic leukemia and brain tumors. Findings from these research studies suggest the efficacy of the stimulants on parent and teacher ratings of attention and putative tasks of attention and executive functioning such as reaction time and learning.
5. Cognitive Remediation The goal of cognitive remediation strategies is to restore neuropsychological functioning following an injury to the brain by assisting the survivor in relearning or strengthening the skill or behavior affected.

(continued)

Table 18.7 (Continued)

6. Cognitive Remediation Program (CRP)[12,18,19]
- Employs a skills acquisition model that focuses on improving cognitive abilities in areas of focusing attention, memory recall, learning, school behavior, and self-esteem, via extensive practice.
- Involves brain exercises, learning strategies, and cognitive-behavioral therapy with the goal of teaching the child new learning strategies that will generalize to real world settings such as the classroom and home environment.
- Frequently utilizes a trained individual therapist who works with the child for 20 two-hour sessions of attention training.

7. Computer-based Cognitive Training
- Provides computerized cognitive exercises designed to restore impaired neurocognitive functioning.
- Targets specific skills such as attention, working memory, processing speed, cognitive flexibility, and/or executive function.
- Frequently consists of a series of tasks that increase in complexity.
- Can provide immediate feedback about performance and progress.
- Designed to be entertaining and engaging.
- Can be completed at home, office, or school setting under minimal supervision.

Table 18.8 Examples of Approaches Used in Cognitive Remediation Programs (CRP) for pediatric cancer survivors[18,19]

Strategies from brain injury rehabilitation
- When capable, child is required to focus for 15 minutes on a learning task.
- Following the learning task, the child then engages in interesting activities such as computer administered Solitare software, card games and memory matching games.

Comprehensive cognitive remediation treatment strategies from special education and educational psychology:
- Metacognitive strategies are employed that address task preparedness, task approach, on-task behavior and generalization strategies.
- Examples of task preparedness activities include:
  - Magic/special words—three words serve as cues to motivate children to perform their best.
  - Soup breath—a brief relaxation exercise.
  - Game face—help the child visualize themselves working hard.
- Examples of on-task activities include:
  - Talk to myself—encourages the use of self-encouraging and self-alerting internal dialogues.
  - Mark my place—helps child find his/her place on a complex visual task.
  - Start at the top, 1 row at a time—instructs child to begin at top left corner and proceed one row at a time when completing visual-spatial tasks or activities.
- Examples of posttask activities include:
  - Check your work—instructs the child on ways to check for errors to make sure work is correct.
  - Ask for feedback—encourages the child to ask for performance feedback.
  - Reward yourself—rewards for effort.

(continued)

Table 18.8 (Continued)
General Approaches from Clinical Psychology: • Are based on cognitive behavioral therapy. • Improve resistance to distraction. • Help children learn to coach themselves through challenging activities. • Practice an appropriate internal dialogue in an overt and covert manner.

Psychopharmacologic Interventions

Stimulants

- Targets difficulties with attention, concentration, executive function, and working memory, similar to those of children with attention deficit hyperactivity disorder (ADHD).
- Treatment with methylphenidate demonstrated short-term and 1-year improvement on computerized measures of sustained attention; parent, teacher and self-report ratings of attention; and, parent ratings of social skills or behavioral problems. Stimulant drug treatment did not demonstrate an impact on academic measures.[14]
- Children who receive the most intensive radiation therapy (24 Gy) and the most intensive doses of chemotherapy (i.e., methotrexate) may demonstrate a poorer response to stimulant medication relative to children who received less intensive radiation therapy and chemotherapy.
- Adverse effects associated with the stimulants are equivalent to those experienced by their healthy peers with ADHD (e.g., irritability, anxiety, sleep and appetite disturbances, and behavioral rebound). However, a greater frequency of adverse side-effects occur with higher doses of stimulants as compared to lower doses of medication.[20] Female gender and lower IQ also are associated with greater frequency of adverse effects.[20]

Summary

The significant strides made in cancer treatment have resulted in cognitive late effects associated with this treatment. As a result, over the past decade, there has been a great deal of research designed to assess and manage these cognitive late effects. The end result has been the promulgation of assessment standards and the development of interventions designed to manage these late effects including cognitive remediation approaches and the use of psychopharmacological approaches. We anticipate that this will enhance the quality of life of these children as they grow into adulthood.

References

1. Daly BP, Kral MK, Brown RT. Cognitive and academic problems associated with childhood cancers and sickle cell disease. *School Psychology Quarterly.* 2008;23(2):230–242.
2. Ellenberg L, Liu Q, Gioia G, et al. Neurocognitive status in long-term survivors of childhood CNS malignancies: a report from the Childhood Cancer Survivor Study. *Neuropsychol.* 2009;23(6):705–717.
3. Mulhern RK, Palmer SL. Neurocognitive late effects in pediatric cancer. *Curr Probl Cancer.* 2003;27(4):177–197.
4. Maddrey AM, Bergeron JA, Lombardo ER, et al. Neuropsychological performance and quality of life of 10 year survivors of childhood medulloblastoma. *J Neurooncol.* 2005;72(3):245–253.
5. Robinson KE, Kuttesch J, Champion J, et al. A quantitative meta-analysis of neurocognitive sequelae of pediatric brain tumors. *Pediatr Blood Cancer.* 2010;55(3):525–531.
6. Campbell LK, Scaduto M, Sharp W, et al. A meta-analysis of the neurocognitive sequelae of treatment for childhood acute lymphocytic leukemia. *Pediatr Blood Cancer.* 2007;49(1):65–73.
7. Peterson CC, Johnson CE, Ramirez LY, et al. A meta-analysis of the neuropsychological sequelae of chemotherapy-only treatment for pediatric acute lymphoblastic leukemia. *Pediatr Blood Cancer.* 2008;51(1):99–104.
8. Reddick WE, Glass JO, Palmer SL, et al. (2005). Atypical white matter volume development in children following craniospinal irradiation. *Neuro Oncol.* 2005: 7(1);12–19.
9. Mulhern RK, White HA, Glass JO, et al. Attentional functioning and white matter integrity among survivors of malignant brain tumors of childhood. *J Int Neuropsychol Soc.* 2004;10(2):180–189.
10. Moore IM, Hockenberry MJ, Anhalt C, et al. Mathematics intervention for prevention of neurocognitive deficits in childhood leukemia. *Pediatr Blood Cancer.* 2012;59(2):278–284.
11. Patel SK. Parent-directed Intervention for Childhood Cancer Survivors with Neurobehavioral dysfunction. Paper presentation at the Biennial NCI/ACS/CDC Cancer Survivorship Research Conference Washington, DC. June 2010.
12. Butler RW, Copeland DR, Fairclough DL, et al. A multicenter, randomized clinical trial of a cognitive remediation program for childhood survivors of a pediatric malignancy. *J Consult Clin Psychol.* 2008;76:367–378.
13. Hardy KK, Willard VW, Bonner MJ. Computerized cognitive training in survivors of childhood cancer: A pilot study. *J Pediatr Oncol Nurs.* 2011;28(1):27–33.
14. Conklin HM, Reddick WE, Ashford J, et al. Long-term efficacy of methylphenidate in enhancing attention regulation, social skills, and academic abilities of childhood cancer survivors. *J Clin Oncol.* 2010;28(29):4465–4472.
15. Landier W. *Educational Issues Following Treatment for Childhood Cancer.* Health Link (Educational Issues, Version 2.0). Arcadia, CA: Children's Oncology Group (COG) 2006. http://www.survivorshipguidelines.org/pdf/EducationalIssues.pdf. Accessed Aug 8, 2013.

16. Embry L, Annett RD, Kunin-Batson A, et al. Implementation of mulit-site neurocognitive assessments within a pediatric cooperative group: Can it be done? *Pediatr Blood Cancer.* 2012;59(3):536–539.

17. Nathan, PC, Patel SN, Diley K, et al. Guidelines for identification of, advocacy for, and intervention in neurocognitive problems in survivors of childhood cancer: A report from the Children's Oncology Group. *Arch Pediatr Adolesc Med.* 2007;161(8); 798–806.

18. Butler RW, Sahler OJZ, Askins MA, et al. Interventions to improve neuropsychological functioning in childhood cancer survivors. *Dev Disabil Res Rev.* 2008;14:251–258.

19. Spencer JS. The role of cognitive remediation in childhood cancer survivors experiencing neurocognitive late effects. *J Pediatr Oncol Nurs.* 2006;23(6): 321–325.

20. Conklin HM, Lawford J, Jasper BW, et al. Side effects of methylphenidate in childhood cancer survivors: A randomized placebo-controlled trial. *Pediatrics*. 2009;124(1);226–233.

Chapter 19

Psychotherapeutic Interventions

Barbara Sourkes, Anne E. Kazak, and Lori Wiener

Referral for Psychological Treatment

The question often arises of when a child with cancer or the child's siblings or family might benefit from a more specific or intensive psychological treatment. There are many potential options for treatment, including individual therapy or cognitive behavioral therapy (CBT) for the child, family therapy for members of the family (with or without the child), support groups, or a combination of approaches. Other therapeutic approaches include online interventions, camps, and recreational activities. Although not all families want or need such services, they may add crucial dimensions to comprehensive care.

Reasons for Referral

- Symptoms of depression, anxiety, trauma (see Chapter 12, Anxiety and Depression).
- General poor coping with the illness and treatment (as perceived by the child, parents, and/or team). These may include persistent difficulties with procedures and side effects of treatment (e.g., hair loss).
- Nonadherence to treatment.
- Preexistent stressors or vulnerabilities that are exacerbated by the illness (e.g., psychiatric history in child or family member; recent geographical move, loss of employment, divorce, death of family member).
- Parental distress (symptoms of depression, anxiety, trauma that are persistent or appear to be interfering with daily functioning) or evidence of other concerns (e.g., substance use).
- Marital/relationship distress.
- Other family concerns/problems that cannot be addressed in the medical setting.
- As a preventive measure by families who want additional support.

Role of the Mental Health Professional, Confidentiality, and Making a Referral

In general, most children and families ultimately cope quite well with the extraordinary stressors associated with their illnesses and treatments. However, some difficulties are to be expected. Seeking help to promote well-being and addressing problems early is important.

- Children, adolescents, and family members are often closely attuned as to whether healthcare providers think that they are coping well.
- Children and families respond best to psychological help when the rationale is presented as routine and recommended directly by the key members of the healthcare team.
- It is important to talk directly to the child and family about psychological concerns and the potential benefit of individual or family therapy. Statements to the effect of this being "normal," "understandable" and "helpful to many other families I've treated" are useful in normalizing the referral.
- There are many types of mental health specialists (e.g., social workers, psychologists, psychiatrists, counselors, therapists). People are often not aware of potential differences and families may benefit from assistance in ascertaining who may be most helpful to them. Referral should be to licensed/credentialed professionals who are *experienced* in the psychological care of children with serious medical conditions.
- If the child or family has a current or past therapy relationship with a provider in their community, discussion as to whether that person could be helpful is indicated. Communication between the community therapist and a hospital mental health professional may be beneficial to ensure consistency and coordination of care.
- The patient/family may not respond affirmatively to the idea of therapy when initially presented. It is helpful to acknowledge their reservations and consider re-opening the conversation at another time if the reasons for referral persist.

The following points apply whether the child/family is referred for counseling with a therapist within the oncology team, or to a mental health professional in the medical center or in the community:

For Young Children

- Use simple nonthreatening terms (e.g., "the talking doctor"). Provide a functional description that distinguishes the mental health professional from the rest of the medical team (e.g., no physical examination).
- Explain that all children who are ill have worries and that these feelings are an understandable response to what they are going through.

- Introduce the concept of confidentiality in developmentally appropriate terms (e.g., "private conversations") while explaining how some information may be shared with the parents and the team.

For Adolescents

Adolescents may express concerns about the stigma of seeing a mental health professional, as well as resistance to admitting the need for assistance. Psychological treatment may be viewed as further confirmation of their vulnerability and dependence at a time when they already feel physically and emotionally exposed by the illness.

- Explain psychotherapy as an empowering process in their desire for more autonomy and control (e.g., "a private time and space apart for you to discuss personal issues").
- The boundaries of confidentiality must be delineated with exquisite clarity regarding what—if anything—will be communicated to the parents or the medical team.

Logistics

Psychological interventions vary in terms of the length of sessions and the number of sessions provided. Patients and families should expect that a therapist could give them an *estimate* of the length of treatment, although this often changes once treatment begins. Delivering psychosocial health care in a medical setting, or treating children and their families in active treatment, requires flexibility from all involved. Traditional expectations for consistency in of time and place (e.g., weekly one-hour meetings in the same setting) must be replaced with flexibility in terms of scheduling around medical appointments, using space in oncology clinics, seeing patients in their hospital rooms, etc. Relative to many medical procedures, therapy sessions take more time, particularly during phases of assessment and early treatment when it may be important to devote an hour or so to a session.

Factors that May Affect the Framework of Psychotherapeutic Intervention are:

- The child's current clinical status (both medical and psychological).
- During hospitalizations, sessions may be scheduled frequently as an integrated part of the child's care plan, although their duration may vary greatly. A common drawback is the limited opportunity for privacy in the hospital setting.
- When the child is an outpatient, coordinating psychotherapy appointments with scheduled clinic visits (whenever possible) consolidates medical and psychological care. This also supports families already burdened by rigorous appointment schedules (and/or geographical

distance) who are attempting to maintain some semblance of normalcy in their daily life.

- Therapists can utilize telephone contact with the children and parents to bridge time between sessions.

Types of Interventions

A number of interventions can facilitate the emotional growth and monitoring of social functioning in a child who has endured the psychosocial challenges, disruptions, and isolation that can be incurred by cancer and its treatment. Patient and family interventions that can assist during and following treatment are described below.

Individual Therapy (Child/Adolescent)

- Most children with cancer enter psychotherapy because of the stress engendered by their illness, rather than more general concerns.
- Individual child psychotherapy facilitates psychological adjustment by providing the children a protected framework for emotional expression, and, at a profound level, the opportunity to explore all facets of the illness experience.
- Through words, play, and drawings, children convey the experience of living with stress and uncertainty.
- Psychotherapy may be the sole intervention or it may be combined with psychotropic medication and cognitive or behavioral symptom-management techniques.
- CBT is a type of therapy that focuses on modifying thoughts (cognitions), assumptions, beliefs, and behaviors, in order to change behavior.
- CBT treatments are often fairly short in duration and their use in pediatric populations for a broad range of psychological difficulties is well established.[1]

Involving Parents

- Most therapists who work with children involve parents in their work.
- An ongoing alliance from the outset between the child's psychotherapist and the parents optimizes the outcome of the work.
- The range and depth of the psychotherapeutic intervention with parents can vary greatly, from a concentrated focus on child-management issues, to the impact of the child's illness on their marriage and the family.
- A crucial aspect of the work with parents is discussion of the well siblings. Both parents and professionals often underestimate the concerns and vulnerabilities of these children unless they present with symptomatic behavior.

Adolescents

- Adolescents often use psychotherapy to discuss quandaries around identity and planning for the future.
- Previous educational and career goals may now be subject to question.
- Vulnerability around present and future intimate relationships, including concerns about sexuality and fertility, often emerge.
- Adolescents who are striving for autonomy and control in their lives must contend with the enforced dependence imposed by the illness.

Themes in Psychosocial Treatment

The Illness and Its Treatment

Core issues include:

- The child's comprehension of the diagnosis and its implications.
- Adaptation to physical changes (both temporary and permanent); body image.
- Coping with painful treatments, procedures, clinic visits, and hospitalizations.
- Facing subsequent milestones in the illness of either a positive nature (e.g., completion of treatment) or a negative nature (e.g., recurrence).

Impact of the Illness on the Normal Life of Family, School, and Peers[2]

- Children's longing to return to their "normal" life, or their "life from before" is counterbalanced by their growing realization that the profoundly "abnormal" presence of cancer cannot be erased nor its impact reversed.
- Within the intertwined spheres of family, school, and peers, children must create and pursue new pathways that include and are not limited by the illness. These processes of re-entry and re-integration pose extraordinary challenges in combination with all the usual developmental tasks of childhood and adolescence.

Awareness of the Life-threatening Nature of the Illness and Implications for the Future

Children's awareness is a fluid process, not a static state and depends on several factors including:

- Current medical status and knowledge about the illness.
- Their "wisdom of the body."
- The urgency and intensity of treatment.
- The emotions of family and caregivers.
- Family communication style.
- Encounters with other children who are ill.

Expressions of anticipatory grief range from the implicit to explicit; the most powerful disclosures are children's references to the possibility or actuality of their own dying. In this context, even young children may discuss concerns around quality of life. Psychotherapy can give children an opportunity for the expression of profound grief and for the integration of all that they have lived in their abbreviated lifespan.[2]

Counseling and Support for Parents

The distress experienced by parents is well established. Parents often express more overt distress than their child and, in addition to professional psychological intervention, may benefit from support groups and from the informal support provided by healthcare providers.

- Problem-solving therapy has been shown to be effective for mothers of children with cancer during treatment, as it provides a structured way for parents to think about their cancer-related concerns and begin to formulate steps to address their worries.[3]
- It is unquestionable that a diagnosis of cancer in a child will have an impact on the relationship of the couple (the child's parents). How parents cope with stress can strengthen or weaken their relationship and may exacerbate existing vulnerabilities or difficulties in the couple relationship.
- In an ongoing study,[4] parents reported that it is optimal to begin counseling to address relationship issues at the time of the child's diagnosis with continuity through the treatment phase.
- Important areas to address in couples therapy include: strengthening the couple's mutual problem-solving skills; building effective communication, and coping "as a unit' under stress.

Family Interventions

Families may benefit from referrals for family therapy. A family approach is particularly helpful to encourage conversation about the impact of cancer and its treatment on the family and to maintain developmental "normality" in the face of the illness. It also provides a forum in which the healthy siblings can find expression. In the case of underlying concerns such as behavioral issues or emotional difficulties, a family therapy approach is also helpful in facilitating a common family solution to problems. As with individual therapy, the way in which the idea is presented and a referral is made to an appropriate provider is essential. Parents often agree that getting help for the whole family is important. They tend to respond well to the idea that helping the entire family can enhance the care of the child. This explanation often overrides their insistence on an exclusive focus on the ill child, as well as objections based on the availability and time constraints of other family members.

Camps

Many pediatric oncology centers make referrals to or have access to established specialized summer camps. These camps combine the fun of summer camp with access to specialized medical care. Some camps also offer therapeutic and educational programs for siblings, young adults, and family activities throughout the year.

Camp for the Child/Adolescent

- Provides an opportunity for children who have or have had cancer to interact with their peers in an informal, recreational environment.
- Tends to appeal to children who are confident, active, and able to separate from parents, and to parents who encourage independence and new experiences.
- Children with chronic or life-threatening illnesses have been found to leave camp programs more independent and knowledgeable about their self-care.[5] Many campers choose to return as counselors.

Sibling Camps

- Healthy siblings who attended specialized sibling camp programs have demonstrated decreased anxiety, lower stress, improved social competence, and greater knowledge about cancer and cancer treatments that were sustained at camp follow-up, demonstrating its effectiveness as an intervention strategy in supporting sibling adjustment.[6]
- Siblings whose parents reported behavioral problems with the onset of the cancer diagnosis seem to benefit from this type of program. No substantial negative effects were found regardless of the camper age, adaptational status or previous camp experience.[7]

Integrated Therapeutic Approaches

One size does not fit all in terms of providing psychosocial treatments for children and families. Sometimes the family does not agree to treatment, even when the concerns and options have been carefully presented. Additional complications in making referrals may result if psychological treatment has negative connotations culturally (e.g., mistrust of disclosure to "strangers").

When families have difficult or conflicting relationships with the healthcare team, a successful referral is unlikely. Approaches to facilitate the family's involvement with key staff members are particularly important when there is conflict with the team (e.g., parents who express distress through anger, threaten lawsuits, or constantly quiz individual team members). Interventions may include structured plans and regular updates and meetings to address the family's concerns.[8] (See Chapter 25, Special Considerations in Working with Families.)

- Support comes in many forms, from an openness to listen and answer questions, to regular visits at expected times, to creative art and play activities that allow the child expression of feelings and concerns.
- There are many instances when a child or family may not necessarily need intensive psychological treatment. The challenge, under these circumstances, is to provide thoughtful emotional support for the child and family in a carefully planned manner with existing resources.
- On some occasions, as the treatment team comes to know the child and family better, it becomes apparent that the original "presenting problem" (e.g., a sad patient) reflects parental conflict or other family strains.
- The initial attempts to engage the family in treatment may not have been targeting them optimally. Creative approaches to joining with the family around their concerns and supporting their problem solving abilities throughout the disease trajectory is important.
- Concerns about payment for psychological services are realistic for many families. Charges for services are likely to vary across treatment settings and providers and can be a barrier to families considering, initiating, and receiving psychosocial services. Oncologists can play an important role by writing a letter of medical necessity, if needed.
- Families may find it easier to make decisions about seeking treatment if provided with information about what services are covered by insurance or offered at no cost, what costs may be incurred by outside providers, and what financial options are available at their treatment center, including grants, "prompt pay," discounts, and costs adjusted on a sliding scale.

Additional approaches include:

- Educate the parents about normal and expectable reactions, as well as "red flags" in the functioning of children, including healthy siblings. Keep the dialogue open and ongoing. Provide the parents with written and appropriate online resources for themselves and for the children.
- Take into account the child's level of comfort in relationships with members of the team, or closeness with one particular individual. That person may be "designated" as a resource for the child, with efforts to ensure consistency of contact between them. This designated individual can consult with the mental health professional on the team for guidance and approaches.
- Child life specialists are particularly skilled in facilitating children's expression of emotion through play and creative arts.
- Involve school personnel. With education about the illness experience, and collaboration with the team, school counselors and teachers can play a vital role for the child.
- Explore resources in the community such as support groups and summer camps for children with cancer.

Considerations for the Cancer Care Team

On a cautionary note, there are risks when untrained or inadequately skilled personnel attempt to undertake a psychotherapeutic role beyond their training. These include:

- Misinterpretation of disclosures or opening up too much emotion, leading to increased distress in the child.
- Promises of confidentiality that may be impossible to maintain, resulting in the child feeling betrayed.
- Overinvolvement with the child on the part of a staff member beyond therapeutically optimal boundaries. Parents may feel that they are "competing" for their child, when they are already threatened by the possibility of loss through death. Vigilance on the part of the entire team is essential in these instances.
- Although exceptionally rewarding, clinical work with seriously ill children and their families can be intense and enormously challenging. The cumulative effects of multiple losses can lead to increased sadness, anxiety, depression, and burnout. Secondary traumatic stress is common across helping professionals of all disciplines who are exposed repeatedly to the traumatic experiences of others.
- Unresolved losses, overinvolvement, or a blurring of boundaries can impact the provider relationship.
- The use of online social networking forums has become a primary way to communicate and stay connected with others. Yet communicating with patients or their family members on social media sites can cross professional-patient boundaries, risking patient confidentiality, exposing patients to inappropriate details of providers' personal lives, and jeopardizing therapeutic relationships. (See Chapter 32, Social Media and Healthcare.)[9]
- In addition to standard recommendations for self-care (e.g., fostering personal fulfillment outside of work, building and using supportive relationships, recognizing and addressing symptoms of burnout), there are interventions that may reduce work-related distress among practitioners. Staff support sessions and moderated meetings that provide for discussion of the emotional aspects of one's work can be helpful for both highly experienced staff and trainees alike.

References

1. Spirito A, Kazak A. *Effective and Emerging Treatments in Pediatric Psychology.* New York, NY: Oxford University Press; 2006.
2. Sourkes B. *Armfuls of Time: The Psychological Experience of the Child with a Life-threatening Illness.* Pittsburgh, PA: University of Pittsburgh Press; 1995.
3. Sahler OJZ, Fairclough DL, Phipps S, et al. Using problem-solving skills training to reduce negative affectivity in mothers of children with newly diagnosed cancer: report of a multisite randomized trial. *J Consult Clin Psychol.* 2005;73(2):272–283.

4. Wiener L, Vasserman-Stokes E, Battles, H, Loucas, C, Muriel, A. How helpful is dyadic coping to parents' relationship during the pediatric cancer experience? International Psycho-oncology Society 15th World Congress, *Psycho-Oncology*. 2013;22(Suppl. 3).

5. Klee KM. Benefits of a mainstreamed summer camp experience for teens with ESRD. *Adv Perit Dial*. 1992;8:423–425.

6. Sidhu R, Passmore A, Baker D. The effectiveness of a peer support camp for siblings of children with cancer. *Pediatr Blood Cancer*. 2006;47(5):580–588.

7. Sahler OJ, Carpenter PJ. Evaluation of a camp program for siblings of children with cancer. *Am J Dis Child*. 1989;143(6):690–696.

8. Rourke J. Social accountability in theory and practice. *Ann Fam Med*. 2006;4(Suppl 1):S45–48.

9. Wiener L, Crum C, Grady C, Merchant M. To friend or not to friend: The use of social media in clinical oncology. *J Oncol Practice*. 2012;8:103–106.

References—General

Brown M, Sourkes B. Psychotherapy in pediatric palliative care. *Child Adolesc Psychiatr Clin North Am*. 2006;15(3):585–596, viii.

Kazak A, Alderfer M, Streisand R, et al. (2004). Treatment of posttraumatic stress symptoms in adolescent survivors of childhood cancer and their families: a randomized clinical trial. *J Fam Psychol*. 2004;18(3):493–504.

Kazak A, Simms S, Alderfer M, et al. (2005). Feasibility and preliminary outcomes from a pilot study of a brief psychological intervention for families of children newly diagnosed with cancer. *J Pediatr Psychol*. 2005;30(8):644–655.

Murray JS. Self-concept of siblings of children with cancer. *Issues Compr Pediatr Nurs*. 2001;24(2):85–94.

Packman W, Greenhalgh J, Chesterman B, et al. (2005). Siblings of pediatric cancer patients: the quantitative and qualitative nature of quality of life. *J Psychosoc Oncol*. 2005;23(1):87–108.

Shaw R, DeMaso D. *Clinical Manual of Pediatric Psychosomatic Medicine: Mental Health Consultation with Physically Ill Children and Adolescents*. Washington DC: American Psychiatric Association; 2006.

Sourkes B. *The Deepening Shade: Psychological Aspect of Life-threatening Illness*. Pittsburgh, PA: University of Pittsburgh Press; 1982.

Sourkes B. Psychotherapy. In: Holland J, ed. *Psycho-oncology: Part XII. The child with cancer*. New York, NY: Oxford University Press; 1998:946–953.

Sourkes BM. Psychological impact of life-limiting condition on the child. In: Goldman A, Haines R, Liben S, eds. *Oxford Textbook of Pediatric Palliative Care*. London: Oxford University Press; 2006:95–107.

Wiener LS, Hersh SP, Kazak AE. Psychiatric and psychosocial support for the child and family. In: Pizzo PA, Poplack DG, eds. *Principles and Practices of Pediatric Oncology*. 5th ed. Philadelphia, PA: Lippincott Williams & Wilkins; 2005:1414–1445.

Chapter 20

Electronic Interventions

Kristina K. Hardy and Martha A. Grootenhuis

Use of Electronic Resources to Support Children and Families

As an increasing number of families of children with cancer use communication technologies, there has been interest in developing intervention tools that can be delivered or supported using the Internet, computers, tablets, cell and smartphones, and other electronic devices. There has similarly been growth in interventions delivered via telephone or via video (e.g., Skype, FaceTime). Over three-quarters of individuals aged 15 and older in the United States have access to smartphones or the Internet, and 84% of those 3 and older have access to a computer at home.[1] This rapid growth in access to the Internet has contributed to significant changes in the provider-patient relationship, as families no longer must rely on clinicians as a primary means of information about their diagnosis, treatment, and support.[2] Of concern to providers, however, many patients and families will have difficulty discerning the quality, objectivity, or accuracy of web-based information. As such, it is recommended that the oncological team discuss the use of electronic resources with families early in the treatment process. To better inform these efforts, the following chapter provides an overview of electronic resources targeted on supporting mental health.

E-mental health (EMH) is the use of information and communication technologies to improve psychological education and care and has many different applications. We present general types of electronic resources that may be appropriate for use with a variety of individuals to promote increased mental health-related knowledge and coping or psychosocial functioning. We included categories of EMH interventions that have been defined by Barak and colleagues[3] in order to be clear about the range and scope of possible tools (see Table 20.1). This chapter also describes examples of childhood-cancer-specific interventions, some of which are not yet available to providers in the United States, and a technology-based approach that will likely become more widely available in the short term. Despite the rapid pace of development in the field, electronic mental health interventions are in their infancy in terms of feasibility and efficacy, particularly in the pediatric oncology population.

Table 20.1 Types of Electronic Products

Resource type	Description	Feedback/Support
Web-based education Interventions	Provide lay descriptions of cancer-related psychosocial outcomes and treatment options, in order to improve patients' understanding and awareness.	Ranges from no feedback to some automated or human feedback.
Online health screening tools	Short, self-directed questionnaires designed to screen for specific mental health difficulties or coping styles and skills.	Feedback is typically automated, but customized to individual responses.
Self-guided Web-based therapeutic interventions	The user-directed program is designed to treat or prevent psychological difficulties with structured information focusing on making behavioral or cognitive changes.	Users may receive automated feedback or reminders that are usually individually tailored.
Human-supported Web-based therapeutic interventions	Content is designed to treat or prevent psychological difficulties with structured information focusing on making behavioral or cognitive changes.	Support and feedback is provided via bulletin-board postings, chat-room moderation, and/or e-mailed, phone, or face-to-face, usually by a mental health professional, but sometimes by a peer supporter.
Online counseling	Supportive services are provided by an online counselor, either in an individual or group format. Communication can either be "synchronous" (i.e., in real time) via chat rooms, instant messaging, etcor "asynchronous" via email, messaging boards, blogs, etc.	Support and feedback can be individualized and provided through several electronic communications media, often by a mental health provider.
Internet-operated therapeutic software	The software may simulate a therapeutic program through use of artificial intelligence programs, robotic simulations, gaming, and three-dimensional virtual environments.	Usually there is automated feedback, that may be very specific to the individual.
Other online activities	Web-based or downloadable activities focused on education, cognitive training, or support.	Users may receive automated feedback that is specific to the program, but usually there is no human feedback other than technical support.

Advantages and Disadvantages of EMH Resources

For many adults and children the use of the computer and Internet is an important aspect of their daily lives. EMH tools make it possible to reach more family members, bridging the distance between hospital and the household. Other advantages of EMH tools include:

- These tools often provide greater access to care with reduced cost (many EMH tools are low to no-cost) and increased convenience (mobile technology allows for access to care at the user's convenience rather than the provider's).
- Electronic resources are often interactive, meaning that information can be both given and received by users, and the type or quantity of information can be adapted to the needs of individuals. Importantly, electronic resources can usually be referenced repeatedly in order to enhance comprehension and retention of skills and information.
- Some studies have shown that effective therapeutic alliances can be formed and preserved with online therapists, suggesting that EMH tools may provide some of the same relational benefits enjoyed by individuals participating in face-to-face therapy.[4,5]
- EMH tools can complement and enhance information provided by the child's medical or psychosocial support team. There is also evidence indicating that providers may benefit when their patients utilize electronic resources, particularly when patients or families share and discuss information about their disease or treatment approaches.[6]
- Many EMH resources emphasize psychoeducation about skills to promote adaptive coping and or self-management.

Despite these advantages, many EMH interventions focus on adults, and may not be developmentally appropriate for children. Other disadvantages include the following:

- Although there is evidence that EMH interventions are helpful,[7] particularly for those with symptoms of anxiety and depression, the efficacy of many EMH tools have not been empirically tested, which can make it difficult for patients, families, and providers to select effective electronic resources.

Many EMH tools do not provide emergent access to human providers, making them inappropriate for individuals with significant mental health issues. In particular, the ability to respond to crisis situations (e.g., suicidal or homicidal ideation) in real time may be severely limited or lacking entirely.

- There may be increased risk for violations of confidentiality, from service providers, other users, or even from outside individuals gaining access to personal information when resources are accessed through a shared computer. Conversely, some electronic resources may allow a user to access content anonymously. Although this may be advantageous in some respects (e.g., increased privacy, neutrality of individual status, and power), it may contribute to more negative outcomes, such as feeling invisible and behaving in a more disinhibited manner in some contexts.

- There is some evidence of low adherence to Internet-based interventions, particularly when they are fully self-directed. Providers who recommend EMH tools should still carefully monitor individuals who use them.
- Although there is evidence that most patients use the Internet to access information and other resources about their health conditions, relatively few patients disclose this to their providers in face-to-face interactions;[6] they do not reveal how they are using e-health tools during the cancer experience.
- When recommending EMH tools, providers should also consider the patient or family member's level of technical ability and literacy, given that some electronic resources (especially online counseling, chat rooms, or instant-messaging) may be more appropriate for users with good written communication skills.

How to Decide When an EMH Tool May Be an Appropriate Resource

Providers should refer to Chapter 19, Psychotherapeutic Interventions, for more general recommendations on how and when to provide therapeutic support to children with cancer and their families. In general, EMH tools are most appropriate for children and families who are largely coping appropriately with their diagnosis and treatment, but who request or require some additional resources or support. Specifically, EMH resources should be considered in the following circumstances:

- To educate patients and families about typical responses to stressors commonly experienced by children undergoing cancer treatment, and strategies to cope successfully with those stressors.
- To support individuals who request additional psychosocial resources and who are perceived by themselves or providers to be generally coping adequately.
- To complement or supplement intervention being delivered by a member of the institution's psychosocial support team, particularly when more comprehensive psychosocial services are unnecessary, impractical, or declined by the family.
- To promote coping in families who demonstrate preexisting stressors that are likely to be exacerbated by the cancer experience.

It is critical to note that *EMH tools should never be substituted for face-to-face assessment*. Intervention with a mental health professional should be provided when clinically significant mental health disorders have been diagnosed or are suspected. Electronic resources may still have a role in supporting traditional mental health services for individuals with significant psychopathology, but these should be recommended in the context of a provider who is more directly intervening and monitoring the patient's psychiatric health.

How to Identify and Recommend Resources to Families

The identification of applications, websites, and other tools may be difficult given that the technology behind the tools is rapidly evolving and individual products, websites, or applications can emerge or disappear frequently. The sheer number of electronic options may make it difficult to decide on which resource is best for a given individual or family. Thus, we will focus on providing general information about the types of tools that may be helpful to children and families, distinguishing between applications that focus on diminishing mental health symptoms in the psychosocial domains (cancer-related distress, self-esteem, quality of life) for both children and parents, and those interventions that focus on cognitive domains (memory, attention). Some specific EMH tools are mentioned in the following section.

Cognitive Interventions

Treatment of some childhood cancers, particularly acute lymphoblastic leukemia (ALL) and brain tumors, affects the CNS, which has been associated with neurocognitive late effects in a percentage of survivors. Affected skills include attention, memory, processing speed, and executive function. In recent years, increasing interest has been placed on identification and evaluation of electronic cognitive rehabilitation programs. Such programs offer advantages over traditional cognitive remediation programs given that children can complete intensive skill-based practice from the convenience of their homes, often with phone-based "coaching" support to facilitate motivated and efficient training.

Computerized cognitive training programs are largely derived from traditional neurorehabilitative strategies use for decades with traumatic brain injury patients. Consisting of child-friendly, game like exercises, most programs target core neurocognitive processes such as attention, working memory, and processing speed. Preliminary support has been published for three programs for survivors of pediatric cancer: *Captain's Log*,[8] *Cogmed*,[9] and *Lumosity*.[10] It should be noted that there are also a large number of other electronic cognitive training programs that are web based, or made for handheld gaming devices, smart phones, or tablets. To date, only the three programs just named have published findings specifically for the population of pediatric cancer survivors (Table 20.2).

Table 20.2 Electronic Cognitive Interventions that have been used with Survivors of Pediatric Cancer

Program	Domains Addressed	Format and Length	Study	Results
Captain's Log (www.braintrain.com)	Sustained attention, working memory, visual motor skills, processing speed, memory, etc.	Game-like exercises that are customized and monitored by a trained provider or available for independent home practice; no fixed training period	Hardy, Willard, & Bonner, 2011 (n = 9; single-arm study)	Improvements in performance-based and questionnaire measures of attention after training
Lumosity (www.lumosity.com)	Attention, working memory, processing speed, executive functioning	Web-based exercises that can be accessed through a license fee ("membership"); no fixed training period. No clinical monitoring is provided with this program.	Kesler, Lacayo, Jo, et al., 2011 (n = 23, single-arm study)	Limited performance-based improvements, but increased activation in brain areas associated with attention and working memory
Cogmed (www.cogmed.com)	Short-term and working memory	12 game like exercises with phone-based coaching support by a trained provider; training period is 25, 30–34 minute training sessions	Hardy, Willard, Allen, et al., 2012 (n = 20, randomized study)	Improvements in performance-based and questionnaire measures of working memory after training

Elements of Electronic Cognitive Interventions

Although the evidence for efficacy of cognitive interventions is still emerging, there is currently no evidence that cognitive training is harmful, or that it is contraindicated for concurrent use with other therapies or supports aimed at improving or compensating for survivors' cognitive impairments. In this way, some families may wish to pursue cognitive training in addition to other therapies or supportive programs such as school-based services or medication. We caution that the decision to pursue cognitive training be made after consultation or evaluation with a psychologist or neuropsychologist, who are best able to identify survivors who may benefit from training programs, and who can also offer additional, evidence-based recommendations to support the survivor's functioning. When making specific recommendations about cognitive training programs, providers should also consider the economic and psychosocial resources of the family. For example, some survivors will be able to complete a cognitive training program successfully with little parental or provider oversight, whereas others will benefit from professional coaching and monitoring to maximize benefit, trouble-shoot any problems with motivation, and provide age-appropriate feedback to children who may continue to struggle cognitively.

General guidelines for cognitive training programs are as follows:

- Programs should be *adaptive* in nature (i.e., tasks get increasingly difficult with correct responding)
- Programs should train cognitive domains known to be affected for survivors of pediatric cancer (i.e., working memory, attention, processing speed, executive functioning)
- Programs should involve massed-practice drills (i.e., exercises are practiced repeatedly)
- Programs should provide feedback on a trial-by-trial basis, so that trainees are made aware when they have responded correctly or incorrectly.

Psychosocial Interventions

Applications and Websites for General Psychosocial Distress

- Online resources are widely available to address the following, commonly reported difficulties experienced by children and adolescents with cancer. Because many EMH resources lack empirical support as stand-alone interventions, it may be prudent to utilize these tools as supplemental sources of support or skills practice to interventions that children are receiving from a mental health or psychosocial support team member. Providers looking for specific resources may wish to consult the website https://beacon.anu.edu.au/, which provides a large list of EMH websites, applications, or support groups, accompanied by an evidence-based rating of each tool provided by an independent panel of experts. General or procedural anxiety (e.g., progressive muscle relaxation (PMR) scripts as applications or websites, visual thermometers for children to indicate the level of experienced anxiety)

- Coping with pain (e.g., online pain diary, body maps for children to indicate areas of the body where pain is present, PMR scripts).
- Psychosocial distress (e.g., psychoeducation websites, cognitive-behavioral therapy tools such as applications for tracking pleasurable activities or automatic thoughts or journaling).
- Desire to connect with other individuals coping with the same illness (e.g., online support groups, disease-specific chat rooms or discussion boards).
- Other areas that may be of relevance or interest to children with cancer and their families (e.g., nutrition, physical activity, positive psychology).

Cancer-Specific Electronic Tools

Online Support

Several programs are available with information or the possibility to connect with similar others. Examples include:

- Starbright world (https://www.starbrightworld.org/) an online social network for teens with chronic and life-threatening medical conditions, and their siblings. Members are able to connect globally with others experiencing similar medical issues.
- 2bMe (http://lookgoodfeelbetter.org/2bMe), part of the Look Good Feel Better for Teens program created for adolescents, aged 13–17, with cancer. The program provides on-site support group services for teens, but the website provides education and tips to help adolescents deal with changes to their appearance, social relationships, and physical activity.
- Based on an in-person therapeutic program, onco online (www.opkoersonline.nl) is a Dutch chat room intervention for adolescent survivors of cancer.[11] It includes information and registration forms for *OK Onco Online*, a secured chat room for the weekly sessions. The main goal of *OK Onco Online* is to prevent and/or treat psychosocial problems of adolescents successfully treated for childhood cancer, by teaching active use of coping skills.
- "ReCaPTure LiFe" (**R**esilience and **C**oping skills for young **P**eople and their families **T**o **L**ive well **F**ollowing cancer) is an online intervention targeted toward cancer survivors aged 15–25. Based on the Adolescent Resilience Model,[12] Recapture Life involves six weekly, small-group sessions, delivered online by a psychologist using innovative video-conferencing technology. Early data indicate that Recapture Life is acceptable to AYAs who

have recently finished cancer treatment and is feasible to deliver to AYAs living far apart, across different time zones and states.

- Caring Bridge (www.caringbridge.org) is a website that helps patients, family, and friends connect with each other or with others experiencing a similar diagnosis. Therapeutic content is limited, but the website provides resources, such as online journaling, that are often included as elements in cancer-focused support groups.

Computer-Based Games to Promote Disease Education and Coping

- Remission (http://www.re-mission2.org/): Re-Mission 2 is a collection of online games that help young people with cancer fight their disease. Each game puts players inside the human body to defeat cancer, using weapons like chemotherapy, antibiotics, and the body's natural defenses. The games are designed to motivate players to stick to their treatments by boosting self-efficacy and positive emotions and by shifting attitudes about chemotherapy.

Online Support for Parents

The **Cascade program**[13] (cope-adapt-survive) is an intervention for parents shortly after end of the treatment of their child with cancer. The program aims to improve QoL and reduce distress and fear of cancer recurrence in parents of children aged <15 years. The program is delivered by a psychologist in three, weekly, 2-hour videoconferencing modules, with 3–5 parents/carers per group. First results show that Cascade is acceptable to parents of children recovering from cancer and is feasible to deliver. Sessions are delivered through video conferencing software (WebEx, by Cisco).

Patient Reported Outcomes in Clinical Practice

- www.hetklikt.nu: In the Netherlands, KLIK has been developed which is a web-based program using electronic Patient Reported Outcomes (ePROs) to systemically monitor and discuss Health Related Quality of Life (HRQOL) in clinical practice. This is effective in increasing discussion about emotional and psychosocial functioning[14]: Promis: www.nihpromis.org: In the future, the Patient-Reported Outcomes Measurements Information System (PROMIS) item banks can be used for screening. PROMIS aims to develop self-reported item banks using Computerized Adaptive Tests (CAT) and Item Response Theory (IRT) that are applicable to patients with a wide variety of chronic disorders.

Conclusion

Electronic mental health resources are rapidly increasing and may be useful to children with cancer and their families to provide education, coping skills, cognitive training, or support. Families may use EMH tools to supplement services being provided by their medical or psychosocial team, or to become better informed and empowered to self-manage stressors associated with the cancer experience. Although further study is needed, EMH tools in adults have shown to be effective for a wide range of common mental health difficulties such as anxiety and depression[7,15,17]; there is considerably less evidence regarding the use of EMH tools in children.[18] They may be particularly appealing for families with limited access to traditional mental health providers, or for institutions that are unable to offer program-based psychosocial support.

Despite numerous features that make EMH tools appealing to providers and families, the availability and proliferation of electronic resources has far outpaced the science demonstrating their efficacy. More information is needed about how accessible and efficacious these tools are for children and adolescents in general, and for children with cancer in particular. Electronic strategies for improving neurocognitive late effects experienced by survivors of pediatric cancer are clearly understudied and the extent to which training-based gains generalize to improvements in real-world functioning is unclear. As a result, it is difficult to derive clinically useful information from much of the field as a whole. Currently, a number of investigations have been evaluated with small samples over a relatively short time frame; thus, the long-term efficacy of many treatments across a diverse group of survivors is unknown.

References

1. File T. Computer and Internet use in the United States. In: *Current Population Survey Reports*. Washington, DC: US Census Bureau, 2013:20–568.
2. Proudfoot JG. Computer-based treatment for anxiety and depression: is it feasible? Is it effective? *Neurosci &Biobehav Rev.* 2004;28:353–363.
3. Barak A, Klein B, Proudfoot JG. Defining Internet-supported therapeutic interventions. *Ann Behav Med.* 2009;38:4–17.
4. Cook JE, Doyle C. Working alliance in online therapy as compared to face-to-face therapy: Preliminary results. *CyberPsych & Behav.* 2002;5:95–105.
5. King R, Bambling M, Reid W, Thomas I. Telephone and online counselling for young people: a naturalistic comparison of session outcome, session impact and therapeutic alliance. *Counsel & Psychotherapy Res.* 2006;6:175–181.
6. Russ H, Giveon SM, Catarivas MG, Yaphe J. The effect of the Internet on the patient-doctor relationship from the patient's perspective: a survey from primary care. *Isr Med Assoc J.* 2011;13(4):220–224.
7. Spek V, Cuijpers P, Nyklicek I, Riper H, Keyzer J, Pop V. Internet-based cognitive behaviour therapy for symptoms of depression and anxiety: a meta-analysis. *Psycholog Med.* 2007;37:319–328.
8. Hardy KK, Willard VW, Bonner MJ. Computerized cognitive training in survivors of childhood cancer: A pilot study. *J Pediatr Oncol Nurs.* 2011;28(1):27–33.

9. Hardy KK, Willard VW, Allen TM, Bonner MJ. Working memory training in survivors of pediatric cancer: a randomized pilot study. *Psychooncol.* 2013;22(8):1856–1865.
10. Kesler SR, Lacayo NJ, Jo B. A pilot study of an online cognitive rehabilitation program for executive function skills in children with cancer-related brain injury. *Brain Injury.* 2011;25 (1):101–112.
11. Maurice-Stam H, Scholten L, De Gee, EA, et al. Feasibility of an online cognitive behavioral-based group intervention for adolescents treated for cancer: a pilot study. *J Psychosoc Oncol.* In press.
12. Sansom-Daly UM, Wakefield CE; Bryant RA, Ellis SJ, Doolan EL, Cohn RJ. Online group-based cognitive-behavioural therapy for adolescents and young adults after cancer treatment: A multicenter randomised controlled trial of Recapture Life-AYA. *BMC Cancer.* 2012;12(1):339.
13. Wakefield CE; Sansom-Daly UM; Ellis SJ; Doolan EL; Cohn RJ. Cope, adapt, survive: trialling an online psychological intervention for parents after their child's cancer treatment, *PsychoOncol.* 2013;(Issue Supplement s3):100.
14. Haverman L, van Rossum MA, van Veenendaal M, et al. Effectiveness of a web-based application to monitor health-related quality of life. *Pediatr.* 2013;131(2):e533–e543.
15. Andersson G, Cuijpers P. Internet-based and other computerized psychological treatments for adult depression: a meta-analysis. *Cognit Behav Therapy.* 2009;38(4):196–205.
16. Barak A, Hen L, Boniel-Nissim M, Shapira N. A comprehensive review and a meta-analysis of the effectiveness of internet-based psychotherapeutic interventions. *J Tech Hum Serv.*, 2008;26(2/4):109–160.
17. Reger MA, Gahm GA. A meta-analysis of the effects of internet- and computer-based cognitive behavioral treatments for anxiety. *J Clin Psych.* 2009;65(1):53–75.
18. Cushing CC, Steele RG. A meta-analytic review of eHealth interventions for pediatric health promoting and maintaining behaviors. *J Pediatr Psychol.* 2010;35:937–949.

Chapter 21

Integrative Oncology

Olle Jane Z. Sahler, Hilary McClafferty, and Marilyn A. Rosen

What Is Pediatric Integrative Oncology?

Pediatric integrative oncology combines and coordinates conventional and evidence-based complementary medicine therapies in the treatment of childhood cancer.

Integrative medicine (IM) differs from "alternative" medicine. To highlight the differences, the National Center for Complementary and Alternative Medicine (NCCAM) defines alternative medicine as practices not supported by evidence, and falling outside the mainstream biomedical model. Alternative therapies will not be covered in this chapter.

Who Is Using IM in the Pediatric Oncology Population and Why?

Many families turn to IM to help support their child during and after treatment. Prevalence studies reveal that 17–84% of pediatric cancer patients use one or more types of IM treatments.[1,2] The number of hospitals and cancer programs offering these services continues to increase.

Reasons for the use of complementary therapies include a desire to improve overall health and to minimize fatigue, stress, fear, anxiety, depression, pain, nausea, vomiting, drug toxicity, and mucositis. Desire to explore all possible treatment options and to offer all possible comfort and support measures are other important factors.

Why Is the Popularity of Integrative Medicine Increasing?

Complementary therapies are seen as supporting the natural healing process and as less invasive than conventional therapies. They are often also seen as less costly, although lack of insurance reimbursement may be an issue. Unfortunately, consumer interest in complementary therapies has outpaced education and training provided in conventional medicine curricula. For example, although a survey of 90 pediatric oncologists revealed that 99% felt it was important to know what complementary therapies were being used, <50% actually asked their patients. Reasons given for not asking were that they lacked knowledge about the modalities and did not have time. This reticence to ask because they felt uneducated is particularly notable because many had concerns about possible harm especially from dietary supplements and chiropractic treatment.[3]

Recently, education and progress in the field of IM in the United States has been supported by better-defined research priorities,[4] increased research funding, and the development of organizations such as the 50-member Consortium of Academic Health Centers for Integrative Medicine, which promotes educational, research, and clinical programs.[5]

What Are the Core Principles of IM?

- Focus on the individual's innate healing response.
- Emphasize the therapeutic relationship between patient and provider.
- Consider the whole person (body, mind, and spirit), and all elements of lifestyle.
- Emphasize health promotion.
- Use all appropriate evidence-based therapies, both conventional and complementary.

Why Do Estimates of Prevalence of Use Vary So Widely?

One explanation is lack of standard definitions. To reduce confusion, the NCCAM classifications in Table 21.1 will be used in this chapter. See also Table 21.2.

Why Is Open Communication about Use Important?

Open communication helps avoid unintended drug-supplement interactions, and may identify additional therapies available to support the patient during conventional treatment. Addressing facts as well as uncertainty and accurately assessing the risks and benefits of the proposed therapy help family and practitioner reach a mutually informed decision.[3]

Providers should ask about integrative therapies at each patient encounter, including reasons for use, types of therapies, positive effects, and side effects. Providers should have ready access to reliable resources and to IM consultants. The NCCAM site, http://nccam.nih.gov/timetotalk, provides downloadable "Time to Talk" pages that include evidence-based tip sheets for various topics such as: "5 tips on safety of mind and body practices for children and teens" and "5 things to know about dietary supplements and children" to facilitate open communication.

Table 21.1 NCCAM Classifications of Complementary Therapies with Examples

Practice	Examples
Whole medical systems	Homeopathy, naturopathy, ayurveda, traditional Chinese medicine
Mind-body medicine	Meditation, prayer, mental healing, creative arts therapy (art, music, dance)
Biologically based practices	Dietary supplements, botanical medicine
Manipulative and body-based practices	Chiropractic, osteopathy, massage
Energy Therapies	Biofield therapies (Qi gong, Reiki), Bioelectromagnetics (electromagnetic fields)

Table 21.2 The 15 Most Frequently Used Complementary Therapies in Pediatric Oncology[6]

Prayer	Megavitamins/minerals	Music therapy
Relaxation/imagery	Homeopathy	Alternative providers*
Dietary supplements	Special diets	Chiropractic
Massage	Therapeutic touch	Chinese medicines
Herbal medicines/teas	Lifestyle/exercise	Aromatherapy

*Includes spiritual advisors and culturally specific healers (e.g., Native American healers).

What Kind of Training Do Conventional Physicians Specializing in IM Receive?

Within the definition of their scope of practice, physicians may provide complementary therapies such as nutritional counseling, herbal medicine, biofeedback, and hypnotherapy. In addition, there are a number of fellowship programs in IM. Board certification has been available since 1996.

What training and oversight Do Nonphysician Complementary-Medicine Providers Receive?

Training, credentialing, and licensing of complementary-medicine providers vary. Families and physicians should consider the following issues when selecting a practitioner:[7]

- Does sufficient evidence exist to suggest a particular modality has therapeutic benefit specific to the patient's condition?
- What are the practitioner's qualifications and scope of practice?
- What is the duration of the proposed treatment?
- Who will facilitate communication and coordination of treatment?

See Table 21.3.

Table 21.3 Credentials of Selected Complementary Practitioners as Recognized in the United States

Practitioner	Credentials
Acupuncturist	Diplomat in Acupuncture (Dipl. Ac.); licensed in some states (L.Ac.)
Medical Acupuncturist	Physician trained in acupuncture
Aromatherapist	No form of aromatherapy "certification" is recognized in the U.S.; not regulated by any governmental body
Ayurvedic practitioner	No legal licensing requirements needed to practice Ayurveda (system of traditional medicine native to the Indian subcontinent)
Chiropractor	Chiropractic National Board; licensed in most states; pediatric training is highly variable
Clinical Hypnotist	American Society of Clinical Hypnosis; training available for MD, DO, DDS, and some other licensed health professionals; full certification available
Healing Touch	American Holistic Nursing Association certification
Herbalist	Professional herbalist designations are conferred by the American Herbalists Guild, the National Certification Commission for Acupuncture and Oriental Medicine, and the National Institute of Medical Herbalists
Homeopathic practitioner	No diploma or certificate from any school or program is recognized as a license to practice
Massage therapist	National Certification Board for Therapeutic Massage and Bodywork (NCBTMB)
Creative Arts therapist (e.g., music, art, dance, writing, drama)	Board Certification through respective specialty board; licensed in some states
Naturopathic doctor	Naturopathy National Board; licensed in some states
Nutritionist (nonregistered dietician [RD])	Master's degree in Nutrition available at some schools; certification of attendance at holistic health courses
Traditional Chinese medicine practitioner	Diplomate of Chinese Herbology (Dipl. C.H.M.); may include acupuncture
More information about complementary practitioners can be found at: nccam.nih.gov	

Framing an Integrative Medicine Approach to the Pediatric Oncology Patient

Research evidence supporting IM in adults is growing steadily; fewer studies are available in children. However, several IM therapies can help support children by improving nutrition and quality of life, goals that align well with the Children's Oncology Group 2013 blueprint for research.[8] See Table 21.4.

Table 21.4 Elements of an Individualized Integrative Approach May Include One or More of the Following Modalities

• Nutrition	• Spirituality	• Whole medical systems approaches
• Dietary supplements	• Sleep	• Environmental exposures
• Mind-body medicine	• Physical activity	• Relationships/social support

The following sections provide an overview of selected integrative pediatric oncology treatment approaches.

Nutrition

The primary goals of an integrative nutrition plan are to focus on the highest quality foods the patient is able to consume for maintenance of existing body stores of healthy tissue, minimization of wasting due to illness and treatment side effects, support of age-appropriate growth, reduction of inflammation, and maintenance of good quality of life.[9]

Challenges include presence of a hyper-metabolic, pro-inflammatory state due to tumor metabolism, anorexia and cachexia, hormonal or other metabolic disruptions, infection, surgical procedures, pain and stress, treatment regimen, original body weight, and individual susceptibility to malnutrition. Unfortunately, the effects of a hyper-metabolic state are often not reversible even with adequate caloric supplementation.[9]

Malnutrition may occur in as many as 50% of children and adolescents with cancer. Inadequate nutrition decreases survival rate, response to treatment, and quality of life, and increases time in the hospital.[9,10]

Children with solid tumors such as neuroblastoma, Wilms tumor, or Ewing sarcoma are at higher risk of undernourishment compared to children receiving high-dose steroids or cranial radiation, who are at increased risk for fat accumulation, insulin resistance, and possible metabolic syndrome. Multimodal treatment regimens add to the complexity of nutrition management because each treatment may result in different or overlapping toxicities such as hepatic or pancreatic toxicity or vomiting, diarrhea, or mucositis.[9]

Dietary Supplements

According to the 2007 National Health Interview Survey, dietary supplements (nonvitamin, nonmineral natural biologically based products including dietary supplements taken by mouth, herbs, and botanical preparations) are the most commonly used complementary therapies.[11] Typical reasons for use include to cure or fight the cancer, provide symptomatic relief, and support conventional therapies.[12]

In a study published in 2013, only 50% of patients disclosed use of a dietary supplement or botanical to their doctor.[1]

There are three primary concerns about the use of dietary supplements: (1) little evidence-based data to guide safe use; (2) potentially harmful drug-herb interactions; and (3) antioxidant activity in some supplements may interfere with the anticancer properties of conventional therapies such as anthracyclines, platinum-containing agents, and alkylating agents, and radiation therapy, which act against cancer cells by generating free radicals. A comprehensive review of antioxidant supplementation in cancer patients concluded that insufficient evidence exists currently to broadly recommend antioxidant therapies.[13]

To enhance disclosure of supplement use, the Society of Integrative Oncology Clinical Practice Committee[14] identified 10 of the most commonly used supplements. Table 21.5 provides background information, proposed mechanism of action in cancer, safety and side effects, dosage recommendations, and drug interactions and cautions.[15] Note that this information is largely based on adult data.

Mind-Body Medicine

Some of the best-studied mind-body modalities in pediatrics include clinical hypnosis and guided imagery, meditation, mindfulness, massage therapy, yoga, creative arts/expressive therapy (music, art, dance, writing, drama),[19] and biofeedback and neurofeedback.

A 2007 U.S. study identified mind-body therapies as the second most common modality used by people <18 years old.[20] Mind-body therapies are used most frequently to treat pain, nausea, vomiting, stress, and sleep disturbance, and to reinforce resiliency, self-control, and confidence.[21,22]

Hypnosis and Imagery

Clinical hypnosis, which often includes imagery, is a state of focused relaxation. Examples of successful use were reported in the 1980s in studies comparing hypnotic versus nonhypnotic techniques for pain management in children undergoing such painful procedures as bone marrow aspiration and lumbar puncture.[23,24] It also helps anticipatory anxiety, nausea, and vomiting. Some suggest that hypnosis should be the first choice in patients interested in mind-body.[21,25]

Meditation and Mindfulness

Mindfulness-based stress reduction (MBSR) is a structured approach to mindfulness involving breath work, relaxation exercises, meditation, and movement exercises.[26] It is generally taught in a 6-to-8-week course format. Although there are no large studies in children, multiple studies of MBSR in adults confirm positive effects on quality of life, mood, mental health, stress symptoms, immune function, and sleep.[27–32]

Massage Therapy

Massage therapy is the systematic, therapeutic stroking, rubbing, or kneading of the skin and underlying muscle and other soft tissue to induce physical and psychological relaxation, improve circulation, and relieve sore muscles.[33] A single session may reduce anxiety, blood pressure, and heart rate; multiple sessions can reduce depression and pain.

Massage can release endorphins and serotonin, which can positively affect mood and block pain signals to the brain. Small randomized controlled trials have shown reduced anxiety and increased sense of well-being in child cancer patients with no reported adverse effects.[32,34] Massage has also been combined with aromatherapy with positive effects and no reported adverse effects.[35] Risk may be increased if platelets are low.

Healing touch is a biofield therapy in which practitioners consciously use their hands and intent to promote health and healing. It can involve actual contact or merely placement of the hands near or over the patient. It has been used in pediatric and adult oncology patients as a gentle supportive therapy associated with stress reduction and reduced heart rate variability.[36–38]

Yoga

Yoga has been studied in children in a variety of clinical applications.[39,40] and has proven to be safe in pediatric oncology patients in small studies. For example, a study showed improvement in perception of gross motor function and overall quality of life in six children with cancer who participated in five yoga sessions over a 2-month period.[41] Another study of 286 young adult survivors showed 32.8% had practiced yoga from time of diagnosis to promote relaxation and maintain flexibility. Average length of practice was 25 months, with a mean of 7 hours of practice per month. No adverse events were reported.[42]

Creative Arts/Expressive Therapy

Music therapy, art therapy, dance therapy, writing, and drama are well accepted and low risk, and offer creative outlets for child and adolescent patients. They have been shown to be effective in reducing anxiety and pain during procedures.[43]

Music therapy is used extensively for self-calming, and to reduce procedural stress, inspire creativity, facilitate adjustment, and enhance self-image.[44–47] Research is revealing the highly complex nature of the positive effect of music on the neurohormonal and immune systems, and its links to pain perception and emotional processing.[48] Functional neuroimaging (fMRI) indicates that emotions evoked by music appear to modulate limbic areas of the brain.[49] Research on the effect of music therapy in neuroplasticity and auditory–motor coupling in stroke victims,[50] raises intriguing questions about its application in children with neurocognitive deficits after tumor resection or radiation.

Biofeedback

The goal of biofeedback is for the individual to learn to manipulate physiologic processes by inducing a particular psychological state and then observing how these changes affect physiological processes. For example, a person may think about something stressful and observe an increase in heart rate, or think about something relaxing and observe a decrease in heart rate. Processes that can be controlled include brainwaves, muscle

Table 21.5 The 10 Most Commonly Used Supplements

Supplement	Background	Mechanism of Action in Cancer	Safety and Side Effects	Dosage	Interactions and Cautions
Curcumin (diferuloyl-methane)	• Major component of the spice turmeric (Curcuma longa); anti-inflammatory chemo-preventive activities	• Inhibits tumor initiation, promotion, invasion, angio-genesis, metastasis • Interferes with cell signaling pathways • Chemosensitizer & radiosensitizer in some cases • Active against many cancers	• Wide margin of safety • Upset stomach at higher doses • May exacerbate gallbladder disease • Caution in pregnancy due to uterine stimulation	• No clear recommendation; Clinical effect at 500–3000 mg Doses <12 gms show no SAE; NB: titrated dose study in pediatric IBD used <2 gm bid with no AE(16)	• Platelet-inhibiting activity: Use cautiously with anti-coagulants • Possible synergistic antiplatelet effect with ginkgo biloba, garlic, saw palmetto • Combined with cyclo-phosphamide and camptothecin, reduced apoptosis
Glutamine	• Essential amino acid with biologic functions including GI cell growth and regeneration	• Reduces cytokine production; improves GI tract mucosal barrier; reduces mucositis severity and intestinal toxicity • May reduce peripheral neuropathy	• Caution in hepatic and renal impairment • Rarely causes edema, rash, head-ache, flu-like syndrome	• Average dose 10 gm/day (range 5–30 gm/day)	• Inconclusive; may interfere with chemo-therapeutic agents; May interact with anti-seizure medications

Vitamin D	• Pro-hormone that controls calcium, phosphorous, and bone metabolism. Low serum 25(OH)D may be associated with increased risk of breast, prostate, colorectal, and other cancers; Associated with poorer prognosis of various malignancies	• Unclear, research is very active	• Generally safe; very high doses associated with hypercalcemia	• Recommended levels 40–80 ng/mL; IOM recommends 400 IU/d through 12 mos, then 600 IU/d for 1–70 yrs • Recommendations may be conservative (17)	• Metabolized by cyto-chrome P450 hepatic enzyme system; theoretical inter-actions are possible; no interactions reported
Maitake Mushrooms	• Maitake-D fraction is a polysaccharide most frequently studied as an adjunct to radiation and chemotherapy	• Basidiomycetes mushrooms contain polysaccharides exerting anti-tumor action by providing T-cell dependent immune modulation that enhances tumor inhibition. May reduce chemotherapy side effects	Generally regarded as safe. May lower blood sugar	• Safe/effective dose not established	• No known interactions • Caution advised in diabetes due to possible hypoglycemia • Caution advised in patients on immune-modulatory therapies

(continued)

Table 21.5 (Continued)

Supplement	Background	Mechanism of Action in Cancer	Safety and Side Effects	Dosage	Interactions and Cautions
Fish Oil (Omega-3 fatty acids)	• Long chain poly-unsaturated fatty acids eicosapentaenoic acid and docosahexaenoic acid are most commonly used as supplements	• Primarily anti-inflammatory effect • May have beneficial effects on body weight; may inhibit pro-inflammatory cytokines in cachexia	• 2–3 gm/d • Occasional GI side effects; no SAE • May have anti-platelet function; no reported AEs in surgical patients	• Be cautious with anti-coagulants/ anti-platelet drugs with vitamin A • ?? hold fish oil if platelets <50,000	• Use cautiously with anti hypertensive medication due to possible hypotensive effects
Green Tea (Camellia sinensis)	• High polyphenol content (40% is epigallocatechin [EGCG])	• Pro-apoptotic effects, antimetastatic properties, anti-oxidant effects, may enhance activity of some chemotherapy	• Caffeine related side effects possible; some reports of liver toxicity in high doses		• Theoretical concerns about use with anti-coagulants • EGCG in high concentrations could inhibit bortezomib used in multiple myeloma • Inhibits P-glyco-protein, may inhibit CYP450 pathway • Possible interaction with sunitinib, irinotecan or verapamil • May increase tamoxifen bioavailability • May increase side effects of drugs metabolized by uridine 5' diphospho-glucuronosyltransferase • Caution with hepatotoxic drugs

Milk Thistle (Silybum marianum)	• Flavonoids and flavonolignans most active compounds; Used for thousands of years for protection from hepatotoxins and for liver and biliary disorders	• Largely unclear. Case reports of tumor regression • Improves liver function in children with hepatotoxicity during ALL treatment at doses of 80–360 mg/d (18)	• Wide margin of safety	• No clear Recommendation • Clinical studies average 200–400 mg/d in divided doses	• None known
Astragalus membranaceus	• Used in traditional Chinese medicine to tonify Qi; potent immune-modulatory effects; contains isoflavonoids and other active compounds	• Potentiates anti- tumor activity of IL-2 in vitro, improves lymphocyte responses, enhances NKC activity; increased phagocytosis has hepato-protective effects • Directly inhibits tumor growth; has antiangiogenic properties; may enhance effects of platinum-based chemotherapy	• No reported AEs		• Avoid use with immune-suppressants as may antagonize effects

(continued)

Table 21.5 (Continued)

Supplement	Background	Mechanism of Action in Cancer	Safety and Side Effects	Dosage	Interactions and Cautions
Melatonin	• Hormone secreted by pineal gland correl-ates with circadian rhythm/ sleep cycles • Regulates growth hormone; stimulates apoptosis; up regulates antioxidant enzymes; suppresses tumor and endothelial growth factors; down regulates pro-oxidative enzymes	• Cues sleep cycle • Interferes with estrogen synthesis and acts on estrogen receptors as a selective estrogen enzyme modifier. Questions raised about association between nocturnal light exposure and breast cancer	• Safe to use as adjuvant therapy with conventional medicine • May improve survival at 1 yr • AEs not reported	• Dose range for sleep 0.5 to 3 gm/d • Solid tumor adjuvant therapy dose ranges up to 20 gm/d	• Caution if used with CYP1A2 and CYP2C9 metabolized drugs • Luvox increases bioavailability of exogenous melatonin • Caffeine, alcohol, Non-steroidals, beta-blockers, benzodiazapines, calcium channel blockers, and diuretics suppress melatonin production

Probiotics	• Live microorganisms with immune-modulating effects • Benefits mucosal maintenance, nutrient absorption, and defense against bacterial pathogens • Used in prevention/ treatment of antibiotic associated diarrhea	• Treatment of intestinal toxicity during chemotherapy/radiation to reduce diarrhea and gut damage	• Generally safe; some gassiness • Concerns about sepsis in immuno-suppressed patients • Case reports both support use in neutropenia and caution against (case series documented fungemia with *Saccharomyces cerevisiae* in 3 immunosuppressed patients)	• Variable dosages, 10–20 billion cells/d of lacto-bacillus GG (Culturelle) effective in chemotherapy induced diarrhea	• Theoretical discussions about doses of antibiotics and probiotics to maintain efficacy of both products

tone, skin conductance, finger temperature, heart rate, and respiratory rate. Eventually, the relaxation response can be easily induced independent of the feedback provided by the external monitor. A study on preprocedural distress in 12 children with cancer showed the benefit of learning effective relaxation techniques using biofeedback in a four-session intervention.[51] Neurofeedback (i.e., EEG biofeedback) may help to improve cognitive function in children with neurocognitive decline after cancer therapy.[52]

Traditional Chinese Medicine/Acupuncture

Many whole systems of medicine have traditional approaches to cancer treatment dating back thousands of years. For example, Traditional Chinese Medicine (TCM), which includes use of Chinese herbs and acupuncture, is commonly used to treat cancer in China.[53] The search for the active components in TCM oncology treatment is ongoing.[54,55] However, there are few studies of TCM use in pediatric oncology. Small studies have shown benefit to using acupuncture to reduce chemotherapy-related nausea and vomiting.[56,57]

A concern about acupuncture is bleeding due to thrombocytopenia. This problem was studied retrospectively in 32 pediatric patients who underwent a total of 237 treatments by highly trained acupuncturists in an academic oncology center. Platelet counts ranged from <20,000/uL to >100,000/uL. Twenty percent of sessions were done in patients with severe thrombocytopenia, 8% with moderate thrombocytopenia, 19% with mild thrombocytopenia, and 53% with normal counts. No acute or serious side effects were recorded in any session.[58]

Where Will Practitioners and Patients Find Reliable Web-Based Information about Integrative Modalities?

A 2013 Pew Internet and American Life Project showed that 85% of U.S. adults use the Internet and 72% of Internet users search for health information online.[59] They also noted: "...For the first time since the Pew Research Center's Internet & American Life Project began systematically tracking smartphone adoption, a majority [56%] of Americans now own a smartphone of some kind..."[60] They also discovered that 19% of smartphone owners had downloaded an app specifically to track or manage health.

SAFE is an acronym for advising patients and families about judging information they find on the Internet (Box 21.1).

Box 21.1 SAFE

S—STAFF. Who created the site? Usually, there is an "About this site" or an "About" page stating who developed or maintains the site, the board of directors, or a history of the site. What are their credentials? If none are listed, they should explain who they are.

A—ADDRESS. If the domain in the URL address is .org, it is run by an organization, probably not for profit. If it is .edu, it is from an educational institution. A .gov is from the government. A .com is likely commercial and, therefore, trying to sell something. Be wary! Some URLs end with country designations, as in .ca for Canada. An address with a .net may be trustworthy or not.

F—FIT. How "fit" is this site? Do several of the links lead to "page not found?" One or two such dead ends may be tolerable, but more indicates the site is missing its fitness goals. Are there dates at the bottom of pages, and are these current? If a page in a health related site has not been updated in two years, be skeptical about the information. Is the News section current?

E—EVIDENCE. Is the content referenced? Do the authors cite medical journal articles and book chapters or just individual opinions and biases? If there are references, how old are they? Research is expanding so rapidly that being current is crucial. Online support groups, consisting of other families' experiences, may be useful, as long as readers know that the material is personal opinion.

Using PubMed and Other Resources to Do Efficient, Effective, and Reliable Searches

1. Use the *subject filter* "complementary medicine" with any search to include hundreds of terms that refer to modalities as well as herbs/ dietary supplements. Another available subject filter is "dietary supplements"; this filter adds the dietary supplements, including vitamins. A search can also be built using the medical subject heading (Mesh) "complementary therapies." It is not as inclusive as the filter, but can offer different results. Other possible Mesh headings include "dietary supplements," "functional food," "plants, medicinal" or "herbal medicine."
2. "How can you be careful about cancer information on websites, Twitter, YouTube, blogs, Facebook, and e-mail?" National Cancer

Institute: http://www.cancer.gov/cancertopics/cancerlibrary/health-info-online

3. "Evaluating Web-Based Resources" The National Center for Complementary and Alternative Medicine: http://nccam.nih.gov/health/webresources

References

1. Ndao DH, Ladas EJ, Bao Y, et al. Use of complementary and alternative medicine among children, adolescent, and young adult cancer survivors: A survey study. *J Pediatric Hematol Oncol.* 2013;35(4):281–288.
2. Myers C, Stuber ML, Bonamer-Rheingans JL, Zeltzer LK. Complementary therapies and childhood cancer. *Cancer Control.* 2005;12(3):172–180.
3. Roth M, Lin J, Kim M, Moody K. Pediatric oncologists' views toward the use of complementary and alternative medicine in children with cancer. *J Pediatric Hematol Oncol.* 2009;31(3):177–182.
4. Briggs JP, Killen J. Perspectives on complementary and alternative medicine research. *JAMA.* 2013;310(7):691–692.
5. Consortium of Academic Health Centers for Integrative Medicine. 2013.
6. McLean TW, Kemper KJ. Complementary and alternative medical (CAM) therapies in pediatric oncology patients. *J Soc Integrat Oncol.* 2006;4(1):40–45.
7. Gilmour J, Harrison C, Asadi L, Cohen MH, Vohra S. Referrals and shared or collaborative care: Managing relationships with complementary and alternative medicine practioners. *Pediatrics.* 2011;Suppl 4:S181–S186.
8. Sung L, Zaoutis T, Ullrich NJ, et al. Children's Oncology Group's 2013 blueprint for research: cancer control and supportive care. *Pediatric Blood & Cancer.* 2013;60(6):1027–1030.
9. Bauer J, Jurgens H, Fruhwald MC. Important aspects of nutrition in children with cancer. *Adv Nutrition.* 2011;2(2):67–77.
10. Brinksma A, Huizinga G, Sulkers E, Kamps W, Roodbol P, Tissing W. Malnutrition in childhood cancer patients: A review on its prevalence and possible causes. *Crit Revs Oncol/Hematol.* 2012;83(2):249–275.
11. Barnes PM, Bloom B, Nahin RL. Complementary and alternative medicine use among adults and children: United States, 2007. *Natl Health Stat Report.* 2008;10(12):1–23.
12. Bishop FL, Prescott P, Chan YK, Saville J, von Elm E, Lewith GT. Prevalence of complementary medicine use in pediatric cancer: A systematic review. *Pediatrics.* 2010;125(4):768–776.
13. Ladas E, Kelly KM. The antioxidant debate. Explore: *J Sci Healing.* 2010;6(2):75–85.
14. Society for Integrative Oncology. 2013. www.integrativeonc.org/index.php/docguide.
15. Frenkel M, Abrams DI, Ladas EJ, et al. Integrating dietary supplements into cancer care. *Integrat Cancer Therap.* 2013;12(5):369–384.
16. Suskind DL, Wahbeh G, Burpee T, Cohen M, Christie D, Weber W. Tolerability of curcumin in pediatric inflammatory bowel disease: A forced-dose titration study. *J Pediatr Gastroenterol Nutr.* 2013;56(3):277–279.
17. Institute of Medicine of the National Academies. *Dietary Reference Intakes for Calcium and Vitamin D.* Washington, DC: Institute of Medicine; 2010 Nov.

18. Ladas EJ, Kroll DJ, Oberlies NH, et al. A randomized, controlled, double-blind, pilot study of milk thistle for the treatment of hepatotoxicity in childhood acute lymphoblastic leukemia (ALL). *Cancer.* 2010;116(2):506–513.

19. McClafferty H. Complementary, holistic, and integrative medicine: Mind-body medicine. *Pediatr Rev.* 2011;32(5):201–203.

20. Birdee GS, Phillips RS, Davis RB, Gardiner P. Factors associated with pediatric use of complementary and alternative medicine. *Pediatrics.* 2010;125(2):249–256.

21. Kanitz JL, Camus ME, Seifert G. Keeping the balance—an overview of mind-body therapies in pediatric oncology. *Complement Therap i Med.* 2013;Suppl 1:S20–S25.

22. Elkins G, Fisher W, Johnson A. Mind-body therapies in integrative oncology. *Curr Treatment Options Oncol.* 2010;11(3-4):128–140.

23. Olness K. Imagery (self-hypnosis) as adjunct therapy in childhood cancer: Clinical experience with 25 patients. *Am J Pediatr Hematol Oncol.* 1981;3(3):313–321.

24. Zeltzer L, LeBaron S. Hypnosis and nonhypnotic techniques for reduction of pain and anxiety during painful procedures in children and adolescents with cancer. *J Pediatr.* 1982;101(6):1032–1035.

25. Accardi MC, Milling LS. The effectiveness of hypnosis for reducing procedure-related pain in children and adolescents: A comprehensive methodological review. *J Behav Med.* 2009;32(4):328–339.

26. Kabat-Zin J. An outpatient program in behavioral medicine for chronic pain patients based on the practice of mindfulness meditation: Theoretical considerations and preliminary results. *Gen Hosp Psychiatry.* 1982;4(1):33–47.

27. Carlson EA, Sampson MC, Sroufe LA. Implications of attachment theory and research for developmental-behavioral pediatrics. *J Dev & Behav Pediatrics.* 2003;24(5):364–379.

28. Henderson VP, Massion AO, Clemow L, Hurley TG, Druker S, Hebert JR. A randomized controlled trial of mindfulness-based stress reduction for women with early-stage breast cancer receiving radiotherapy. *Integrat Cancer Therap.* 2013;12:404–413.

29. Anderson SR, Wurtzen H, Steding-Jessen M, et al. Effect of mindfulness-based stress reduction on sleep quality: Results of a randomized trial among Danish breast cancer patients. *Acta Oncologica.* 2013;52(2):336–344.

30. Wurtzen H, Dalton SO, Elsass P, et al. Mindfulness significantly reduces self-reported levels of anxiety and depression: Results of a randomised controlled trial among 336 Danish women treated for Stage I-III breast cancer. *Euro J Cancer.* 2013;49(6):1365–1373.

31. Zainal NZ, Booth S, Huppert FA. The efficacy of mindfulness-based stress reduction on mental health of breast cancer patients: A meta-analysis. *Psychooncol.* 2013;22(7):1457–1465.

32. Post-White J, Fitzgerald M, Savik K, Hooke MC, Hannahan AB, Sencer SF. Massage therapy for children with cancer. *J Pediatr Oncol Nurs.* 2009;26(1):16–28.

33. National Center for Complementary and Alternative Medicine (NCCAM). Massage therapy. www 2013Available from: URL: http://nccam.nih.gov/health/massage

34. Mehling WE, Lown EA, Dvorak CC, et al. Hematopoietic cell transplant and use of massage for improved symptom management: Results from a pilot randomized control trial. *Evidence-Based Complementary Altern Med.* (eCAM) 2012;ID 450150:1–9.

35. Fellowes D, Barnes K, Wilkinson S. Aromatherapy and massage for symptom relief in patients with cancer. *Cochrane Database of Systematic Reviews.* 2004;2(CD002287).

36. Kemper KJ, Fletcher NB, Hamilton CA, McLean TW. Impact of healing touch on pediatric oncology outpatients: Pilot study. *J Soc Integrat Oncol.* 2009;7(1):12–18.

37. Wong J, Ghiasuddin A, Kimata C, Patelesio B, Siu A. The impact of healing touch on pediatric oncology patients. *Integr Cancer Ther.* 2013;12(1):25–30.

38. Danhauer SC, Tooze JA, Holder P, Miller C, Jesse MT. Healing touch as a supportive intervention for adult leukemia patients: A pilot investigation of effects on distress and symptoms. J Soc Integrat Oncol. 2008;6(3):89–97.

39. Birdee GS, Yeh GY, Wayne PM, Phillips RS, Davis RB, Gardiner P. Clinical applications of yoga for the pediatric population: A systemic review. *Academ Pediatr.* 2009;9(4):212–220.

40. Galantino ML, Galbavy R, Quinn L. Therapeutic effects of yoga for children: A systematic review of the literature. *Pediatr Phys Therapy.* 2008;20(1):66–80.

41. Geyer R, Lyons A, Amazeen L, Alishio L, Cooks L. Feasibility study: The effect of therapeutic yoga on quality of life in children hospitalized with cancer. *Pediatr Phys Therapy.* 2011;23(4):375–379.

42. Park CL, Cho D, Wortmann JH. The impact of Yoga upon young adult cancer survivors. *Complement Therapies Clin Practice.* 2013;19(2):77–82.

43. Klassen JA, Liang Y, Tjosvold L, Klassen TP, Hartling L. Music for pain and anxiety in children undergoing medical procedures: A systemic review of randomized controlled trials. *Ambul Pediatrics.* 2008;8(2):117–128.

44. Robb SL, Clair AA, Watanabe M, et al. A non-randomized [corrected] controlled trial of the active music engagement (AME) intervention on children with cancer. *Psychooncol.* 2008;17(7):699–708.

45. Hilliard RE. Music therapy in pediatric oncology: A review of the literature. *Soc Integrat Oncol.* 2006;4(2):75–78.

46. O'Callaghan C, Barry P, Thompson K. Music's relevance for adolescents and young adults with cancer: A constructivist research approach. *Support Care Cancer.* 2012;20(4):687–697.

47. O'Callaghan C, Dun B, Baron A, Barry P. Music's relevance for children with cancer: Music therapists' qualitative clinical data-mining research. *Social Work Health Care.* 2013;52(2-3):125–143.

48. Leardi S, Pietroletti R, Angeloni G, Necozione S, Ranalletta G, Del Gusto B. Randomized clinical trial examining the effect of music therapy in stress response to day surgery. *Br J Surg.* 2007;94(8):943–947.

49. Koelsch S. Towards a neural basis of music-evoked emotions. *Trends Cogn Sci.* 2010;14(3):131–137.

50. Rodriguez-Fornells A, Rojo N, Amengual JL, Ripolles P, Altenmuller E, Munte TF. The involvement of audio-motor coupling in the music-supported therapy applied to stroke patients. *Ann NY Acad Sci.* 2012;1252:282–293.

51. Shockey DP, Menzies V, Glick DF, Taylor AG, Boitnott A, Rovnyak V. Preprocedural distress in children with cancer: An intervention using biofeedback and relaxation. *J Pediatr Oncol Nurs.* 2013;30(3):129–138.

52. de Ruiter MA, Schouten-Van Meeteren AY, van Mourik R, et al. Neurofeedback to improve neurocognitive functioning of children treated for a brain tumor: Design of a randomized controlled double-blind trial. *BMC Cancer.* 2012;12:581.

53. Li X, Yang G, Li X, et al. Traditional Chinese medicine in cancer care: A review of controlled clinical studies published in chinese. *PloS One.* 2013;8(4):e60338.

54. Mohd FF, Koutsoukas A, Lowe R, et al. Chemogenomics approaches to rationalizing the mode-of-action of traditional Chinese and Ayurvedic medicines. *J Chem Inform Model.* 2013;53(3):661–673.

55. Gundeti MS, Sisodia BS, Marlewar S, Reddy RG. Consultative workshop on integrative approach to cancer. *J Ayurveda & Integrat Med.* 2012;3(4):230–231.

56. Jindal V, Ge A, Mansky PJ. Safety and efficacy of acupuncture in children: A review of the evidence. J Pediatr Hematol Oncol. 2008;30(6):431–442.

57. Gottschling S, Reindl TK, Meyer S, et al. Acupuncture to alleviate chemotherapy-induced nausea and vomiting in pediatric oncology—a randomized multicenter crossover pilot trial. *Klinische Padiatrie* 2008;220(6):365–370.

58. Ladas EJ, Rooney D, Taromina K, Ndao DH, Kelly KM. The safety of acupuncture in children and adolescents with cancer therapy-related thrombocytopenia. *Support Care Cancer.* 2010;18(11):1487–1490.

59. Pew Research Center's Internet & American Life Project. Pew Internet: Health. www 2013Available from: URL: http://www.pewinternet.org/commentary/2011/november/pew-internet-health.aspx

60. Pew Research Center's Internet & American Life Project. Smartphone Ownership 2013. www 2013Available from: URL: http://www.pewinternet.org/reports/2013/smartphone-ownership-2013.aspx

Section V

Communication and Supportive Care Considerations

Chapter 22

Talking to Children and Adolescents about Cancer

Joanna Breyer

Introduction

Working in pediatric oncology requires open, honest, and sensitive communication with parents and with children appropriate to their age and understanding[1] to:

- Establish trust with the medical team.
- Enlist parents as partners.
- Decrease child's anxiety.
- Explain to child why unpleasant treatments are necessary.
- Increase likelihood of cooperation from child.
- Facilitate optimal end-of-life care.

This chapter will address age-appropriate communication in the pediatric oncology setting relevant to:

- Diagnosis, treatment and referral for psychosocial services.
- Difficult decisions.
- End-of-life care.

In all instances, the cultural, religious, humanistic, and spiritual values of the family need to be understood by the medical team and may affect the manner and the nature of what is communicated to the child. It is important to remember that despite a remarkable blossoming of pediatric palliative care services across the globe[2] and an international trend towards fuller disclosure, many cultures have different beliefs, values, and practices that may affect what doctors disclose and what patients or families want disclosed about cancer[3,4]

Diagnosis, Treatment, and Referral for Psychosocial Services

We will discuss children's developmental readiness to receive information of varying complexity and review age-appropriate ways of talking with children and adolescents about their diagnosis of cancer, its treatment and the use of psychosocial services.

In institutions in which a psychologist, social worker, or psychiatrist is not routinely part of the child's medical team, referral for specialized consultation with mental health professionals is indicated in the following situations:

- If the child or adolescent appears depressed, anxious, agitated, angry, or has other concerning psychological symptoms:
  - is exhibiting or expressing high levels of unrelenting anxiety with medically required procedures.
  - is non-compliant taking medications.
  - is behaving dramatically differently from behavior before diagnosis.
  - If parents are having difficulties with each other, with the medical team or in dealing with their child and they appear depressed, very anxious or have other concerning psychiatric symptoms or behaviors.
- If parents report siblings are having difficulties:
  - at home.
  - at school.
  - with peers.
- If the child relapses or his or her prognosis worsens and family stress is evident.

Examples of explanations of medical terms and procedures and ways to introduce psychosocial services to children at different stages and their parents are provided next.

Ages 2–5 Years

Children in this age group are characterized by egocentrism, magical thinking, impulsivity, increasing verbal skills, dependency on primary caregivers for order, direction, self-esteem, and an increasing differentiation between self and others. They have a limited conception of time or capacity to distinguish fact from fantasy. They have wonderful imaginations.

Communication with this age group needs to be:

- Simple, direct, clear.
- Delivered in small portions.
- Repeated often and then checked for what has actually been heard.

Since the concept of time is not developed, only deliver information that will affect the child immediately or in the very near future.

The explanations should be tailored to the individual child and circumstances of the specific treatment (e.g., "you are getting this medicine to help the lump get smaller").

Leukemias

"Your blood is not working right and we need to fix it."

Solid Tumors

"A lump is growing in your _____ and we need to make it go away."

Cause

- No one knows.
- Nothing you did or said caused this to happen.
- Not catching (contagious).

Treatments

Given the limited conception of time for this age group, the explanation for each stage of treatment and side effects are most appropriately given just before or as they begin to happen. "We will tell you what we need to do and answer any questions you have before we do it."

Chemotherapy

"Right now we will give you some medicine that will... (help your blood get better)."

Radiation

"Now you will need to lie still on a special bed while a machine like a big camera shines a special light on your body that you won't feel. The light will help..."

Surgery

"Now we will help you go to sleep so you will not feel anything and then we will take out what is left of the lump. When you wake up, it will be gone and you will have a bandage over where the lump was."

Amputation

"You are going to have a special operation. Do you know what an operation is?" Explain anesthesia and not feeling anything. "During that operation the doctors will take off the bottom part of your leg, the part with the lump in it. They have to do that because they hope it will stop the lump growing anywhere else in your body." Encourage questions. Give simple description of prosthesis if appropriate: "A special metal/plastic leg that will help you walk, run, and get around so you will be able to play with other kids."

Bone Marrow or Stem Cell Transplant

"You will need to stay in hospital for a while in a special room and get medicine that will help... Your mommy or daddy will be able to stay with you."

Side Effects

Hair loss—as it is beginning to fall out. "We hope the medicine will help you get better but it also makes your hair fall out. Your hair will come back later." "Would you like us to cut your hair shorter so there is less to come out?" "Some kids like to wear a wig when they don't have hair. Would you like to get one?"

Other Side Effects

Respond only when a child has a particular side effect because:

- Side effects vary widely between children.
- Some children are quite suggestible and you do not want to predict a side effect that might not occur.

For example, if a child is vomiting, "We will try to help you feel better with some new medicine."

If child is having tantrums while on steroids, "Sometimes the medicine can make you feel upset and it's hard to control yourself, but we still cannot let you hit people."

Introducing Psychosocial Services

To Parents (by oncologist):

- "Getting cancer is obviously confusing and upsetting for preschoolers. It is not unusual to see major behavior changes particularly at first. Sometimes, through playing and talking with children, a psychosocial clinician can find out what in particular is worrying or bothering a child and can make a plan to help."
- Understand how parents are viewing the presenting problem.

  "Having a young child with cancer is extraordinarily stressful. Sometimes meeting with a psychosocial clinician to discuss [presenting problem] can be very helpful."

To Child (by psychosocial clinician):

- Directly to child: "I talk and play with children in the hospital who are [presenting problem, e.g., feeling sad, getting pokes, taking medication...]. We can talk, have fun, and plan how to make things go more easily."
- Indirectly: "I have someone here I'd like you to meet (animal puppet). He's shy and doesn't like [presenting problem, e.g., getting shots, being in the hospital, taking medicine...], but maybe he'll talk to you."

Ages 6–11 Years

Children in this age group are increasingly concrete, verbal and interested in and capable of understanding more biological facts. They may still use magical thinking and wonder if they or something else "caused" the illness. They are learning new skills and are interested in interacting with and obtaining the approval of peers as well as parents and siblings. Communication with this age group can include somewhat fuller biological explanations about their illness and treatment.

Leukemias

"Our blood is made up of red and white blood cells and platelets." Explain function of each. "Your body is making too many white cells that are crowding out the other cells and stopping them from doing their jobs."

Treatments

The concept of time will still be limited, particularly for the 6–8-year-old group, so give some advance notice of treatments but do not overwhelm the child with too much information about the full course of his treatment in advance unless he asks.

- Encourage questions and respond to them fully.
- Give choices when possible.

Chemotherapy

"The medicine we will give you will, hopefully, stop the white cells growing so fast and give the red cells more room to do their job" (or "make your lump get smaller").

Introducing Psychosocial Services

To Parent (by oncologist):

- See previous introduction to psychosocial services, add, "Also it is sometimes hard for children this age to miss or go back to school and keep up with friends."

To child (by psychosocial clinician):

- "Many kids your age do not like being sick and having to [presenting problem, e.g., have medical procedures, go back to school...]. I talk and play with children your age and we work together to figure out ways to help things go more easily."

Ages 12–17 Years

Adolescence is a time of upheaval and change that involves the development of new skills and capacity for abstract thought, as well as emotional vulnerability, increased peer involvement, and mood fluctuations. Control and increased independence are major issues for this age group.

Communication should be clear, straightforward, and include as full a medical explanation as the adolescent indicates he or she wants. They need to be included as partners in a joint enterprise and given choices whenever possible. Depending on age and maturity, as well as the clinical situation, adolescents can be told their illness is very serious, even life-threatening, but with the treatments there is a (very) good chance they can be cured.

The full course of their treatment should be described to them from the start. Common immediate side effects can be described in general terms so they are not blindsided. For example, "Different people have different reactions to the medicines you are taking. Some feel tired or sick or get mouth sores. Tell us what you notice about what you are feeling. We will give you medications that we hope will help you feel more comfortable."

Possible Late Effects

The older and more cognitively mature adolescent can be told, "There may be some long-term effects from the treatment; some are more likely than others. Would you like to hear about them now or later?"

To parent (by oncologist):

"This is a hard age to get cancer. It's an age when adolescents want control, independence, and are very aware of how they look. Sometimes it can be helpful to have somebody outside the family available to talk with them. What do you think?"

To adolescent (by psychosocial clinician):

"I've talked with a lot of kids your age who have cancer. They've told me some things that were hard and some things that helped." [Give examples.] "Some of these may or may not be true for you." "What's been hard for you so far?" "What has helped?"

Difficult Decisions

See Chapter 29, Ethical Issues in Pediatric Oncology. Treatment decisions should be in the best interest of the child. Difficult decisions occur most often when parents and medical caregivers, and perhaps the child, do not agree about what is in the child's best interest.[5]

Examples:

- Parents want aggressive treatment whereas the medical team feels the risks of harm to the child considerably outweigh the potential benefit.
    - Giving an aggressive treatment with likely toxic effects to a terminally ill child.
- Team wants a treatment that the parents oppose.
    - Blood transfusion opposed by parents on religious grounds.
    - Stem cell transplant with 60% likelihood of success versus palliative chemotherapy.
    - Increasing pain medication for a terminally ill child when the medical team perceives the child to be suffering, whereas the parents want their child awake and alert.
- Child refuses to get treatment or to complete a treatment that is underway.
- Parents refuse to let the medical team discuss the illness or treatment with their child.

Disagreements between Medical Team and Family about Treatment

Careful and sensitive communication is critical in resolving or avoiding such situations. Efforts should include the following steps:

- Medical team must clearly state their views and the reasons for a particular treatment recommendation. Ascertain that the parents have understood what is being communicated.
- Staff must try to understand reasons behind the parents' or child's wishes (for or against a treatment) such as fears, concerns, family history, barriers, and cultural traditions.

- Team should consider if accommodations can be made to meet parents' or child's concerns and wishes.
- Team can request medical ethics or mental health consultation to help gain perspective or clarify issues and to suggest additional ways to communicate with the family.
- Team can go to court in order to obtain temporary guardianship to administer or not administer a particular treatment.[6]

If an adolescent should refuse potentially life-saving treatment against the wishes of his parents and the medical team, the medical team can:

- Give greater deference to the wishes of an older and more mature adolescent. In the United States some adolescents can be declared "emancipated minors" and can sign consent forms in place of their parents.
- Give the adolescent the relevant medical information (published studies showing risk, impact on likely survival, etc.).
- Check he/she has accurately understood the information.
- Probe further to understand the parents' position and reasons for resistance (family, religious beliefs, side effects).
- Mobilize additional relevant resources (mental health professionals, ethics consultants, teachers, and religious counselors, key family members) to address his/her resistance.
- Consider treatment compromises that could be made that would offer less risk to adolescent.

If an adolescent continues to refuse treatment and parents are unwilling to force him, the medical team can decide whether to go to court for temporary guardianship. The reality is that few medical centers are prepared to physically restrain an adolescent in order to give treatment. Very rarely an adolescent may run away rather than face a treatment he abhors but, more typically, if all the steps have been taken that are outlined above, the adolescent will agree to complete treatment or a minimally modified version of it.

Communication about the Illness

If parents tell the medical team not to give a child any medical facts, it is important to thoroughly understand family history; religious, spiritual, or cultural beliefs; and what the parents fear if the child is told. In some cultures in which disclosure and transparency are not the norm, the doctors and the family may think they have a greater duty to protect the patient from bad news than to inform the person accurately about the condition,[4,7,8] especially when the patient is a child.

The medical team can:

- Try to address parents' fears.
- Explain the benefits of open communication.
- Explain that the child may find out anyway or may already know.
- Suggest parents may come to feel differently over time.
- Explain that the medical team cannot lie to the child but they will do their best to respect the parents' wishes.

- Explain that if a child asks a question that the team is constrained from answering, the child will be told that his parents have asked them not to answer that question and the child should discuss it with the parents.

The older and more mature the child, the more isolated he or she may feel in this situation. Additional approaches to be considered are discussions with other family members or religious counselors of the same faith or to request an ethics consult. It is important to keep the lines of communication open and to respect parents' autonomy and their wish to protect their child.

End-of-Life

See Chapter 26, Spiritual and Religious Considerations, and Chapter 30, Integrating Palliative Care.

This section includes:

- Communication with families when cure of the child is no longer possible.
- How to introduce a Do Not Rescucitate order (DNR).
- How to respond when a child suddenly becomes terminally ill.

Communication

Often a child's journey to the terminal phase has been a gradual, heart-breaking rather than sudden process. The child may have experienced:

- Several relapses.
- One or two bone marrow or stem cell transplants.
- Several experimental treatments.

Objective of communication to the child:

- To give honest/accurate information on illness progression appropriate to the child's age and cognitive understanding[9] while preserving and sustaining hope for as long as possible;[10,11] understanding that the object of hope may change with time (cure/delay/quality of life/no pain/participation in family or peer event/wish to be remembered).[12]
- Being responsive and attuned to the child's questions and parents' wishes and level of understanding.[13]

Communication models have been designed to improve the ease and sensitivity of communication in pediatric palliative and end-of–life care.[14,13] The following 10 sections encompass these models and consider what contributes to effective communication with patients and families facing the death of their child.

1. Cultural, Religious, Spiritual and Humanistic Values of the Family and the Wishes of the Parents

In the United States, there is a wide spectrum of religious, spiritual, and humanistic views. There are also striking differences between ethnic groups in their wish to be informed of details of a cancer diagnosis and even more so of a terminal prognosis.[8,15] So it is hardly surprising that many parents are initially very reluctant to communicate to the child the severity of his or her condition. Frequent concerns and how to address them are listed in Table 22.1.

2. Age and Developmental Maturity of the Child

Various authors have noted correctly that a child (patient or sibling) exposed to death or the likelihood of death may have an earlier awareness about the finality and irreversibility of death than the child not so exposed. However a basic understanding of the stages through which a child views death is essential to allow age-appropriate communication. The stages are described in the first two columns of Table 22.2.

3. Importance of Ongoing and Sensitive Communication Through Illness

Encourage parents and convey to the child that it is all right to raise questions about death and what, if anything, happens after death.

- Build an atmosphere of trust and openness.
- Always check what the family's understanding of the illness is before giving new information.
- Take the time to discover the assumptions, values, and priorities of the family.[16,13] Take the opportunity to talk about beliefs, God, an afterlife

Table 22.1 Barriers for Parents Communicating Severe Condition to Child

Barriers and Beliefs	Alternative Views
Unwilling to accept prognosis themselves	It is likely to comfort child to know and not have to imagine what is happening to their body.
Speaking of it will make it happen	Reverse is true. Speaking of it will make what will happen more manageable not more likely. It can clarify misconceptions, allow meaningful communication, and allay some fears.
Signifies giving up hope	It may allow realistic transfer of hope.
Signifies abandoning child	It may allow child to feel less alone.[14]
Child will "give up" if told	Resilience of children is remarkable.
If child is not "giving up," how can parent?	Accepting is not "giving up."
Must trust God will not let their child die	Care needed here. This deep belief may be allowing parents to function. Respect faith but give accurate medical information.
Could not speak of it without crying	OK to show feelings.
Will not know what to say	Parent can share their view of an afterlife or beliefs about what, if anything, happens after death. Psychosocial clinicians can help parents think through what they want to say to the child and how to initiate the conversation.

Table 22.2 Child's Understanding of Death and Signs of Fear of Death During Illness			
Cognitive & Stage Characteristics	**Concept and Causality of Death**	**Emotional State**	**Behaviors/ Actions**
Ages 0–2 years Infant/Toddler			
• Sensory/motor stage • Nonverbal • No concept of time • Reacts to behavior of caregivers and internal sensations	• Separation = death No cognitive concept of causality • Responds physically and emotionally	More related to internal sensations and reactions of caregivers than to fear of death	Response to internal sensations and caregivers' reactions May seem to withdraw as death approaches
Ages 3–5 years Preschooler			
• Preoperational • Magical thinking, blurs fantasy and reality • Egocentricity • Reacts to emotions of caregivers	• Temporary • Reversible • Happens to others (usually) • Confused between separation and death	• Separation anxiety • Fear • Loneliness • Anger	• Cries a lot • Protests • Fights/acts out Hyperactive Withdraws • Denies events • Play shows death fears • Difficulty sleeping
Ages 6–11 years, School Age			
• Concrete operational • Reacts to emotions and behavior of caregivers of others • Limited to increasing concept of time • Interest in biological processes	• Permanent • Irreversible • Universal (almost) • It happens; it can happen again "Did I cause it?" "Did X cause it?" • Personification • Usually can avoid for self perhaps can't avoid it for others What process caused it?	• Sad, anxious • Bodily fears, angry, confused • Guilty	• Crying, insomnia • Nightmares • Withdraws • Interest and questions about death • Denies events • School phobia, fears • Lower grades • Less concentration • Avoids discussion • Fights • Is "too nice"

(continued)

Table 22.2 (Continued)

Cognitive & Stage Characteristics	Concept and Causality of Death	Emotional State	Behaviors/ Actions
Ages 12–17 years—Adolescence			
• Formal operational • Abstract thinking • Fluctuations between cognitive and emotional understanding • Attuned to cognitive and emotional reactions of family and peers • Wish for independence/ control	• Death final • Irreversible • Universal (cognitive) • But I am immortal (emotional) • Questions cause (Who, how, what, why) • Don't want to talk (with you) about cause	• Sad, anxious • Angry, confused • Guilty • Isolated • Alone	• Cries a lot • Impulsive/takes risks • Tantrums, fights • Argues a lot • Insomnia • Avoids family • Seeks out peers Less concentration Lower grades Nightmares • Interest in death • Denies events Withdraws

or how people are remembered, whether there is an afterlife as openings arise through treatment. For example, follow up on a child's earlier questions about death to discover his or her views about what happens after death that can then be referenced should the child become terminally ill. Sometimes, difficult conversations about death are, at least initially, easier to have, with parents and children, if they are made hypothetical and do not occur during a medical crisis.[13]

- A strong alliance built with the patient and family throughout treatment is the foundation that allows "difficult" conversations to occur when cure is not an option—in which family values and priorities can be incorporated into the revised goals of care.[8]

With a parent: "We hope your child will get better, but we are worried the treatments may not work. If that were the case, what would be most important to your child and family?"
With a child: "If you were to get very sick:

- Would you want to be at home or in the hospital?"
- Anything you would really want your parents to know? What about your friends?"

Pre-adolescent children, because of their concreteness, their imagination, and their suggestibility often find it comforting to believe that death is like a journey,[17] at the end of which they will meet familiar people who have died, like grandparents. This may also be an idea encouraged by the child's parents, and it is important to inquire about the family's faith beliefs (see Chapter 26, Spiritual and Religious Considerations).

Adolescents whose religious beliefs and values are likely to be more in flux and who are less suggestible may find this a less comforting idea. Adolescents can be encouraged to develop their own spiritual beliefs, through discussion, reading, and conversations with peers or adults they respect. They can be asked about their fears about death. Some adolescents close to their death may decide to whom they want to leave personally meaningful possessions, may call friends and family to say goodbye, and may even plan their funerals. (See Chapter 30, Integrating Palliative Care.) Some adolescents will speak with their peers, even through social media, not with parents or therapists, about their approaching death. (See Chapter 32, Social Media and Healthcare.) Some adolescents will delay any discussion or acknowledgment of likelihood of death until the last possible moment. Others will refuse to acknowledge it at all.

4. Use of Language

How language is used can make a significant difference in talking about dying.

Some parents may find it more tolerable to use words other than "death" or "dying" to explain to their child what is happening. An Asian father, who previously had refused to discuss the possibility of his son's death, asked the doctors, "Is he getting ready to leave us?" then asked the team to use that phrase when talking with his son.

5. The Importance of Hope

Caregivers must respect the role of hope in communicating with children and families about end-of-life. For some parents, it is hope that sustains them in their daily life with their dying child.[10,11] It allows them to function with their child and not be overcome with grief. One parent described hope "almost as a religious belief."[11] Hope is not incompatible with the knowledge of likely death and must be distinguished from denial. As one wise teenager who had been given a terminal diagnosis remarked, "I need to hope for one thing and prepare for another."

A caregiver must give accurate medical information while feeling out where the family's hopes (which cannot be for cure any more) might now be directed. Helping a family shift their hopes to different objectives like comfort or how a child wants to be remembered is a sensitive and difficult but invaluable task. A caregiver must not fall into the trap of feeling the need to repeat bad news because the parent or patient's hopefulness misleads her. As one parent remarked "I do not need to be told twice that my child will die" and a patient said, "I think she thinks I do not understand because I am choosing to focus on my one-in-a-thousand chance to survive."

6. Expect Fluctuations in Ability to Discuss Death

Expect fluctuations in the capacity to face the idea of the child's death when communicating with the child and with the parent. The Dual Process Model of Grief[18] is helpful in anticipating the death of a child.[19] Both the child and parents are facing the dual tasks of dealing with the child's likely death while continuing to function in the world. Different family members may have different foci, and caregivers should expect—indeed encourage—a back-and-forth quality in conversations, thoughts, and actions, with patient, siblings, and parents. Usually these fluctuations do not constitute a denial of the imminent death, rather, as with hope, it allows the child, parent, and sibling to live their lives in a more positive way until the time of death.

- For parents, these fluctuations may enable them to be with their child in the present.
- Everyday life would be unbearable if they were solely focused on the child's imminent death.
- For a sibling, gradual recognition of the declining health of a brother or sister may be coupled with an increased wish to spend time with friends.
- For the child, a brief excursion into the subject of death may be all that can be tolerated or needed before returning to the reality of his or her current life.
  - A teenager may plan for her funeral one week and, the following week, plan the courses she wants to take next semester.
  - A 12-year-old may talk in quick succession about his likely death, his worry about how his parents will manage, and how his local baseball team is doing.
  - A terminally ill 8-year-old describes how sad a baby dinosaur is because his mother has died, but notes that he will be all right because he will remember his mother and have his father with him. He then ends the intense play session saying, "That's enough of that, now let's play a game."

7. Denial, Avoidance or Indirect Acknowledgment of Imminent Death

There are many reasons that parents of terminally ill children may not discuss with their child their imminent death.

For religious, cultural, and individual reasons:

- Some parents may not believe their child will die.
- Some parents believe they are protecting their children by not telling them.
- Some parents may only acknowledge the death as it is happening, which may preclude saying good-bye explicitly.
- Some children may not believe it.
- Some children may not want to discuss it.
- Some children will want to protect their parents by not discussing it.

Some of these children may say goodbye more indirectly but equally meaningfully:

- An adolescent who talked little about her imminent death bought an after- shave lotion for her boyfriend called "Eternity."
- An 11-year-old boy asked to have an ice cream party for his friends.
- Another child used his "Make a Wish" money to buy presents for his friends and family two days before his death.

For some parents and children, the quality of the patient's life and death, adequate pain management, being at home, or achieving a particular goal may be most important. Also, reminiscing about treasured family moments or the patient's achievements, making a photograph book, expressing love verbally or nonverbally may serve as valuable substitutes for an explicit acknowledgement of a child's imminent death.

8. Expressions of Death-Related Anxiety in Child or Siblings

It is important for parents to feel they have responded to their child's needs for open communication[20] and, therefore, caregivers and parents should be aware of direct and indirect ways in which children may feel and express death related anxiety at different stages and be prepared to follow their lead.

Table 22.2 describes a child's understanding of death by developmental stage and the emotional states and behaviors that may indicate fears about death at each stage.

Babies and toddlers may show different behaviors (increased crying, more difficulty sleeping) as they become sicker, which more likely reflect changes in internal sensations caused by their illness or external events that effect their internal sensations (parents' sadness, anxiety, changes in routine, etc.) than a specific fear of death.

When the child is exhibiting emotions or behavior suggesting fears about dying, either a parent or a psychosocial clinician, with a parent's permission, can gently probe the child's concerns and worries or can speak with the child about what other children in similar situations might worry about. With younger children, an animal puppet expressing similar concerns to the child can be a wonderful therapeutic tool to identify concerns and strategize about solutions. A clinician can offer a safe, open environment for discussion, follow a child's lead, help identify a child's wishes and goals, and encourage parents to do the same.

9. Additional Modes of Communication about Fears of Death

See Chapter 22, Talking to Children and Adolescents about Cancer. Direct or indirect verbal communication is not the only way to probe for feelings related to death. For children, adolescents, and siblings, drawings may be another powerful mode of communication.[21] For some children, poetry or journal writing may be another mode. This artwork or creative writing may be an end in itself or may be a springboard for more direct verbal communication between family members and their clinician.

10. How to Communicate About Death

Ages 2–5

Description of Death

- Body stops working.
- Body does not breathe, talk, or move anymore.
- But spirit may live on in different ways according to family's belief.

Likely Questions and Possible Responses

- Am I going to die?
  - "What are your thoughts about that?
  - "Do you feel you are dying?"
  - 1st relapse: "We don't think so. Doctors have very good treatments to make children with leukemia better even if it has come back once."
  - 3rd relapse: "We hope not, but we cannot be sure. We are giving you medicine to slow it down and see that you are comfortable... Ask us again if you are worried, and we will tell you what is happening."
- What happens when I die?
  - "No one knows exactly."
  - "Some people believe..."
  - Family beliefs... A journey... Heaven... Meet other family members again.
  - "What do you think happens?"
  - "What do you think heaven is like?"
  - If the child believes heaven is a place where one sees people who have already died:
    - "Who might be there waiting for you?"

Ages 6–11

Description of Death

- Add more physical details.
- Elaborate on how spirit may live on if appropriate.

Likely Questions and Possible Responses

- Am I going to die?
  - "What are your thoughts about that?"
  - "Why are you asking now?"
  - If untreatable relapse: "Right now we don't have any more medicine that will cure your cancer. We hope we can slow it down. We can make you as comfortable as possible and help you do what you want to do."
  - "You are not dying right now but it could happen down the road. If you did get that sick, what would you worry about? Would you want to know? What would you want us to know?"
- How will I die?
  - "How are you thinking it might happen?"
  - Give as matter-of-fact, least anxiety provoking, accurate answer as possible.
- What happens after I die/after someone dies?
  - Explore child's own beliefs.
  - Encourage child to expand on them.

Ages 12–17

Description of Death

- Adolescents are likely to be aware of the universality, irreversibility, and finality of death and its physical manifestations.

Likely Questions and Possible Responses

- Am I going to die?
    - "Can you tell me what you have been thinking about this?"
    - "Do you feel like you are dying?"
    - If in a terminal phase: "We are worried. Right now we don't have medicine that can cure your cancer, but we can see that you are comfortable and can do some things that you might want to do."
    - "What do you understand is happening?"
    - "If we can't stop the cancer from growing, you are likely to die—not right now, but at some point…"
    - "If that does happen what is important for us to know about what you would want."
- How will I die?
    - If questions are not asked, caregiver can ask, "Do you have any questions about how it might happen?"
    - Give as matter-of-fact, least anxiety provoking, accurate answer as possible.
- When will I die?
    - (Difficult question to answer.) Encourage more general than specific response such as, "months not years" or "weeks not months." "Would you like us to tell you if we think it is close?"

Do Not Resuscitate (DNR)

Discussions about resuscitation status are frequently delayed until a time of crisis because of the shared reluctance by caregivers and parents to have such discussions. This does not need to be the case.[22] Ideally, as a child nears death, the medical team will gently prepare the parents for how the child might die and describe legal constraints. In the United States, different states have different versions of a Do Not Resuscitate order. It may be called a DNR order, a Do Not Attempt Resuscitation (DNAR) order, a DNAR verification form, an Allow Natural Death (AND) order, or a Comfort Care form. The important fact to know is that if the relevant order has not been signed by the parent, and the child has a medical crisis at home or in the hospital, the responding medical team is legally required to take aggressive and invasive measures to preserve life including performing chest compressions and intubation. Parents often feel that agreeing to a DNR order represents giving up on their child or as if they are signing a death warrant. These misconceptions have to be addressed before many parents are prepared to sign a DNR order.[23]

Steps to consider in discussions with the parents include the following:

- Ascertain that maximizing comfort is a valued treatment goal for parents in their child's end-of-life care.
- Ask if child has indicated directly or indirectly what his or her wishes are as death approaches. For example, "to have no pain" or "to be at home," and, if so, how these wishes might influence parents' decisions about DNR and comfort care.
- Discuss advantages of careful advanced planning that can minimize the child's suffering and avoid parents having to make major decisions during the stress of a medical crisis.

- Check that parents understand the disease process is not reversible.
- Clarify that the Comfort Care form or DNR order need *only* exclude extraordinary measures likely to cause suffering like chest compressions and intubation, whereas measures that can increase comfort temporarily like oxygen will still be provided.
- Explore the idea that aggressive measures may not only inflict suffering but may also lead to maintaining life artificially with minimum quality and no hope of recovery.
- Emphasize that once parents have a Comfort Care form at home, they can put it away and still choose whether to show it to medical personnel in an emergency.
- Clarify that DNR orders can be revoked and changed at any point at parents' request.

Sudden Death

Paced, sensitive, and honest communication about the child's likely death can allow time for preparations, anticipatory grieving, planning for comfort and gradual acknowledgment of inevitability of death,[12]—all ingredients that may help in bereavement. Unfortunately, sometimes a child may have an unexpected, sudden medical complication related either to his illness or to his treatment that may be immediately life-threatening and allow less time for preparing the parents and the child for the likelihood of the child's death. The medical team should still keep in mind the considerations previously described in talking with the family while remembering there may be little time left for any conversations to occur. In this situation, parents are likely to:

- Be in a state of shock.
- Rely upon their basic cultural, spiritual, religious beliefs. (Some families may show increased openness to caregiver suggestions, other families the opposite.)

The Medical team's role in this situation is to:

- Be sensitive to and respectful of the parents and child's emotional reactions.
- Provide accurate medical information to parents.
- Help parents provide physical and emotional comfort to the child.
- Encourage parents to respond to child's' concerns in a way compatible with the family's spiritual values.
- Facilitate conversations about child's likely death at request of parents.
- Encourage parents to keep siblings informed and involved in saying goodbye to their brother or sister directly or indirectly.[23]

Conclusion

Children diagnosed with cancer face an uncertain future and difficult treatments to endure. Their parents and siblings often have to change their lives to accommodate the child's medical and emotional requirements.

Accurate, paced, sensitive, age appropriate communication between the medical team, the parents, patient, and siblings beginning at diagnosis can ease the family's path, help in making difficult decisions, and, if necessary, allow conversations to occur that will help the family face the tragedy of the child's death together and ease the bereavement process afterward.

References

1. EAPC Taskforce Steering Committee. IMPaCCT: Standards for pediatric palliative care in Europe. *Eur J Palliat Care.* 2007;14(3):109–114.
2. Knapp C, Madden V, Fowler Kerry S. *Pediatric Palliative Care: Global Perspectives.* London, New York: Springer; 2012.
3. Mitchell JL. Cross-cultural issues in the disclosure of cancer. *Cancer Pract.* 1998;6(3):153–160.
4. Parsons SK, Saiki-Craighill S et al. Telling children and adolescents about their cancer diagnosis, cross cultural comparisons in the US and Japan. *Psycho-oncol.* 2007;16(1): 60–80.
5. Oppenheim D, Brugieres L, Corradini L, Vivant F, Hartmann O. An ethics dilemma: when parents and doctors disagree on the best treatment for the child. *Bulletin Du Cancer.* 2004;91(9):735–738.
6. Ridgway D. Court-mediated disputes between physicians and families over the medical care of children. *Arch. Pediatr. Adolesc. Med.* 2004;158(9):891–896.
7. Gupta VB, Willert J, Pian M et al. When disclosing a serious diagnosis to a minor conflicts with family values. *J Dev Behav Pediatr.* 2008;29(3):231
8. Evan E, Cohen H. Child relationships. In Wolfe J, Hinds PS, Sourkes BM. *Textbook of Interdisciplinary Pediatric Palliative Care.* Philadelphia, PA: Elsevier; 2011.
9. Masera G, Spinetta JJ, Jankovic M, et al. Guidelines for assistance to terminally ill children with cancer: a report of the SIOP Working Committee on psychosocial issues in pediatric oncology. *Med Pediatr Oncol.* 1999;32(1):44–48.
10. Summer LH. Pediatric hospice and palliative care. In Ferrell BR, Coyle N, eds., *Oxford Textbook of Palliative Nursing.* 3rd ed. New York, NY: Oxford University Press; 2010; 997–1017.
11. O'Shea, ER., Bennett Kanarek, R. Understanding pediatric palliative care—what it is and what it should be. *J Pediatr. Oncol Nurs.* 2013; 30(1):34–44.
12. Kane J, Joselow M, Duncan J. Understanding illness experience and providing anticipatory guidance. In Wolfe J, Hinds PS, Sourkes BM. Textbook of Interdisciplinary Pediatric Palliative Care. Philadelphia, PA: Elsevier; 2011.
13. Mack JW, Hinds, PS. Practical aspects of communication. In Wolfe J, Hinds P, Sourkes B, eds.,Textbook of Interdisciplinary Pediatric Palliative Care. Philadelphia, PA: Elsevier Saunders; 2011; 179–189.
14 Beale EA, Baile WF, Aaron J. Silence is not golden: communicating with children dying from cancer. *J Clinical Oncol.* 2005; 23:3629–3636.
15. Linnard-Palmer L. *When Parents Say No: Religious and Cultural Influences on Pediatric Healthcare Treatment.* Indianopolis: Sigma Theta Tau International; 2006.

16. Levetown M. Communicating with children and families: from every-day interactions to skill in conveying distressing information. *Pediatrics.* 2008;121, e1441–e1460. doi:10.1542/peds.2008-0565

17. Jankovic M, Spinetta JJ, Masera G, et al. Communicating with the dying child: an invitation to listening—A report of the SIOP Working Committee on psychosocial issues in pediatric oncology. *Pediatr Blood Cancer.* 2008;50(5):1087–1088.

18. Stroebe MS, Schut H. Models of coping with bereavement: A review. In: Stroebe MS, Hansson RO, Stroebe W, Schut H, eds., *Handbook of Bereavement Research: Consequences, Coping and Care.* Washington, DC: American Psychological Association; 2001:375–404.

19. Breyer J, Sanfeliz A, Cieurzo, CE, Meyer, EA. Loss and grief. In: Brown RT, ed., Comprehensive Handbook of Childhood Cancer and Sickle Cell Disease: A Biopsychosocial Approach. New York, NY: Oxford University Press; 2006:358–380.

20. Kreichbergs U, Valdimarsdóttir U, Onelöv E, Henter J, Steineck G. Talking about death with children who have severe malignant disease. *N Engl J Med.* 2004;351(12):1175–1186.

21. Muriel A, Case C, Sourkes B. Children's voices: the experience of patients and their siblings. In Wolfe J, Hinds P, Sourkes B, eds.,*Textbook of Interdisciplinary Pediatric Palliative Care* Philadelphia, PA: Elsevier Saunders; 2011: 179–189.

21. Zinner SE. The use of pediatric advanced directives—a tool for palliative care physicians. *Am J Hosp Palliat Med.* 2009;25(6):427–430.

22. Baker J. Resuscitation. In Wolfe J, Hinds PS, Sourkes BM. *Textbook of inter-disciplinary pediatric palliative care.* Philadelphia, PA: Elsevier Saunders; 2011.

23. Davies B. *Shadows in the Sun: The Experiences of Sibling Bereavement in Childhood.* Philadelphia, PA: Brunner/Mazel; 1999.

Chapter 23

Coping with Pediatric Cancer

Mary Jo Kupst and Andrea Farkas Patenaude

Psychosocial care in pediatric oncology often involves assessment of the coping skills of a patient or family member and provision of interventions to ensure appropriate support. Coping may be defined as the cognitive and behavioral efforts to manage the demands and situations which are appraised as a challenge or a threat[1] These are voluntary efforts as opposed to involuntary reactions to stress.[2] (See Chapter 19, Psychotherapeutic Interventions, and Chapter 24, Impact of Cancer on Family and Siblings.)

Coping and resilience are relatively stable concepts. The field has recently expanded, however, with more studies of coping in non-Western populations[3,4] and more studies of interventional approaches to support positive coping. Increased attention has been drawn to factors such as gender, socioeconomic status[5] or being a "lone" or single parent[6] as affecting coping. Technological advances can make it easier to deliver and/or evaluate interventions related to coping in children with cancer or family members.[7] Regardless of whether these methods are utilized, repeated assessment of coping, first at diagnosis and later at least at transitional points in the child's care, is essential to determining needed psychosocial and other services.

It is challenging to fully evaluate how children with cancer and their parents cope with the stresses of the child's diagnosis and treatment. It is each parent's worst nightmare to have a child who has cancer and, thus, initially at least, parents feel overwhelmed and scared. How they respond and deal with the stresses of pediatric cancer can vary widely, influenced by personality, prior experiences, family, or cultural factors. To understand coping, it is important to consider what parents and children must "cope with" in order to be effective in helping them manage the stressors involved in the diagnosis and treatment of pediatric cancer.

Coping Tasks

Diagnosis and Early Treatment

Parent Tasks

- Assimilate a large amount of medical and treatment information.
- Make treatment decisions quickly.

- Manage emotional reactions—for example, shock, feeling overwhelmed, anxiety, fear about child possibly dying from cancer or cancer treatment.
- Learn practical tasks related to hospital and clinic routines.
- Balance hospital stays and visits with demands of home, family, work, school.
- Deal with changes in relationships, financial stresses, communication issues.
- Sometimes may need to deal with their own or spouse's medical or mental health conditions, which complicate their own responses.
- Support child who may be (a) undergoing painful or frightening procedures, (b) having to take medicines with very unpleasant side effects, (c) feeling moody or sad, uncooperative, angry or aggressive. (d) cognitively altered from normal state.
- Obtain and use available support (family, social, hospital).

Early Patient Tasks

- Deal with painful or distressing procedures (lumbar punctures, bone marrow aspirations, needle sticks).
- Cope with physical symptoms and side effects (nausea, vomiting, fatigue).
- Adjust to interruptions of school, social life, activities.
- Meet new staff, learn about and adjust to hospital environment, new medical routines.
- Manage emotional reactions to diagnosis and treatment, for example, anxiety, sadness, anger.
- Cope with separation from parents, siblings, and peers and feelings of loneliness when hospitalized.

Middle to Later Treatment

Parent Tasks

- Manage emotional reactions, which may increase as families settle into routine visits, hospitalizations, and have more time to think and process what they have experienced.
- Deal with fatigue as demands on time continue.
- Seek and utilize available supports.
- Possibly return to work and balance work and home and hospital-based demands, especially challenging because of ups and downs of child's health.

Patient Tasks

- Deal with side effects of treatment (physical changes, temporary and permanent).
- Adhere to treatment regimen.
- Try to maintain academics, work, friendships, communication with close friends and relatives.

Ending Treatment

Parent and Patient Tasks

- Manage conflicting emotional reactions: happy that treatment is over, but loss of "safety net" of treatment and support of cancer team.

- Reorganizing life without clinic and hospital schedules.
- Child may need to make adjustment to be seen as and treated as a healthy child rather than a "cancer patient"; loss of "special status."
- Siblings may increase demands on parents as ill child's routine normalizes.

Survivorship

Parent and Patient Tasks

- Acknowledge concern over relapse or recurrence but maintain optimism.
- Learn to live beyond cancer—increased ability to focus on the future and make future life plans.

Parents: Change focus from this child to more inclusion of other children, family, responsibilities.

Child and Adolescent Tasks

- Adhere to continued medical follow-up: Attend late effects/long-term follow-up clinic.
- Deal with late effects of treatment.
- Regularly agree to assessment of neurocognitive and psychosocial functioning; seek treatment for distress, if needed.
- If needed, receive special school accommodations for school problems secondary to late effects and continuing nononcologic medical and cognitive problems.
- Undergo vocational or educational counseling, if needed.
- Seek additional medical subspecialist for consultation and treatment.
- Learn to make healthy behavior and lifestyle choices.
- Learn how to inform new friends about cancer history.

Relapse or Recurrence

Parent and Patient Tasks

- Manage emotional reactions that are sometimes even more intense than at diagnosis.
- Learn and begin new routine of treatment, medications, procedures.
- Manage change in balance among demands from hospital, home, work, school.
- Utilize available psychosocial supports.
- Maintain optimism.

Dying and Death

- Accept change in focus and decisions about moving child from active treatment to palliative care.
- Deal with emotional reactions, for example, helplessness, anger, anticipatory grief about loss.
- Involve siblings, grandparents, and friends in meaningful ways in saying their goodbyes to the child.
- Make decisions about pragmatic matters, for example, home versus hospital; code versus no-code, funeral arrangements with the patient, if possible.
- Utilize available support.

Coping Strategies

In stressful situations, people tend to use ways of coping that have worked for them in the past. Sometimes they may need help in learning or using different strategies because old ways of coping no longer work. There are many ways to cope and, depending on the situation, people may use different strategies over the course of the child's disease and treatment.[8]

Assessment of a Child's or Family's Coping

Assessment of Current Coping Tasks

- What is being asked of the person in this moment?
- How does the person appraise the stressor?
- Is the threat changeable or not?
- Are there misunderstandings or distortions in the person's view of what is required that can be corrected to reduce distress?
- How hopeful is the person about the outcome of the present treatment or other threat?
- What emotional or social resources does the person have?
- What does the person do to try to live with the threat?
- Variables that have been found to affect coping include developmental level, coping style (active or passive), changing aspects of the situation, coping of other family members, and the presence or absence of good social support.

Types of Coping Strategies

- **Outer-directed coping** (behavioral, primary control, problem-focused "approach" strategies): Generally more likely to be helpful when the situation can be changed, for example, when confronting a stressor. Problem-focused coping, including information-seeking and planful problem-solving, may be more helpful later and after treatment, as focus shifts beyond the immediate demands of treatment.
- **Inner-directed coping** (cognitive, secondary control, emotion-focused, or avoidant): Attempts to change the way one attends to or interprets a stressor; helpful if a situation can't be changed, for example, denial, avoidance, positive reappraisal. Avoidance/distancing, may be helpful early in treatment, especially in coping with procedures such as lumbar punctures and bone marrow aspirations. There is also some evidence that the ability to manage emotional responses is related to better overall adjustment in children and adolescents.[2]

Information Preference

Another aspect of coping involves individuals' preferences for receiving a large amount of medical information versus not wanting to know any more than is minimally essential. Those who seek detailed information are sometimes referred to as "monitors," while those who prefer to avoid anything but the most basic facts are called "blunters."[4] It can be helpful to ask both parents and older children and adolescents how much information they prefer to be given, from whom they prefer to receive medical information, and whether they prefer information to be provided verbally, in written form, or both ways. A challenge for parents and staff is that "monitors," although wanting more medical information, may be quite distressed by it and may require considerable support from psychosocial staff in dealing with what they learn. Psychosocial staff may also be useful in making sure that "blunters," while wishing to avoid detailed medical information, have sufficient information to make informed decisions about the child's status and medical options.

Coping—General Points

- Some people find it helpful to talk about their feelings and seek outside support or help; others prefer to keep feelings private and to work on them individually.
- Some cultures value open discussion of emotions, whereas while others value more self-contained behavior. No one way is superior.
- Knowledge of having survived past adversity can help a family dealing with the challenges of cancer. Families with few previous problems of major significance may be unprepared for adapting to a "crisis mode" and may find it more difficult to believe that they will be able to re-establish emotional equilibrium.
- Coping is a process. How well a child or family copes should not be judged based on a single assessment but on the success they achieve over time in dealing with the many stressful situations that arise in pediatric cancer treatment.
- Within a family, when one person's ways of coping changes, it can be hard for others to adjust. A father may be surprised, for example, when his wife/partner has difficulty with parenting tasks that have previously been easy for her. As he takes on more active parenting roles to try to compensate, their relationship may become a bit contentious as they renegotiate their roles. Conversely, a mother who previously allowed her husband to make all major decisions may develop more independence and confidence through dealing directly with hospital staff. This can cause changes in their relationship that may be difficult for some couples to integrate.
- In some families, parents take turns being the "strong" one (whatever that means in the context of that family) and the other is allowed to rest and be spared difficult conversations or decisions for a period of time.
- Coping skills change over time. Parents who are highly distressed often become more accepting, able to listen to the treatment plan and do what is necessary for their child's treatment. Conversely, parents or children who have coped well initially may encounter situations in which something (not necessarily major) can overburden their coping abilities. They may need intervention to learn new strategies when preferred methods don't work.
- Parents or children may hear and respond to information differently than it was intended by members of the team. Also, parents and patients may react very differently and show different emotions to various members of the healthcare team.

- Frequent communication among staff is critical to be sure the staff 's view of the parents' strengths and vulnerabilities are accurate and that patient and family needs are communicated to relevant staff members.
- Regular care conferences among oncology team members and other disciplines caring for the child and family are useful for facilitating better communication.
- Consider other stressors that parents or children may bring with them besides those brought on by the child's cancer.
- Consultation with a mental health professional can be helpful to the family and team for additional assessment of how the child and parents are coping.

Helping Parents of Children and Adolescents with Cancer

Parents' Responses

- Most parents have coping strategies that have worked for them under other circumstances and will tend to rely on these familiar approaches.
- Some parents believe they should be stoic and not show their emotions, especially in the presence of their child. Staff may worry that these parents don't understand the severity of what is happening (e.g. that they are in "denial") or that they might be distant from their child. However, this behavior may be adaptive as parents may need to avoid fully experiencing their emotions in order to focus on necessary tasks related their child's treatment.
- Some parents are persistently inconsolable, which can complicate the discussions with the team about what is to happen next. The parent may need more time to process the information and may also benefit from consultation with a psychosocial staff member who can help unravel the factors contributing to the parent's overwhelming distress.
- Parents may also respond with anger to the diagnosis, sometimes directing that anger at the hospital or staff. These parents can benefit first and foremost from staff efforts to build positive relationships with the family and encouraging discussion about their concerns and their feelings of helplessness and anger. It often takes time to form these connections and for these parents to trust and accept the help offered.

Interventions for the Parents at Diagnosis

See Chapter 19, Psychotherapeutic Interventions, and Chapter 24, Impact of Cancer on Family and Siblings. Much psychosocial research has indicated the importance of early assessment and intervention with parents. Discussions with mental health professionals as part of the oncology team should be conducted as soon as possible after diagnosis. In centers in which these professionals are not part of the oncology program, referrals should be made to mental health professionals with expertise in psychological issues related to pediatric conditions.

The goal is to help parents tolerate their distress while working to understand the implications of the child's illness and treatment, to support the ill child, and communicate to and comfort healthy siblings and to make necessary arrangements for the care of all family members.

Interventions may include hospital-based parents' groups or referral to community groups like Candle lighters for parents of children with cancer. There have been several empirically supported intervention programs for parents, for example, Kazak et al., 2007,[10] Sahler et al.,[11] which can also serve as examples of ways to help parents early in treatment.

Helping Children and Adolescents Cope with Cancer

See Chapter 19, Psychotherapeutic Interventions, Chapter 22, Talking to Children and Adolescents about Cancer, and Chapter 24, Impact of Cancer on Family and Siblings.

Children's Responses

Like parents, children vary in the ways they cope with the news that they have cancer and need medical treatment. Responses vary depending on age, developmental level, previous experiences, and personality of the child. Recent research[2] indicates that level of cognitive functioning is also a strong determinant of the ability to process and think through a situation and ways to deal with it. Initial strategies may include withdrawal, wishful thinking, becoming very sad or worried, and/or lashing out angrily. Some children try to spare showing their parents their own upset in such situations and may benefit from having someone outside the family to talk to.

Interventions for the Child at Diagnosis

Helping a child better comprehend what having cancer means and how it will affect his or her daily life, and hearing messages of hope through treatment (when appropriate) can be helpful.

- It is important to provide early interventions to help with procedural distress, pain, and anxiety during treatment.
- Siblings may also need help in coping with feelings, as they often feel left out.

It is helpful to talk with children and adolescents to find out their preferred ways of coping:

- "Are you someone who likes to know everything about what's going to happen and when it will happen—the big picture? Or are you someone who likes to know a little bit at a time or, say, just before you need your blood taken, for example?"
- "Does it help you to talk about things that are hard or are on your mind or are you someone who wants to work things out on your own?"

- "Can your friends help you with your feelings or with problems or do you usually try to deal with your feelings yourself?"
- "What is the hardest thing for you right now?"
  - Where possible, help the child/adolescent achieve a sense of control.
    - Within limits, allow some choice on when to take medications, do mouth care, take a bath, etc.
    - Respect the need for avoidance/withdrawal especially during procedures.
  - Provide opportunity for child/adolescent to talk about ways to cope.
  - For adolescents, increase social support.
    - Offer availability of adolescent group if it exists, opportunities to keep up with friends, class connection through the Internet, introduction to other adolescents who have completed treatment.
  - Provide opportunity for teaching relaxation/stress reduction strategies to children and adolescents early in treatment, especially for procedural distress. See Table 23.1.

Research Measures

The following are measures that are frequently used in coping research. Self-report coping measures reveal preferred coping strategies or disposition, but they do not necessarily reflect actual coping under the extreme stresses of pediatric cancer. Observed behavior ratings provide a picture of actual behavior but require trained observers. These may be more appropriate in specific situations, for example, patients experiencing pain, patients undergoing procedures, and work with very young children. It is advisable when selecting a particular coping measure to read the manual and the literature and to consider whether you want self-report or observed behavior ratings. It is also important to remember that coping is a process and one-time assessments may not be accurate indicators of how children or family members cope over time.

Self-Report Coping Measures

ACOPE[13]—Adolescent coping style and behavior: Conceptualization and measurement. This 54-item scale assesses self-reported coping strategies of adolescents (ages 12–18) with 12 factors, for example, Ventilating feelings, Seeking diversions, Developing self-reliance and optimism. It can be completed in 30 minutes. It is available in Arabic, English, French, German, Spanish, and Swedish.

Brief COPE[14]—This tool for assessing coping strategies can be completed in 20–30 minutes. Available in Chinese, English, French, Italian, and Spanish. The author grants permission to translate it into other languages.

Kidcope[15]—This process measure of coping has two forms, one for younger children (ages 7–12) and one for adolescents (ages 13–18). Both frequency and effectiveness of 10 strategies—for example, problem-solving, social support, emotional regulation—are rated, usually related to a

Table 23.1 Issues in Coping Relative to Developmental Level*	
Emotional and Behavioral Issues	**Possible Interventions**
Very Young Children	
• Fears of separation from parents • Painful or frightening medical procedures • Restrictions in play, environmental exploration • Temporary regression in developmental milestones • Yelling, crying, screaming reactions; attempts to control, refusal, tantrums, clinging, aggression, withdrawal	• Parental presence • Distraction techniques • Child-Life interventions • Normalizing the child's behavior for parents • Help parents to learn supportive yet appropriate responses; give control where possible to child
School-age Children	
• Disruption of school • Loss of peer interactions, activities • Greater understanding of seriousness of condition • More seeking emotional and social support; may still show anger, sadness over losses	• Encourage continuation of schoolwork either home-bound or return to school • Encourage continuation of contacts through e-mail, phone, visits/activities if possible • Provide information, discuss, revisit • Supportive counseling from psychosocial staff
Adolescents	
• Disruption of school, peer activities • Dependence versus independence • Intense emotional reactions to situations • Increased use of social support strategies • More focus on existential/identity issues; Humor, self-talk, diversion, positive reappraisal; But also risk-taking behavior	• Help with return to school • Family intervention to help with potential conflicts • Normalize but may need assessment for further psychological intervention • Encourage involvement in social activities including peer support groups • Provide opportunities for discussion with staff, peers, family
Young Adults	
• Similar to adolescents in coping; May need to postpone or interrupt school, work, relationships, marriage • More concern with long-term effects, e.g. fertility, career, financial issues • Complications in roles of parent versus close friend or spouse	• Provide opportunities to meet other young adults with similar conditions • Provide medical information; recommendations, access to specialists • Provide opportunities for discussion, support

* Cf. National Institutes of Health (NIH) table on pediatric development and chronic illness.[12]

stressor determined by the child or adolescent. It can be completed in 10–15 minutes. It is available in English, German, and Spanish.

The Monitoring/Blunting Style Scale[16] (Adolescent or parent)—This scale utilizes 4 hypothetical threat-evoking scenarios to identify individuals in terms of "their distinctive attentional styles." Three scores can be generated, a Monitoring score (0–16), a Blunting score (0–16) and a total difference Score (–16 to +16). It can be completed in 20 minutes and is available in Chinese, Dutch, English, French, German, Hebrew, and Spanish.

Responses to Stress Questionnaire[17] (Adolescents). This scale contains 57 items on three dimensions—voluntary-involuntary responses, engagement-disengagement, primary-secondary control. It is available in English (some versions in Spanish and Chinese).

Ways of Coping[18] (Adolescent or Parent)—This questionnaire measures coping processes— for example, confrontive coping, seeking social support—and can be completed in 10–20 minutes. It is available in Chinese, Dutch, English, French, German, Hebrew, Japanese, Spanish, and Swedish.

References

1. Lazarus RS. *Emotion and Adaptation*. New York, NY: Oxford University Press; 1991.
2. Compas, BE, Jaser, SS., Dunn, MJ, Rodriguez, EM. Coping with chronic illness in childhood and adolescence. *Ann Rev Clin Psychol*. 2012;8:455–480.
3. Banerjee AT, Watt L, Gulati S, et al. Cultural beliefs and coping strategies related to childhood cancer: The perceptions of South Asian immigrant parents in Canada. *J Pediatr Oncol Nurs*. 2011;28:169–178.
4. Li HC, Chung OK, Ho KY, Chiu SY, Lopez V. Coping strategies used by children hospitalized with cancer: an exploratory study. *Psycho-Oncol*. 2011;20(9):969–976j.
5. Gage-Bouchard EA, Devine KA, Heckler CE. The relationship between socio-demographic characteristics, family environment, and caregiver coping in families of children with cancer. *J Clin Psychol Med Settings*. 2013;20(4):478–487.
6. Wiener, L, Pao M, Battles H, et al. Socio-environmental factors associated with long parenting chronically ill children. *Children's Health Care*. in press.
7. Judge Santacroce S, Asmus K, Kadan-Lottick N, Grey M. Feasibility and preliminary outcomes from a pilot study of coping skills training for adolescent-young adult survivors of childhood cancer and their parents. *J Pediatr Oncol Nurs*. 2010 Jan–Feb;27(1):10–20. doi: 10.1177/1043454209340325.
8. Hoekstra-Weebers, JE, Wijnberg-Williams BJ, Jaspers JP, Kamps WA, Wiel, HB. Coping and its effect on psychological distress of parents of pediatric cancer patients: a longitudinal prospective study. *Psycho-oncol*. 2012;21(8):903–911.
9. Miller SM. Monitoring versus blunting styles of coping with cancer influence the information patients want and need about their disease. Implications for cancer screening and management. *Cancer*. 1995;76(2):167–177.
10. Kazak AE, Rourke MT, Alderfer MA, Pai A, Reilly AF, Meadows AT. Evidence-based assessment, intervention and psychosocial care in pediatric oncology: a blueprint for comprehensive services across treatment. *J Pediatr Psychol*. 2007;2(9):1099–1110.

11. Sahler, OJ, Dolgin MJ, Phipps S, et al. Specificity of problem-solving skills training in mothers of children newly diagnosed with cancer: results of a multi-site randomized trial. *J Clin Oncol.* 2013;31(10):1329–1335.

12. Kupst MJ, Bingen K. Stress and coping in the pediatric cancer experience. In Brown RT, ed., *Comprehensive Handbook of Childhood Cancer and Sickle Cell Disease: A Biopsychosocial Approach.* New York, NY: Oxford University Press; 2006: 35–52.

13. Patterson JM, McCubbin HI. Adolescent coping style and behavior: Conceptualization and measurement. *J Adolesc.* 1987;10(2):163–186.

14. Carver, CS. You want to measure coping but your protocol's too long: consider the Brief COPE. *Int J Behav Med.* 1997;4:92–100.

15. Spirito A, Stark LJ, Williams C. Development of a brief checklist to assess coping in pediatric patients. *J Pediatr Psychol.* 1988;13:555–574.

16. Miller, SM. Monitoring and blunting: Validation of a questionnaire to assess styles of information under threat. *J Pers Soc Psychol.* 1987;52(2):345–353.

17. Connor-Smith, JK, Compas, BE, Wadsworth, ME, Thomsen, AH, Saltzman, H. Responses to stress in adolescence: Measurement of coping and involuntary responses to stress. *J Cons Clin Psychol.* 2000;68:976–992.

18. Folkman S, Lazarus RS. *Manual for the Ways of Coping Questionnaire.* Palo Alto, CA: Consulting Psychologists Press; 1988.

Further Reading

Aldridge AA, Roesch SC. Coping and adjustment in children with cancer: A meta-analytic study. *J Behav Med.* 2007;30(2):115–129.

Folkman, S, Moskowitz, JT. Coping: pitfalls and promise. *Ann Rev Psychol.* 2004;55:745–774.

Kupst MJ, Bingen K. Stress and coping in the pediatric cancer experience. In Brown RT, ed., *Comprehensive Handbook of Childhood Cancer and Sickle Cell Disease: A Biopsychosocial Approach.* New York, NY: Oxford University Press; 2006: 35–52.

Patenaude AF, Kupst MJ. Psychosocial functioning in pediatric cancer. *J Pediatr Psychol.* 2005;30(1):9–27.

Chapter 24

Impact of Cancer on Family and Siblings

Avi Madan-Swain and Pamela S. Hinds

A child's cancer diagnosis reverberates throughout the family system leaving no member untouched. The child's adjustment to the cancer diagnosis is dependent on personal characteristics and is influenced by family composition and communication, premorbid psychiatric difficulties, adjustment of family members, and available family and community resources. Additionally, the family's cultural context directly influences how they define and manage their child's diagnosis and medical care. Over the course of the cancer experience and across cultures, the adaptive family develops a cognitive understanding of the disease and treatment demands, is able to manage emotional reactions to the disease and treatment and their implications, and uses available resources to meet its changing situational needs.[1–6]

The majority of families adapt competently to the extraordinary stress associated with learning that one's child has cancer, drawing on their own strengths and social support, and by ultimately finding meaning and purpose in their cancer experience. Although almost all families benefit from some psychosocial assistance, approximately one-fourth to one-third of families demonstrate significant psychosocial difficulties at some point in the course of treatment that call for tailored interventions.[4,6–7]

Predictors of Positive Family Adaptation[1–6]

- Absence of premorbid psychopathology.
- Family cohesion and flexibility.
- Ability to reorganize and balance demands of the illness with family needs and responsibilities.
- Access to economic resources.
- Clear family boundaries.
- Open and effective communication.
- Active coping.
- Strong spiritual belief system.
- Seeking social support from extended family, church, work place, community.

Predictors of Negative Family Psychosocial Response

- Lone or single parent/caregiver.
- Conflicted family relationships.
- Marital or couple discord.
- Financial difficulties (e.g., employment, transportation, child care, and insurance problems).
- Fixed personal beliefs that include blame for self or others related to the cancer experience (see Chapter 26, Spiritual and Religious Considerations).
- Language barriers or cultural differences (between clinicians and patients/families).
- No or very minimal social support.

(See Chapter 25, Special Considerations in Working with Families.)

Ensuring Appropriate Delivery of Services

In an ideal world, families of children would have ready access to a team of professionals who could provide a range of services across the entire course of treatment. Indeed, each of the major behavioral health profession fields (e.g. social work, psychology, psychiatry and nursing) have made important contributions to pediatric cancer care. In addition, child-life specialists, art and music therapists, and chaplains are also key members of the psychosocial team. Representatives of all these disciplines are usually available within children's hospitals, or by referral to providers in the community. However, the number of staff available and the organization and access to services varies. Unfortunately, not all the resources noted in this chapter are available at all hospitals. Recent reports from the Institute of Medicine advocate for cancer-care settings to have mechanisms in place to ensure appropriate delivery of psychosocial services. From the time a child/family enters a cancer-care system, members of the psychosocial team (e.g., social work, psychologist, child psychiatrist, nurse, child life specialist, chaplain) are notified, so ideally the following steps can occur:

- Systematic psychosocial evaluation of the family completed by caregivers as well as psychosocial team members. Empirically based measures include the Distress Thermometer[8] and the Psychosocial Assessment Tool (PAT).[9] Child assessment is also recommended.
- Psychosocial interdisciplinary team members (e.g., social work, child life specialist, chaplain, psychologist) complete structured assessments to identify both family risk and resilience or protective factors.
- During psychosocial team staffing, assessment information from team members as well as from the family is discussed, care goals outlined, and referrals made to link the family, as needed, with available resources/services.

- Individually tailored psychosocial care plans are implemented and periodically reviewed to re-assess adaptation, interventions provided, and need for additional services.
- When possible, newly diagnosed families are paired with parent mentors to help prepare them for their child's cancer journey, including how to understand and interpret some cancer-related experiences.
- Educational material are made available to families in a variety of modalities (e.g., written, videos, online, and CD's) to accommodate for differences in learning/coping styles and educational levels.
- Efforts to pair non-English-speaking families with same-language interpreters to increase comfort.
- Ongoing verbal and written communication between the medical and psychosocial team members should occur throughout treatment regarding child/family adjustment.

The cancer experience may include many transitions (diagnosis and remission, survivorship, or end-of-life and bereavement), each having its own challenges that require adjustments and adaptations on the part of the child and the family. In this chapter, we describe clinical interventions found to be helpful at the different points of transition to parents and siblings who are experiencing cancer of a child/sibling.

Diagnosis/Remission

Parents describe the diagnosis of cancer as a complicated and stressful period. The hallmark of the initial treatment phase is disrupted family life for all family members as the cancer diagnosis and initial phases of treatment become the consuming focus.[7,10–16] Families must learn the complexities of treatment and its side effects, the rationale governing clinical trials, and master medical terminology. Limited English proficiency or low education level can be impediments to learning; an interpreter may be needed to help families effectively overcome the language barrier. Additionally, culture influences healthcare beliefs, practices, healthcare utilization, adherence, and the family's communication and transactions with the clinical-care team, so the team members need to be culturally sensitive and enquire into these areas. (See Chapter 31, Caring for International Patients.) See Table 24.1.

Remission

Treatment is a protracted period lasting from months to years. Most children experience remission or a favorable response to the treatment resulting in a period of illness stabilization. Although this is a relief, parents often remain fearful of the possibility of relapse. Families tend to adapt to the chronicity of cancer but financial considerations and caregiver strain often emerge. During this same period, children and adolescents frequently have to be isolated from peers because of compromised immune systems. They may also miss a substantial amount of school due to their treatment regimen or treatment-related side effects. Please refer to the technology intervention described earlier in "Parental Monitoring of the Well-Sibling Response" to prevent social isolation of the ill child during this time by connecting the ill child, through technology, to the classroom and with caring others in a variety of settings. See Table 24.2.

Table 24.1 Diagnosis and Initial Treatment Interventions for Parents, the Ill Child and Well Siblings

Family Psychosocial Issue	Suggested Clinical Intervention
Parents are shocked by the diagnosis, overwhelmed by the detailed treatment information and must make often urgent treatment decisions	• Be factual and empathic regarding diagnosis and treatment; provide written and verbal information and online materials; support parent requests for discussion of information obtained from the Internet or their own reading; support value of second opinions if parents raise the issue; encourage them to discuss with extended family and friends; expect to repeat treatment information, schedule additional meetings as needed.
Clinicians need to anticipate that treatment consent conferences can evoke high levels of distress and likely contain information upsetting or confusing to family members:	• Include a psychosocial team member in consent conferences to process information with family and inform medical team of relevant issues/ concerns. • If using interpreters with non-English-speaking families, collaborate with the interpreters to identify key treatment concepts that need to be reinforced. When possible, use the same interpreters. Be mindful not to rely on a sibling to serve as the interpreter. • Be knowledgeable about cultural norms and convey respect for family values to further facilitate their understanding of informed consent content. • Encourage parents to ask questions BUT be sensitive to cultural differences in communication styles. For example, "respecto" among some Latino families could be diminished when asking parents if they "have any questions." A more effective method is to prompt them for their views or opinions on a particular issue. (See Chapter 31, Caring for International Patients). • Help family understand the distinction between randomized clinical trial (RCT) and standard treatment, the voluntary nature of research and the right to withdraw. • Encourage caregivers to write their questions down. • Discuss a plan for sharing information with other family members including siblings—who will do the sharing, how much is to be communicated depending on the age of the siblings, etc.
Parents likely lack information on psychosocial aspects of childhood cancer (See Chapter 6, Tumors of the Central Nervous System, and Chapter 18, Cognitive Sequelae).	• Introduce family to psychosocial team members and describe their roles. • Provide family with written and verbal material on hospital and other resources. • Discuss common psychosocial responses and invite discussion of their feelings.

(continued)

Table 24.1 (Continued)

Family Psychosocial Issue	Suggested Clinical Intervention
	• Identify pressing concrete needs (e.g., transportation, insurance, lodging), ability of caregivers to comprehend and process information, and stressors in past year. Construct a psychosocial care plan. • Encourage parents to advocate for themselves and their child. • If child's medical treatment includes central nervous system treatment (i.e., brain tumor, leukemia), refer for baseline neuropsychological evaluation if testing materials are language-appropriate for the ill child. Neurocognitive screening may also be recommended for children prior to bone marrow transplantation. (See Chapter 18, Cognitive Sequelae.)
Parental need to be able to manage their own emotional responses (e.g., may experience increased symptoms of depression, anxiety, sleep disturbance and uncertainty about the prognosis)	• Identify and normalize common responses and provide empathy. • Educate parents regarding children's developmentally appropriate responses to treatment. • Assess each individual's coping styles and strategies; they may differ among family members (e.g., information seeking versus avoidant). Encourage use of adaptive coping for heightened distress. If a seeming match with parent coping style, consider teaching problem-solving skills, a six-step process that begins with establishing a relationship with the parent, explaining the purpose of the problem-solving strategies, having the parent identify a specific problem, doing the problem analysis together, asking the parent to carry out the plan to address the problem, and then following up.[17–18] • Remind parents that they have to take care of themselves (i.e., time to rest, exercise, eat as best they can) in order to be able to care for their child. • Ask if they would like to be introduced to families with children who have a similar diagnosis or participate in mentoring program. • Prepare parents for a possible delay in their own emotional reactions to the diagnosis. • Help family members identify areas in which control can be exercised (visitors to the home or hospital room) and areas in which they will have shared (nutrition) or little (cancer backbone therapy) control. • Alert couples to the likelihood that they may cope differently from each other during their child's illness and its treatment.

(continued)

Table 24.1 (Continued)

Family Psychosocial Issue	Suggested Clinical Intervention
Parental seeking of assurances that their child will survive and searching for meaning in the cancer	• Parents may ask, "(i.e., "*Why did this happen to me?*" or "*What caused my child to have cancer?*"). Family members looking for a cause may blame themselves or others or question their faith. • Be sensitive to cultural norms and a family's belief systems. • Encourage family members to meet with their own minister or hospital chaplain to discuss their feelings and further explore specific religious and/or cultural beliefs that offer explanation and meaning. (See Chapter 25, Spiritual and Religious Considerations.)
Strained family relationships (i.e., marital; parent-child, etc.):• Marital/ couple strain from being geographically separated during acute periods during their ill child's treatment	• Altered communication patterns and coping styles may occur because of • physical separation, desire to protect spouse from feelings of fear, uncertainty and exhaustion. • Strained feelings can also occur between other family members such as grandparents or step-parents. • Encourage parents to talk openly with each other about their feelings and coping style. • Offer referral to psychosocial clinicians to help them deal with marital/couple stress or to facilitate communication amongst other family members such as grandparents. • Monitor individual parental emotional reaction because they affect the ability of spouses/partners to support each other. May need to make referrals to the psychosocial clinicians if differences in parental coping styles are at risk of contributing to poor family functioning.
Parental need to provide emotional support to their ill child/adolescent and to be able to speak to the child's questions about dying (See Chapter 22 on Talking to Children and Adolescents about Cancer).	• Encourage parents to honestly share information with their ill child regarding diagnosis and treatment. • Educate parents about common age-related ways children understand illness and express and handle emotions. • If child/adolescent experiences procedural distress, behavioral intervention (e.g., desensitization, anxiety-management strategies such as deep breathing, guided imagery, etc. can be used). • Discuss overprotection and how it is particularly disruptive of normal child, and particularly teen development. • Encourage parents of adolescents to support age-appropriate autonomy of their ill child. • Encourage consistency in discipline to avoid behavioral difficulties.

(continued)

Table 24.1 (Continued)

Family Psychosocial Issue	Suggested Clinical Intervention
	• Medical and psychosocial team members meet individually with the ill child to offer brief, age-appropriate discussions using terms familiar to the child. Discuss chemotherapy and safety limitations imposed by the treatment. Allow time for questions. Emphasize that there are different types of cancer and encourage the ill child to ask about their kind of cancer. If an adult family member has died from cancer, clarify that adult cancer is different from pediatric cancer. Make an optimistic statement that everything possible is being done to make the ill child better. • During hospitalizations, encourage parental caregivers to choose one or more methods of communication with the clinical care team such as the whiteboards in their child's room, asking for parent/clinician care conferences, asking for bedside consultations, and other methods that each setting offers, and work collaboratively with the clinical care team to develop daily goals.
Parental need to assist ill child/ adolescent in handling physical aspects of diagnosis and treatment	• Assist parents to anticipate physical side effects. • Encourage parental involvement in medical care. • Encourage parents to nurture and comfort their ill child. • Encourage parents to involve their child in school and extracurricular activities. Monitor school attendance to assess for reluctance to attend due to physical changes (e.g., hair loss) or being behind academically.
Parental need to monitor well sibling response • Siblings will sense that something is "wrong" because of parents' anxiety, but may not understand or be adequately informed of the diagnosis. • The well sibling may feel responsible for the ill child's cancer, i.e., worry that they "wished" the illness on the sibling by prior angry thoughts. • Expect siblings to experience shock, sadness, fear and confusion over what to expect during the course of the illness.	• Encourage parent to bring sibling(s) in to tour the clinic, meet with medical team (e.g., oncologist, nurse practitioner) and ask questions. • Identify with the parents a person who can consistently serve as the source of treatment information for the well sibling. Explain the cancer diagnosis to the well sibling/s and make sure they understand that they are not responsible. Often the child life specialist, psychologist or social worker on the team can be of assistance in working with siblings. • Encourage parents to set aside some special time with the healthy sibling so that they do not feel unloved, abandoned or isolated. Consider using commercially available technology (e.g., Skype, face time, web cams) as a way to allow the well sibling to communicate with the ill sibling and caretaker parent.

(continued)

Table 24.1 (Continued)

Family Psychosocial Issue	Suggested Clinical Intervention
• Anticipate well sibling to feel lonely, less valued in the family or jealous of the attention the ill child is receiving when parental roles are altered to include a dominant focus on the ill child. • Anticipate emotional reactions to disruptions in the well child's routines and having other people care for them.	• Encourage parents to normalize their well child's feelings and provide written, videos, online (http://www.lls.org/resourcecenter/helpfulorganization/patientcaregiverresources/ch; (Leukemia & Lymphoma Society); http://www.acco.org/Information/Resources/Books.aspx; (American Cancer Society); http://www.cancer.net/coping/relationships-and-cancer/Siblings-and-cancer; (Cancer.Net); http://www.alexslemonade.org/childhood-cancer/resources (Alex's Lemonade Stand Foundation) and other forms of materials designed for children to understand cancer or for parents to use to help guide their well child. Alert parents to hospital-based resources such as sibling groups or special camp activities. • Advocate and utilize support activities for siblings of children with cancer (e.g., www.supersibs.org). • Discuss how the family roles and responsibilities shift as the family accommodates the demands of cancer treatment. • Encourage parents to avoid placing difficult caregiving demands upon the well sibling. • Offer to contact teachers of both the ill child and the sibling to make sure they are aware of the ill child's health status. Offer informational materials that the parents can send to the school. • Encourage supportive individual counseling and/or family therapy.
• Anticipate school difficulties including decline in academic performance, acting out or withdrawal • Well sibling may inhibit expression of own worries to avoid causing parents more anxiety.	
Parental need to balance needs of all family members	• Help parents anticipate needs of individual family members. • Assist parents with developing strategies to balance their competing demands. • Encourage parents to talk with a social worker about making practical arrangements such as for childcare, transportation, and jobs. For example, a social worker can assist with writing a letter to an employer for Family Medical Leave Act (FMLA).

(continued)

Table 24.1 (Continued)

Family Psychosocial Issue	Suggested Clinical Intervention
Parental need to obtain and maintain social relationships and support outside the immediate family	• Specifically inquire about types of outside support used by parents. • If there is available extended social support, encourage the parents to access it. Encourage parents to make a list of tasks/activities they need assistance with and give it to a designated family member (e.g., grandparent, aunt, uncle, close friend, etc.) who can disseminate to others. • Refer to psychosocial team to help family set up care team through their church or local community. • Suggest family consider setting up a webpage (CarePages, CaringBridge) in order to keep family and friends informed of their child's progress.

Table 24.2 Remission

Family Psychosocial Issue	Suggested Clinical Intervention
Chronicity of disease and living with uncertainty	• Monitor family functioning and refer to social work, psychology if there is any change in reported concrete needs and stress/distress, or observed behavioral changes. • Reinforce family strengths and encourage use of problem solving to address any issues that arise. • Encourage rest and respite for parents. • Whenever possible, provide child with sense of control by offering choices. • Encourage the child/adolescent with cancer and the well sibling/s to attend school regularly. Refer to psychologist, child life therapist, or education liaison on the psychosocial team to develop a school reentry plan and assist child/adolescent in dealing with peer reactions, academic and peer pressures, fostering independence and autonomy. • Assist parents in preparing the well sibling/s to handle questions from friends or others about the ill sibling.[12,15–16] • Encourage parents to ask their well child/children about their thoughts, emotions and worries[12,15–16] • Encourage parents to seek assistance from family members and friends to ensure well siblings' are able to attend their extra-curricular activities[12,15–16] • Monitor physical activity. Many teenagers avoid outside activity when instructed not to participate in contact sports. Encourage daily exercise to maintain strength and endurance through fun activities (e.g., Wii).

(continued)

Table 24.2 (Continued)

Family Psychosocial Issue	Suggested Clinical Intervention
Parent role in assisting the ill child in dealing with treatment side effects, self-esteem, body image and changes in personal aspirations	• Increase child/adolescent's active coping by encouraging continued contact with hospital-based therapist or, if desired, refer to psychologist in the community for supportive counseling. Monitor sleep patterns and provide sleep hygiene information when necessary. • Assess body image changes (e.g., hair loss, skin discoloration, scars). • In particular, youth with amputations or limb salvage procedures who can no longer function in areas of previous interest to them (e.g., on the football team) need to be closely monitored for distress and helped to develop alternative interests and activities. (See Chapter 5, Sarcomas and other Solid Tumors.)
Clinicians need to monitor parental and the ill child/adolescent's adherence to medical treatment. (See Chapter 17, Medication Adherence.)	• Identify and address practical barriers to treatment adherence. • If additional treatments are planned once the child is in remission, educate child/adolescent and family about the additional procedures (e.g., radiation therapy, bone marrow transplant) and refer to child life specialist to provide further education through medical play to decrease anxiety. • Encourage parents to help their child/adolescent to interact with other patients, become involved with support groups, or attend camps for children with cancer. Even more important, is to encourage their reintegration with peer group outside the hospital. • Monitor child/adolescent's medication adherence. Problem solve potential barriers and work with psychosocial team to implement behavioral program to ensure adherence. • Encourage teens to take responsibility for taking medications, BUT reinforce that parents are ultimately responsible to ensure medication compliance. • Repeat/adapt/provide new information as child progresses through stages of cognitive development. Cancer diagnosis and treatment takes on new meaning as the child matures and understands potential treatment late effects.

Completing Treatment and Survivorship

As treatment draws to an end, parents report feeling relief that the treatment is over and also feeling concern about relapse and reduced contact with hospital staff. The hallmark of this phase is the presence of mixed emotions.[19] (Chapter 33, Pediatric Cancer Survivors.) Additionally, sibling adjustment needs to be closely monitored given literature indicating presence of cancer-related posttraumatic stress symptoms (Table 24.3).[12,20]

Disease Recurrence and Death

Recurrence of a child's cancer poses immediate and long-term emotional risks for the patient and family. Parents of children who have relapsed experience significantly higher levels of depression and anxiety. Studies show biologic indicators of a strong stress reaction in parents of children with cancer recurrence that suggest different interventions may be needed at the time of recurrence.[21] (Chapter 30, Integrating Palliative Care; Table 24.4).

Table 24.3 Completing Treatment and Survivorship

Family Psychosocial Issue	Suggested Clinical Intervention
Prepare family members and ill child for the emotions associated with completion of treatment	Family: • Educate the family about common feelings including uncertainty, ambivalence, anxiety, and sadness regarding decreased contact with clinic and medical staff, and fear of relapse. Prepare family for these possible emotions and indicate benefit of supportive counseling to cope with these emotions. Ill Child: • Educate and assess ill child/adolescent's emotional response. Stress need to change perspective from "patient" to "survivor."
	• Provide education on actual or potential disease/treatment effects.
Adjusting to treatment late effects	• If child's treatment included central nervous system treatment, follow-up neuropsychological testing should be done at regular intervals. (See Chapter 18, Cognitive Sequelae.) Well Sibling • Educate and prepare family about possible adjustment difficulties sibling may experience including anxiety and cancer related posttraumatic stress symptoms and indicate benefit from supportive therapy to cope with these emotions.[12, 20] • Educate siblings about any actual or potential disease/treatment related side effects[12, 20]

(continued)

Table 24.3 (Continued)

Family Psychosocial Issue	Suggested Clinical Intervention
Anticipate family desire to return to "normal" • Sometimes at the end of treatment feelings emerge about the treatment and about rational and irrational feelings related to the experience. Can be a difficult time emotionally for parents individually and within the marital couple. Also may experience disappointment that things do not immediately return to the way they were before diagnosis and treatment.	• Monitor family adjustment during follow-up visits. • Educate family about unrealistic expectation of returning quickly to "normal." Emphasize that this is a time of transition for all family members.
Maintaining appropriate medical follow-up care (See Chapter 33, Pediatric Cancer Survivors.)	• With family permission, communicate with the child's pediatrician or other significant health care providers to clarify follow-up care guidelines. • Schedule an end of-treatment conference to discuss issues, concerns and follow-up plan. • Provide the family with a record of medical care. • Assess and address any barriers to follow-up.

Table 24.4 Recurrence

Family Psychosocial Issue	Suggested Clinical Intervention
Intense emotional reactions • Frequently shock and disbelief followed by increased symptoms of psychological distress including anxiety, anger and depression	• Listen to parents and acknowledge reactions including anxiety, fears, anger, sadness and depressive feelings as being normal. Monitor these symptoms and offer the availability of social work or psychology or possibly psychiatry if symptoms are severe or reactivate a previous mental illness. If a parent is reluctant to see a professional counselor, assess for other sources of support and encourage the family to regroup their social network and share their feelings, fears and concerns with a trusted friend, religious leader, or other individuals who could respectfully hear their concerns. • Alternative forms of therapeutic interventions (e.g., journaling) can be useful in the expression of feelings/fears/concerns. • Identify and respect parental preferences for obtaining treatment-related information including how they prefer information to be provided to the child.

(continued)

Table 24.4 (Continued)

Family Psychosocial Issue	Suggested Clinical Intervention
• An urgency to confirm that other curative treatment options exist including second opinions	• Openly discuss treatment options (e.g., Bone Marrow Transplant (BMT), Phase I trials) including the family's exploration of a second opinion from other treatment centers and alternative medical cures. • When indicated medically, shift medical focus from "cure" and start open discussion with family regarding "palliation" or symptom control. • Carefully balance additional treatment with quality of life for the child. Encourage hope for what is possible and align with the family with this hope. • When appropriate, make referrals to hospice. The transition can be smoothed when families understand that they will not be cut off from the treatment team with whom they have developed a close relationship over the years. (See Chapter 30, Integrating Palliative Care.)
• Possible changes in communication between parent and patients around recurrence and implications	• Refer for supportive family therapy to help maintain family communication and relationships and avoid detachment. • When age appropriate, include patients in discussion to make sure their wishes are heard. (See Chapter 30, Integrating Palliative Care.)
Coping with child's emotional reaction to disease progression and approaching death	• Provide developmentally appropriate information regarding prognosis. Answer child's questions honestly, while respecting parental wishes. • Refer for supportive therapy if psychological distress increases. • Offer choices/sense of control (e.g., being at home versus being in the hospital, using more or less pain medication, etc.). • Facilitate closure activities (such as funeral planning, giving away toys, taking final trips etc. as requested by child, as needed. Consider using "Voicing My Choices" to help child/teen express their wishes/desires.[22] • Encourage the family to keep the child as active and engaged as possible. • Encourage family to work with art therapist to create a "legacy" art piece
Siblings' response to disease progression and approaching death Sibling response to BMT	• Sibling will benefit from meeting with members of the medical team to understand reasons for this new treatment phase and what it entails for their ill brother/sister • Inquire if the parents and siblings would like their teacher notified of the change in the ill sibling's medical status.

(continued)

Table 24.4 (Continued)

Family Psychosocial Issue	Suggested Clinical Intervention
	• Offer sibling psychosocial support from team. • Member of the medical team to meet with sibling and educate them about HLA typing.[23] • Sibling donor assessment completed by independent member of the psychosocial team (e.g., child-life specialist, psychologist) to ensure that sibling understands what is being asked of them and that they don't feel coerced.[23] • Close monitoring of several issues including fear of being chosen, fear they will not be a match, and guilt if transplant is unsuccessful.[23] • Siblings need to be provided with complete and honest information throughout the transplant journey; particularly if the transplant is not successful.[23] • Encourage parents to assign specific task to sibling to support family structure. This is viewed positively by well sibling(s) as being included in the family experience.

Bereavement

The anticipated and actual death of the child or adolescent with cancer is a dynamic, painfully intense experience. Grief is multifaceted and includes psychological, physical, behavioral, spiritual, existential, and social dimensions.[24–25] Literature indicates that parental health during bereavement is quite fragile and providing support early is critical. In fact, if parental health is not attended to, the likelihood of having a first psychiatric hospitalization or having to leave employment is statistically significantly greater for bereaved parents than for parents who have never experienced the loss of a child.[26–29] (Chapter 22, Talking with Children, and Chapter 30, Integrating Palliative Care; Table 24.5).

Table 24.5 Bereavement	
Family Psychosocial Issue	**Suggested Clinical Intervention**
Need to learn about choices when treatment is not curative	• Openly and respectfully explore options with the family (e.g., in-hospital palliative care program or hospice). Reassure the family that regardless of their decision, contact with the medical team will be maintained.
Need to monitor family functioning	• Inform parents that differences in coping style may result in their feeling intermittently close to or distant from each other through and after their child's dying. • Acknowledge and normalize parent's feelings of intense sadness. If death is protracted, the emotional burden can be draining. Monitor parental report of sleep difficulties, feelings of fatigue, mood problems including feeling easily overwhelmed, irritable, withdrawn or even "emotionally numb" and make appropriate referrals to psychologist, chaplain, nurse, social worker, or possibly a psychiatrist. • Provide information to family members about how to prepare emotionally and cognitively for issues related to end-of-life (e.g., funeral arrangements, death, grieving).
Need to assist siblings around death	• Encourage parents to be open with siblings and provide accurate and developmentally appropriate information to reduce fears. • Refer to psychosocial team to contact sibling's teacher and/or visit the school to process the death with peers. • Refer for supportive therapy (e.g., psychologist, hospital chaplain, grief counselor, bereavement groups such as Compassionate Friends). • Provide reading materials for sibling, parent and community members regarding adjusting to/dealing with the loss of a child. • Encourage establishment of "death anniversary" remembrances/rituals.
Need for family to learn how to cope in the days, months, and years after the loss of a child	• Contact parents and assure them that support is available to them after the loss of their child. The National Quality Forum recommendation is to follow families following the loss of a child for 13 months.[22] • Staff may wish to attend the child's funeral, which is most often viewed as supportive and respectful but can also be intrusive and distressing to some families. A team discussion with close friends or family may illuminate how best to proceed. • Develop a plan among members of the healthcare team whereby a team member is charged with coordinating contacts with the bereaved family in the short-term period following the child's death. • Prepare family members that their friends, relatives, community members may have difficulty speaking of the deceased child. • Provide bereavement support for parents, siblings, grandparents or refer the family for such services.

(continued)

Table 24.4 (Continued)

Family Psychosocial Issue	Suggested Clinical Intervention
	• Provide selected, age appropriate reading materials about bereavement to parents, siblings, grandparents, classroom teachers and others who were closely involved with the child. • Prepare family members for the likelihood that each may have individual ways of expressing grief and that they may, at times not be able to comfort one another. • If available, offer participation in annual memorial service held for oncology patients to provide sense of closure. • Offer information on how to connect with other families who have lost a child, if desired. • Helpful to have a psychosocial team member call the family 1-year after child's death to check-in on them, and if needed, to make additional referrals for psychological services

References

1. da Silva FM, Jacob, E, Nascimento LC. Impact of childhood cancer on parents' relationships: a systematic review. *J Nurs Scholarship*. 2010;42(3):250–261.
2. Kupst MJ, Bingen K. Stress and coping in the pediatric cancer experience. In: Brown RT, ed., *Comprehensive Handbook of Childhood Cancer and Sickle Cell Disease: A Biopsychosocial Approach*. New York, NY: Oxford University Press; 2006:35–52.
3. Long KA, Marsland A. Family adjustment to childhood cancer: A systematic review. *Clin Child Fam Psych*. 2011;14(1):57–88.
4. Alderfer MA, Kazak AE. Family issues when a child is on treatment for cancer. In: Brown RT, ed., *Comprehensive Handbook of Childhood Cancer and Sickle Cell Disease: A Biopsychosocial Approach*. New York, NY: Oxford University Press; 2006:53–74.
5. Khoury MN. Lebanese parents' experiences with a child with cancer. *Eur J Onc Nurs*. 2013;17:16021.
6. Woznick LA, Goodheart CD. *Living with Childhood Cancer: A Practical Guide to Help Families Cope*. Washington, DC: American Psychological Association; 2002.
7. Kazak AE, Rourke MT, Crump TA. Families and other systems in pediatric psychology. In: Roberts MC, ed., *Handbook of Pediatric Psychology*. 3rd ed. New York, NY: Guilford Press; 2003:159–175.
8. Haverman L, van Oers HA, Limperg, PF, et al. Development and validation of the distress thermometer for parents of a chronically ill child. *J Pediatr*. 2013;163(4):1140–1146.
9. Kazak A, Barakat L, Ditaranto S, et al. Screening for psychosocial risk at cancer diagnosis: The psychosocial assessment tool (PAT). *J Pediatric Hematology/Oncology*. 2011;33:289–294.

10. McGrath P. Findings on the impact of treatment for childhood acute lymphoblastic leukaemia on family relationships. *Child Family Social Work.* 2001;6(3):229–237.
11. Sahler OJ, Roghmann KJ, Mulhern RK, et al. Sibling adaptation to Childhood Cancer Collaborative Study: The association of sibling adaptation with maternal well-being, physical health, and resource use. *J Dev Behav Pediatr.* 1997;18(4):233–243.
12. Alderfer MA, Long KA, Lown EA, et al. Psychosocial adjustment of siblings of children with cancer: a systematic review. *Psycho-Oncol.* 2010;19:789–805.
13. Houtzager, BA, Grootenhuis MA, Hoekstra-Weebers JEHM, Caron HN, Last BF. Psychosocial functioning in siblings of paediatric cancer patients one to six months after diagnosis. *Euro Cancer.* 2003;39:1423–1432.
14. Houtzager BA, Grootenhuis MA, Caron HN, Last BF. Quality of life and psychological adaptation in siblings of paeditric cancer patients 2 years after diagnosis. *Psycho-Oncol.* 2004;13:499–511.
15. Long KA, Marsland AL, Alderfer MA. Cumulative family risk predicts sibling adjustment to childhood cancer. *Cancer.* 2013;119:2503–2510.
16. Spinetta JJ, Jankovic M, Eden T, et al. Guidelines for assistance to siblings of children with cancer: a report of the SIOP working committee on psyhosoical issues in pediatric oncology. *Med & Pediatr Oncol.* 1999;33:395–398.
17. Sahler OJ, Dolgin MJ, Phipps S. et al. Specificity of problem-solving skills training in mothers of children newly diagnosed with cancer: results of a multisite randomized clinical trial. JCO. 2013:31(10):1329–1335.
18. Sahler OJ, Fairclough DL, Phipps S, et al. Using problem-solving skills training to reduce negative affectivity in mothers of children with newly diagnosed cancer: report of a multisite randomized trial. *J Consult Clin Psychol.* 2005;73:272–283.
19. Keene N, Hobbie W, Ruccione K. *Childhood Cancer Survivors: A Practical Guide to Your Future.* Sebastopol, CA: O'Reilly & Associate; 2003.
20. Lund LW, Winther JF, Cederkvist L, et al. Hospital contact for mental health disorders in survivors of childhood cancer and their siblings in Denmark: a population-based cohort study. *Lancet Oncol.* 2013;14(10):971–980.
21. Hinds PS, Birenbaum LK, Pedrosa A, Pedrosa F. Guidelines for the recurrence of pediatric cancer. *Semin Oncol Nurs.* 2002;18(1):50–59.
22. Wiener L, Zadeh S, Battles H, et al. Allowing adolescents and young adults to plan their end-of life care. *Pediatrics.* 2012;130(5):1–9. Voicing My CHOICES Advance Care Planning Guide is found at: http://www.agingwithdignity.org/voicing-my-choices.php
23. Pentz RD, Alderfer MA, Pelletier W, et al. Needs of siblings of pediatric stem cell transplant recipients: role for an advocate. *Pediatrics.* In press
24. American Cancer Society (ACS). *Coping with Grief and Loss.* Atlanta, GA: ACS; 2001. http://documents.cancer.org/6036. Revised Jul 23,2001. Accessed Oct 22,2008.
25. Kriecbergs UC, Lannen P, Onelov E, Wolfe J. Parental grief after losing a child to cancer. Impact of professional and social support on long-term outcomes. *J Clin Oncol.* 2007;25(22):3307–3312.
26. Jalmsell L, Onelov E, Steineck G, Henter JI, & Kreicbergs U. Hematopoietic stem cell transplantation in children with cancer and the risk of long-term psychological morbidity in bereaved parents. *Bone Marrow Transplant.* 2011;46(8):1063–1070.

27. Jalmsell, L, Kreicbergs, U, Onelov E, Steineck G, & Henter JL. Anxiety is contagious-symptoms of anxiety in the terminally ill child affect long-term psychological well-being in bereaved parents. *Pediatr Blood Cancer.* 2010;54(5): 751–757.

28. Lannen PK, Wolfe J, Prigerson HG, Onelov E, Kreicbergs UC. Unresolved grief in a national sample of bereaved parents: impaired mental and physical health 4 to 9 years later. *J Clin Oncol.* 2008;26(36):5870–5876.

29. National Quality Forum. *A National Framework and Preferred Practices for Palliative and Hospice Care Quality: A Consensus Report.* Washington, DC: National Quality Forum; 2006.

Chapter 25

Special Considerations in Working with Families

Lori Wiener, Steven K. Reader, and Anne E. Kazak

Families are very diverse and the more traditional definitions of family often fall short of capturing the families that we work with in pediatric oncology. In addition, a child may derive physical care (e.g., food and shelter); medical care; and emotional, spiritual and cultural needs from different individuals. Therefore, when considering the child's living situation, it is important to be respectful of variations in family structure. Furthermore, some families may have preexisting challenges such as parental mental illness, substance abuse, or cognitive limitations that may add to the burden of caring for their child. This chapter covers a broad array of considerations in working with families. Chapter 31, Caring for International Patients, addresses unique concerns for parents who travel from outside the United States to receive cancer care for their child. Regardless of the family structure or where their native home may be, it is essential that physicians and nurses work closely with members of the psychosocial team to provide comprehensive, culturally sensitive care.

Family Structure

Foster Parents

Children with cancer sometimes live in foster care. This situation may arise for various reasons, including child abuse and neglect, domestic violence, homelessness, parental substance abuse, and parental mental health problems. Foster care placements may include foster homes, group homes, residential treatment facilities, and juvenile justice facilities.[1] It is, unfortunately, not uncommon for children in the foster care system to have multiple placements, which can create more adjustment issues for the child and challenges for continuity and consistency of medical care. Siblings of the child may be placed in a different foster placement, which can create additional stress for the child. The child's foster home may include other foster children. The frequency of emotional and behavioral concerns is higher in children in foster care,[2] which can lead to increased stress in the home and have an impact on medical adherence.

Considerations for the child with cancer who is in foster care:

- Children in foster care have a higher rate of physical, developmental, and behavioral health concerns, and these concerns are often chronic, under identified, undertreated, and cause significant functional impairment.[1]
- The division of family/social services usually has legal custody of the child and directs and monitors the foster placement, as well as the ongoing medical care of the child.
- State jurisdiction issues may arise that impact coverage of services based on geographic location (e.g., a child in foster care in one state not being eligible for medical services in another state).

A recent initiative led by the American Academy of Pediatrics[1] recommends establishing medical homes for foster care children that can provide comprehensive healthcare, with healthcare providers working closely in coordination with child welfare agencies. These foster care medical homes would include healthcare providers who have additional training and experience with foster care children.[3] Connecting foster care families of children with cancer to such a system of care, if available, would likely enhance overall medical treatment for cancer.

Extended Family

Consistent with our understanding of families as diverse, when working with families of children with cancer it is important to consider other members of the family system. Grandmothers and grandfathers are often involved, either as primary caregivers, as secondary caregivers, or as family members whose role(s) shift dramatically upon diagnosis to assist their children and grandchildren.

- When grandparents are primary caregivers, whether legally or in an informal arrangement, and depending on specifics of the arrangement and the availability and ability of the child's biological parents as caregivers, family roles may need discussion and clarification during treatment.
- Some grandparents may experience powerlessness and injustice as they watch their own children and their grandchild experience the stress and pain associated with the diagnosis, treatment, and uncertainty of disease outcome.[4]
- Some grandparents put their own lives on hold to help retain some normalcy in the lives of their children's families as they play a primary role in helping with other children (siblings of the child with cancer).
- Because of their experience and often being a bit removed from daily parenting, grandparents may have views about the child's coping that differ from parents' perspectives.[5]
- Healthcare team members are often unsure of how to approach grandparents. It is helpful to talk with the family about the role of grandparents and how the family prefers that information be shared.[5]
- Some grandparents are impressed by how their own children manage to handle something so difficult and previously unimaginable to them while

other grandparents may feel resentment about having to take on primary caregiving roles, and may be dealing with their own health issues.
- Grandparents appreciate having their suffering and stress acknowledged and being offered support services available within the medical center or community.

Lone Parenting

In the last 30 years, the proportion of children in two-parent families has decreased significantly. In the United States, over one-fourth of the 75 million children under the age of 18 live in a single-parent family.[6] The most common type of single parent home is one with a mother present; approximately 84% of custodial parents are mothers.[7]

The challenges of single or "lone" parenting for a child with cancer have been outlined.[8] Single parents often struggle to balance work, childcare, a home, and employment while caring for their sick child. With an often more limited support system to share the responsibility of the sick child's care or daily decisions, single parents can be isolated and may experience anger toward former life partners, or those who provide little emotional or financial assistance. Young single parent families and parents who self-identify as a "lone parent" may be at greater risk than some single parents with good support systems.[9]

Psychosocial Considerations for Single Parent Families

- Identify the economic, psychological, social, and support needs early in the child's treatment.
- Learn who will be involved in the child's care and treatment decisions.
- Determine guardianship and custody issues as well as parental visitation arrangements.

Ask to see the official paperwork and then place a copy in the child's medical chart. Problems arise when a noncustodial person gives permission, but the custodial person was not aware of it. (See Box 25.1.)

- Consider the impact of possible remarriage and stepfamily relationships on the child.
- If the child's parents are separated or divorced, work toward keeping both parents informed about the child's diagnosis, treatments, and progress.
- Ask if reassignment of home responsibilities and financial assistance (especially travel and child care costs) is required in order for treatment to be obtained.
- Inquire about the other children in the home: Who is caring for them, and how they are coping?
- Explore extended family and nonfamily supports that may be available through the course of the child's illness.
- Early identification of parents who perceive themselves to be "lone parenting" a chronically ill child can help facilitate appropriate triage when a family enters the medical system, and that early identification can lead to the development and implementation of targeted, evidence-based interventions.

- Consider referral for individual counseling and/or support group to enhance coping skills and to increase the parent's support network.

Gay or Lesbian Families

Families headed by gay or lesbian parents are as diverse as other families. In some cases, they are single-parent families, in other cases two-parent families. Gay and lesbian families also encounter separation but are often not covered by the same legal protections as heterosexual divorced families. Children in gay and lesbian families may be children from prior heterosexual unions of one partner or may be the biological or adopted child of the parents.

Although the majority states allow same sex marriage and/or civil unions, providers should approach families with an openness to encourage disclosure of the nature of the family (e.g., parents may be reluctant to acknowledge their sexual orientation if they worry that they might be treated differently). Legal custody or guardianship may become an issue if one parent is not able to sign for hospital admissions or consent documents. Access to a good support network can make a difference in how well nontraditional families cope in general, but particularly so when in crisis. If a supportive network does not exist, talk to the hospital social worker about other resources.

Unmarried Couples

Unmarried parents might have additional problems with certain legal, insurance, and financial arrangements.

Blended Families

When parents remarry or are repartnered, stepfamily households are created. Blended families refers to a situation in which a child from a previous relationship is included in a family created by a new marriage/union. As more children from different previous relationships are added to the family, the complexity increases. It is critical that the healthcare team assess decision making and communication between biological parents, stepparents, and grandparents or other primary caregivers early in treatment.

Assessment of Blended Family Dynamics/Constellation

- Inquire about and apply the patient's definition of family. ("Who is in your family? Who do you consider members of your family?")
- How long have parents been separated/divorced/remarried? (Adjustment to new family may take several years)
- Explore how family members have adjusted to recent changes in family.
- Identify the support system (don't assume). Depending on custody arrangements and work schedules, stepfathers may have more time at home with the child than stepmothers or biological parents.
- Be inclusive and nonjudgmental.
- Understand that the medical condition may unify and strengthen or separate the family.
- Encourage the family to be sensitive and flexible regarding whom the patient would like present during procedures.

Additional Questions

- Who speaks for the family?
- Who is involved in the daily care and medical care of the patient?
- Are roles in the family clearly defined?
- Who mobilizes the resources?
- Are limits effectively set? (This may impact treatment adherence).
- Who mediates when conflicts arise?

Cultural Considerations

Previous sections of this chapter have illustrated the diversity of family structures that can be encountered by healthcare providers treating children with cancer. Given the increasing ethnic diversity of the population of the United States,[10] it is important to discuss issues of cultural diversity. Cultural groups can differ in terms of the hierarchy in family structure, which can determine the primary person(s) with whom the medical team may need to communicate and consult for decision making. Language barriers point to the critical need to have sufficient language interpreters. It is also important to be open-minded and inquire about family belief and value systems, including spiritual ones that can impact the acceptability of and adherence with treatment options. Assessing availability of social supports may involve asking about religious practices and church organizations, as well as ethnic community organizations. Ethnic minority groups have often faced the adversities of socioeconomic stress[11] and racial discrimination/abuse, which have led not only to health disparities but also distrust of the medical establishment.[12] Helping families address larger life issues such as financial stress, housing, and accessing medical resources through the help of a social worker or community liaison is often a primary need. For some families and cultures, open communication and explanation of the risks and benefits of medical procedures, as well as shared decision making, can help build trust. Cultural competency training for healthcare providers should also be an integral part of health care organizations.[13]

Handling Conflictual Situations with the Treatment Team

Regardless of the structure of a family, at times conflicts will arise between families and the treating team. Factors contributing to these situations include the stress experienced by families and providers, and frustrations in understanding and communicating with multiple team members (e.g., conflicting information received from team members). These situations can be challenging to pediatric oncology treatment teams. When handled successfully, conflicts subside and care is delivered as planned. When conflicts escalate, the outcome can be less favorable for the patient, family, and treatment teams, even to the point of jeopardizing the needed treatment. Approaches that are helpful in these situations include the following:[14]

- Assignment of consistent care providers whenever possible.
- Early proactive involvement of psychosocial-team members.
- Primary oncologist and nurse meeting regularly with the family.
- Assure the family feels "heard."
- Multidisciplinary care conferences.

- Written plans to address psychosocial problems and an outline of how regular contact and communication will be maintained.
- Support for staff who work with challenging families, and assuring staff safety and well-being.

Parental Impairment

Preexisting challenges to parenting can include parental illness, significant intellectual deficits, mental health problems, substance abuse, and legal problems including incarceration. Such impairment adds significantly to the burden of dealing with a child's cancer diagnosis and treatment. Parents may have periods of competent functioning alternating with periods of difficulty and even incapacitation. During times of impairment, parents want to be able to provide care for their children and, most often, do not wish to relinquish custody of their children. However, alternative guardians may be necessary, not only for day-to-day care but also in order to sign consents and make medical decisions when the parent is unable.

Parental Intellectual Vulnerabilities

- Consider whether a parent(s) has intellectual deficits that could impede their ability to understand medical treatments and/or follow-through with appointments.
- Provide a quiet room or office space so that parents will not be distracted or interrupted.
- People with cognitive impairments may need more repetition than others. It can be helpful to ask parents to summarize their understanding of what they heard in order to assess knowledge. Written information or instructions may be helpful, at an appropriate reading level for the parents.
- Identify staff, such as a social worker, to help facilitate the coordination of health, educational, and social services.
- Assess whether parents are relying on the patient or other children to remember medication names/schedules, side effects, and treatment plans.

Parental Mental Illness

- When parental mental illness is perceived to be affecting the child and his or her care, close collaboration between the psychosocial and medical team is important. Parents need to be assured that their privacy will be respected. It is important that reports of parental mental illness are made on accurate information.
- A parent with psychological problems that are well controlled with medication and/or therapy might still benefit from added support and services during the time of the child's cancer diagnosis and treatment. Conversely, a parent with less well-controlled problems or more serious mental illness (e.g., active psychosis) might be unable to participate

fully in the child's treatment and medical decisions. Identification of other family members to provide support is important in this situation.

- If parental mental illness interferes with the child's care, a next step approach might include a referral for treatment. If this is not possible and/or treatment is unsuccessful, a suitable legal guardian might need to be found for the child.
- Children at risk of abuse and neglect due to parental incapacitation are the responsibility of all members of the medical community and relevant professional groups.
- If neglect is confirmed, it is important to engage the family in finding appropriate care for the child. Parents are much less threatened with a shared decision-making process. The staff should document all meetings and interventions in the medical record, continuing to monitor conventionally and be prepared to intervene with a referral to protective (social) services, if required.

Parental Substance Use

- When a parent abuses substances, the child is at greater risk for neglect or abuse. The risk to the child increases in a single-parent household where there is no supporting adult to diffuse parental stress and protect the child from the effects of the parent's problem.
- Parental abuse of alcohol and other drugs impacts all family members and all aspects of their life. The circumstances within chemically involved families can change rapidly and therefore assessment must be ongoing.
- If a parent smells like alcohol and his/her behavior seems likely associated with drugs or alcohol, a team member that the parent trusts should have a direct conversation with the parent in a nonthreatening style as soon as possible.
- Denial of alcohol or other drug abuse is common. Parents may minimize the extent of their drug and/or alcohol use ("My kid has cancer, I just needed something to calm down") or deny any relapses because of fears that their children will be removed from their custody.
- Parental substance abuse is also commonly associated with poor mental health or psychiatric illness, domestic violence, incarceration, poverty, and homelessness.
- If a parent is incapacitated due to substance abuse and deemed legally incompetent, the medical staff will need to engage other family members to fully discuss consent and treatment options. If legal incompetence of a parent has not been established, clinicians should seek help from hospital lawyers in determining who in the family should be involved in choice of treatment and consent for treatment. The staff should document all meetings and interventions in the medical record, continuing to monitor conventionally and be prepared to intervene with a referral to protective (social) services, if required (Box 25.1).

Box 25.1 Guardianship and Custody Options

Extended family

Grandparents, other relatives, the other biological parent, friends, and spouses/partners who are not biological parents are the most commonly appointed guardians.

Standby guardianship

Many states allow parents to retain custody while still ensuring the future legal custody of their children. In standby guardianship, a parent nominates another person to assume complete custody of the child when the parent dies or becomes incapacitated. The authority of the standby guardian does not become operative until the parent dies, is incapacitated, or consents.

Joint guardianship

Joint guardianship allows a parent to name one or more persons to share custody, with equal sharing of rights and responsibilities until one guardian dies or resigns.

References

1. American Academy of Pediatrics. *Fostering Health: Health Care for Children and Adolescents in Foster Care*. 2nd ed., Smithtown, NY 11787: American Academy of Pediatrics; 2005.
2. Szilagyi M. The pediatrician and the child in foster care. *Pediatrics in Review*.1998;19:39–50.
3. Gillaspy SR, Bonner BL. Child Maltreatment. In: Roberts MC, Steele RG, eds., *The Handbook of Pediatric Psychology* 4th ed. New York, NY: Guilford Press; 2009: 556–571.
4. Charlebois S, Bouchard L. "The worse experience": The experiences of grandparents who have a grandchild with cancer. *Canadian Oncol Nurs J*. 2007;17:26–36.
5. Moules NJ, Laing CM, McCaffrey G, et al. Grandparents' experiences of childhood cancer, Part 1: Doubled and Silenced. *J Pediatr Oncol Nurs*. 2012;29:119–132.
6. U.S. Census Bureau, Housing and Household Economic Statistics Division, Fertility & Family Statistics Branch. *America's Families and Living Arrangements: 2010*. http://www.census.gov/population/www/socdemo/hh-fam/cps2010.html. Accessed April 19, 2012.
7. Grall TS. Custodial mothers and fathers and their child support: 2005. United States Census Bureau. http://www.census.gov/prod/2007pubs/p60-234.pdf. Published August, 2007. Accessed August 5, 2008.
8. Brown RT, Wiener L, Kupst MJ, et al. Single parenting and children with chronic illness: An understudied phenomenon. *J Pediatr Psychol*. 2008;33:408–421.
9. Wiener L, Pao M, Battles H, et al. Socio-environmental factors associated with lone parenting chronically ill children. *Children's Health Care*, 2013;42:264–280.

10. Hixson L, Hepler B, Kim, M. *The White Population: 2010* (No. C2010BR-05). Washington, DC: US Census Bureau; 2011.
11. Berry JG, Bloom S, Foley S, et al. Health inequity in children and youth with chronic health conditions. *Pediatrics*. 2010;126:S111.
12. Ely B, Coleman C. Recruitment and retention of children in longitudinal research. *J Specialists Pediatr Nurs*. 2007;12:199–202.
13. Hines J, Mitchell MJ, Crosby LE, et al. Engaging patients with sickle cell disease and their families in disease education, research, and community awareness. *J Prevent Interven Commun*. 2011;39:256–272.
14. Rourke MT, Reilly A, Kersun LS, et al. Understanding and managing challenging families in pediatric oncology. Poster session presented at the American Psychosocial Oncology Society (APOS) 3rd Annual Conference, Amelia Island, FL; 2006, February.

Chapter 26

Spiritual and Religious Considerations

Mary Lynn Dell and Daniel H. Grossoehme

Clinicians, pediatric oncology patients, families, and communities dealing with childhood cancers commonly cite religious and spiritual beliefs as helpful, and often as sustaining. This support occurs across the continuum of initial diagnosis, intensive treatments, remissions, recurrences, through the dying process, death, bereavement, and beyond. Diagnosis of life-altering or life-threatening illness raises key questions at the interface of medicine, palliative care, and spirituality and religion—such as the meaning of life and suffering.

Key Definitions and Concepts

Although spirituality and religion in the pediatric oncology setting are as individualized and personal as each patient, family, and caregiver interaction, the following terms, though common and familiar, may be helpful:

Spirituality—Feelings, thoughts, experiences and behaviors that arise from a search for the sacred; may or may not include elements of traditional religion.[1]

Religion—Specific teachings, beliefs, and practices of established world faith traditions, organized religious groups, or institutions.[1]

Faith—an additional term used in many cultures and religions—may:[2]

- Be an integral, centering process underlying the formation of beliefs, values, and meanings.
- Give coherence and direction.
- Link individuals in shared trusts and loyalties with others.
- Ground personal and communal stances to a larger frame of reference.
- Enable one to face challenges of human life and death and rely on that which is deemed to be ultimate in life.
- Be more inclusive and extend beyond religious faith.
- Be a common feature across human experience.

Characteristics of Healthy and Unhealthy Religious/Spiritual Belief and Practice

Healthy religious and spiritual beliefs can promote attitudes and behaviors that can provide comfort, hope, resilience, and biopsychosocial adaptation in developmentally appropriate ways for all involved—children and adolescents with cancer, siblings, and their parents, and other significant caregivers.

General characteristics of healthy religious/spiritual belief and practice include:

- Comfort with humans making the best medical decisions possible no matter what role they believe God or the Divine has in the healing process.
- The encouragement of age-appropriate personal freedom and responsibility in all aspects of life, including dealing with cancer.
- The encouragement of continued personal growth and encouragement of community support, even in the midst of cancer diagnosis, treatment, and uncertainty about outcome and the future.
- Provision of hope and new alternatives for personal fulfillment.

Alternatively, unhealthy religious and spiritual beliefs can lead to attitudes and behaviors that are distressing to the childhood cancer patient and family, perhaps even hindering treatment adherence and detracting from the emotional and physical stamina helpful in acute care and long-term treatment and recovery.

General characteristics of unhealthy religious/spiritual belief and practice include:

- A punitive morality in which guilt predominates—the patient and/or parents are unable to forgive or be forgiven, regardless of whether the issue at hand is related to the illness. Common examples include believing or being told that the child or adolescent developed or "was given" cancer as a consequence of not praying enough, not having enough faith, or perhaps not attending church services regularly.
- Excessively perfectionistic and unaccepting of human limitations.
- Discourages developmentally appropriate personal freedom, leading to feelings of helplessness.
- Induces or contributes to fear, either in actual cancer-related situations or existentially in personal religious and spiritual matters.
- Discourages or limits alternatives for human growth and expression, especially when such alternatives would be helpful in coping with the challenges accompanying cancer.

Particular manifestations or details of unhealthy religious and spiritual beliefs and practices may be unique to each patient and family in their specific circumstances. However, by being familiar with the general characteristics of healthy and unhealthy religious and spiritual beliefs and practices noted earlier, healthcare professionals are in unique positions to support healthy practices and to identify concerns that need additional exploration and perhaps consultation or referral to a chaplain or other religious professional or mental health clinician, if adversely affecting the child patient (Personal communication, ES Bowman, August 17, 2003).

Spiritual Themes in Child and Family Life—with and without Cancer

Not all children and families identify themselves as spiritual or religious in their world views, nor do they identify spiritual or religious beliefs as influences on their health or adaptation to illness. However, a spiritual/religious orientation or lack thereof may influence many aspects of daily life including the meaning of life, coping, justice/fairness, guilt, altruism, attitudes toward medical care, and beliefs about afterlife.

When a child or adolescent is diagnosed with cancer, the identified patient and all who care about that person may confront other issues involving spiritual or religious beliefs. These include, but are not limited to, the meaning of pain and suffering, value judgments regarding opiate medication and physiological dependency, coping with physical disfigurement, and/or disability and bioethical issues that often arise during the course of illness, treatment, and end-of-life. Although spirituality and religion are normally resources on which people draw, they may also be sources of suffering (e.g., feeling punished by the Divine; abandoned by the Divine or others; etc). Clinicians may need to attend to the role and routine of prayer practices and religious or cultural dietary restrictions that may affect treatment.

Three Common Approaches to Spirituality/Religion by Clinicians

1. Openness and receptivity to spiritual/religious content but no active inquiry.
2. Neutral inquiry into spiritual/religious areas of family life, accompanied by referral/collaboration with chaplain or religious professional.
3. All spiritual/religious concerns referred to chaplain or religious professional.

Regardless of the clinician's preferred approach or style of dealing with religious or spiritual matters in ill and dying children, adolescents, and their families, it may be helpful to think about his/her own religious or spiritual beliefs, attitudes and boundaries. Knowing what one's own beliefs are (or are not) facilitates understanding and discerning patients' spirituality/religion in ways that do not interfere with the support patients and families experience from their own beliefs and practices. For instance, one scenario medical professionals commonly encounter is being invited to pray with families, their friends, and perhaps even visiting clergy at significant points in the child's treatment. Many clinicians find that anticipating these situations in advance, perhaps consulting with colleagues and religious professionals whose advice they trust, can be helpful in navigating these potentially anxiety-laden situations.

Considerations in Working with Families Experiencing Pain and Suffering[3]

- Recognize that the authority of medical professionals is a potent influence in the lives of patients and families.
- Strive to create open, nonthreatening environment for spiritual/religious conversations.[4]
- Maintain appropriate professional boundaries to insure ethical care.
- Listen—simply being present and listening nonjudgmentally can be both therapeutic and appreciated by families.
- Tolerate grief and doubt without false reassurance or platitudes.
- Remain focused on the family member—do not shift focus to yourself.
- Give families time to process events, express emotions, and to draw upon their faith, their faith communities, and other spiritual resources for coping and support.

Spiritual/Religious Understanding of Parents/Caregiver and the Family Unit

Before speaking with children and adolescents about their spiritual/religious beliefs, it is important to speak with the parents first in order to understand the family's background and context. People with spiritual struggles often do not request spiritual care and their pain may go unnoticed.[5] Helpful questions about the family belief system include the following:

- How do family members understand life's purpose and meaning? Have they ever considered or discussed these questions, either before or during their child or adolescent's illness?
- How does the family understand illness, pain, suffering?
- How does the family understand the concepts and relationships of body, mind, spirit, soul, etc.?
- How does the family understand and explain the specific illness of their child?
- Who is the most appropriate person(s) to tend to issues of spirituality and religion in a specific family: family's clergyperson, individual faith community, hospital chaplain, other trusted family member or friend, other treatment team member with good relationship and appropriate professionalism?
- Might the child or adolescent have beliefs and religious experiences that differ from his/her parents? Have the parents and their son or daughter ever talked about these with each other, either before or after the cancer diagnosis?

During this period of significant upheaval and stress, parents of ill and dying children and adolescents may:[6,7]

- Find great comfort, solace, and encouragement from both personal faith and the support of their faith communities.
- Question the existence or the goodness of a God who permits small children to suffer and die.
- Believe that God is punishing them (the parents) for past transgressions.
- Feel angry at God and/or organized religion.
- Feel empty, unable to pray.
- Lose the hope and comfort of spirituality/religion.
- Reject spiritual/religious caregivers.
- Ask, "Why my child?

Spiritual/Religious Understanding of the Child and Adolescent[7,8]

In most situations, clinicians should follow a child's lead. Questions children might ask caregivers or clinicians or that clinicians might follow-up with include the following:

- What happens to me when I die?
- Can I still see what's happening on earth after I'm dead?
- Where is God?
- What is God like?
- Do you ever think about God?
- Why did God let me get cancer? What does God think/feel about it?
- How do you feel about God?

Often when younger children ask these questions, it is because they have already been thinking about their own beliefs and answers. In these instances, reflecting the question back in a caring, gently inquisitive manner can be all that is necessary to begin a discussion: "Hmmm... That's a very interesting (important, thoughtful) question. Where do you think God is?" Following up the children's responses with similarly brief, relevant questions appropriate to their previous comments are often all that is necessary to permit or enable them to express their thoughts of a religious or spiritual nature, and in the process often work out the answers to some of their own questions. Questions about matters that are distressing to the child or adolescent or issues pertaining to beliefs, teachings, and practices of a specific religious tradition may be communicated back to parents to address, referred to the family's religious leader or to hospital chaplains, or a combination of these. Children or adolescents may be told in a gentle, empathic manner that this information will be shared with others. These discussions are often done with the children's participation and can lead to better understanding and communication about this very important area between the children, family members, treatment team, and any religious professionals involved. See Appendix.

Differences in religious/spiritual beliefs and practices of adolescents and their families are quite common among members of all types of families, with and without medical illnesses. With adolescents, or even children as young as eight or nine years of age, one-on-one conversation may be important to ascertain if their parents' spiritual/religious beliefs are similar or different than their own.

What May Siblings Do?[7]

- Fear that same thing will happen to them, other siblings, or parents.
- Show increased or decreased interest in spirituality/religion, practices, rituals.
- Be confused and not know what to believe or do.
- Feel guilt or jealousy or abandoned by God, parents, ill sibling, and faith community.
- Be angry at God, parents, ill sibling.
- Wonder why God is letting the sibling be sick and/or die.

Important to Note Regarding Inquiry about Religious Affiliation

- Affiliations are helpful for identifying common, general beliefs (e.g., burial preferences for orthodox Jews and observant Muslims), but do not assume that all families believe/follow all traditional customs.
- Beliefs and practices of a tradition vary geographically.
- Many interfaith marriages exist in which spiritual/religious beliefs and expressions are highly individualized.
- Many individuals are influenced greatly by faith of grandparents, significant others—these influences may not be tapped by usual questions on religious affiliation.
- *Always ask your patient and family about their individual preferences.*

Indications for Clergy Referral[9]

- Spiritual struggle or questions with spiritual/religious focus.
- Desire for prayer, sacrament, ritual, or worship.
- Patient/family request for any reason.
- Bioethical issue (also refer to bioethics and psychosocial specialists) Consultation regarding religious/spiritual beliefs and practices that may affect treatment, including the identification of unhealthy beliefs/practices contributing to distress or treatment concerns.
- Any other issue arising with spiritual/religious content.

Most hospitals have chaplains who are available, often 24 hours a day. In certain settings, a chaplain makes visits to patients without prompting. When parents have connections with their own clergy, a formal referral to hospital chaplaincy may or may not be necessary. It is recommended that the nature and process of clergy involvement in any pediatric oncology program be shared with patients and families verbally and in written materials when they first visit or are admitted to the program.

Spiritual and Religious Caveats

- Spirituality and religion are not confined to church worship attendance, affiliation, reading sacred writings, traditional prayer or observance of ritual.
- Beliefs and practices of a child and family may be a combination of traditions, influenced to varying degrees by geography, past life experiences, influential persons in their lives, and ethnic, socioeconomic, political, and gender considerations.
- Medical teams should become familiar with hospital and outpatient chaplains and clergy and pastoral counselors in the geographical area in which they practice. Any hospital or outpatient center treating children and adolescents with cancer and hematologic illnesses will be staffed with pastoral caregivers/chaplains or have access to knowledgeable clergy in the community who have experience working with medically ill youth and their families. Just as physicians and other medical providers have working relationships and knowledge of medical professionals in other specialties and spheres of care, so too, hospital chaplains and pastoral caregivers typically have extensive referral networks and contacts. Given the increasing religious diversity in the United States and North America today, locating leaders and other resources in even less common religions has become a common task for hospital and clinic-based religious professionals.

Appendix: Spiritual Assessment of Children and Families

Numerous tools exist to assess the multi-faceted construct of spirituality. Clinicians may find these helpful in initiating conversations with children and parents about spirituality and health care. These tools do not have established psychometrics. Spiritual assessment of children is challenging due to wide developmental range and clinicians must adjust their assessments accordingly.

For Parents/Families[10]

A spiritual history tool developed by Christine Pulchalksi MD and colleagues uses the mnemonic FICA to recall helpful questions. Questions may be reworded so long as they cover the same content.

- **F**aith: Do you consider yourself spiritual or religious?
- **I**mportance: What's the importance of spirituality or religion in your life?
- **C**ommunity: Are you part of any spiritual, religious, or worshipping community?
- **A**ct: How would you like me to account for these beliefs in your healthcare?

Spiritual Struggle: A Screener for Parents/Families[11]

This screener was developed based on research showing that 7–50% of hospitalized adults have spiritual struggle and do not typically self-refer for spiritual care. It was also based on studies showing poorer health outcomes related to spiritual struggle. Indications for "order spiritual assessment" suggest the need for deeper assessment by a chaplain.

1. "Is religion or spirituality important to you as you cope with your illness?" If "yes", ask,

1a. "How much strength or comfort do you get from your religious or spiritual beliefs right now—"
   - All that you need?
   - Somewhat less than what you need? (Refer to chaplain for further assessment.)
   - None at all? (Refer to chaplain for further assessment.)

If "no", ask,

1b. "Has there ever been a time when religion/spirituality was important to you?" (Yes/no; if "yes" refer to chaplain for further assessment.)

2. "Would you like a visit from a chaplain?" (Yes/no; if "yes" refer to chaplain.)

References

1. Shafranske EP, ed. *Religion and the Clinical Practice of Psychology*. Washington, DC: American Psychological Association; 1996.
2. Fowler JW, Dell ML. Stages of faith and identity: birth to teens. *Child Adolesc Psychiatr Clin N Am*. 2004;13(1):17–33.
3 Stuber ML, Houskamp BM. Spirituality in children confronting death. *Child Adolesc Psychiatr Clin N Am*. 2004;13(1):127–136.
4. Griffith JL. *Religion That Heals, Religion That Harms: A Guide for Clinical Practice*. New York: Guilford Press; 2010.
5. Fitchett G, Meyer PM, Burton LA. Spiritual care in the hospital: who requests it? Who needs it? *J Pastoral Care*. 2000;54(2):173–186.
6. Sexson SB. Religious and spiritual assessment of the child and adolescent. *Child Adolesc Psychiatr Clin N Am*. 2004;13(1):35–47.
7. Barnes LP, Plotnikoff GA, Fox K, Pendleton S. Spirituality, religion, and pediatrics: intersecting worlds of healing. *Pediatrics*. 2000;106(Suppl. 4):899–906.
8. Fosarelli P. Children and the development of faith: implications for pediatric practice. *Contemporary Pediatrics*. 2003;20(1):85–86.
9. Dell ML. Religious professionals and institutions: untapped resources for clinical care. *Child Adolesc Psychiatr Clin N Am*. 2004;13(1):85–110.
10. Borneman T, Ferrell B, Puchalski CM. Evaluation of the FICA tool for spiritual assessment. *J Pain Symptom Management*. 2010;40(2):163–173.
11. Fitchett G, Risk J. Screening for spiritual struggle. *J Pastoral Care & Counsel*. 2009; 63:1,2 (accessed August 19, 2013).

Further Reading

Galanti GA. *Caring for Patients from Different Cultures*. 3rd ed. Philadelphia, PA: University of Pennsylvania Press; 2003.

McEvoy M. Culture and spirituality as an integrated concept in pediatric care. *MCN Am J Matern Child Nurs*. 2003;28(1):39–43.

Spector RE. *Cultural Diversity in Health and Illness*. 6th ed. Upper Saddle River, New Jersey: Prentice Hall; 2004.

Chapter 27

School and Peer Relationships

Robert B. Noll and William M. Bukowski

Considerable theoretical and empirical work has highlighted the importance of peer relationships for healthy psychological and cognitive development for all children regardless of health status.[1] Work focusing on children's social reputation (What is the child like?) and social acceptance (Is the child liked?) has demonstrated the stability and predictive validity of peer relationships. Children who are viewed by their peers as being aggressive or isolated and do not have friends are at risk for later academic difficulties, externalizing symptoms, delinquency, negative self-perceptions, depressive symptoms, and dropping out of school.[2] In contrast, friendships in childhood have been demonstrated to be concurrently and longitudinally associated with less loneliness, less depression, and more positive self-concept,[3] and may offer protection against the effects of victimization.[4] Having more best-friend nominations in high school was associated with greater lifetime income 35 years later.[5] Since the long-term prognosis for pediatric cancer has improved dramatically over the past 30 years, the majority of children with cancer will survive. Therefore, peer relationships of children with cancer during and after treatment are especially important.

Reasons Parents or Children Think That Cancer Might Adversely Affect Social Functioning

- Child's altered appearance due to treatment effects.
- Long absence from school.
- Physical limitations related to pain or fatigue.
- Inability to participate in sports or other extracurricular activities.
- General parental protectiveness related to their child with cancer.[6]

What Do We Know about the Social Functioning of Children with Cancer?

- Although parents and children often have the concerns previously listed, the majority of children with cancer want to return to school as soon as possible and have few problems.

- Return to school is a sign of a return to normalcy for children/adolescents—we strongly encourage this step as soon as medically feasible.
- Children without primary CNS involvement typically do well with their peers.[7,8]
    - Children on chemotherapy have less energy and tend to be less aggressive and disruptive than before they were diagnosed.
    - Data from peers shows children with cancer are liked more than typically developing peers.[9]
- Children with brain tumors are at risk for problems with peers.[10] They tend to have fewer friends and are viewed by peers as being sensitive and isolated.[11] It is not clear when these problems begin to emerge or why they occur for this group of children with cancer.

How Do Scientists Assess Social Functioning of Children?

The associations between parent or teacher reports of peer relationships and data from peers are low.[12] The optimal manner to ascertain how children get along with their peers is to ask their peers. Although this methodology provides a significant improvement over parent and teacher reports, it is probably beyond the ability of pediatric oncologists and other clinical staff to complete these types of assessments. Peers observe other children interacting in situations that parents or teachers may not see.

Answers for Clinicians Trying to Send Children Back to School

- After the child is diagnosed with cancer, encourage parents to call their child's school to provide information about their child's diagnosis. Since pediatric cancer is less than 1% of all cancers, most principals, teachers, school nurses, or school psychologists will have no experience; few school professionals will know about the excellent prognosis of many cancer diagnoses.
    - To ease the burden of communication between families and the school, we encourage schools to select one liaison person to work with families and the medical center.
    - To minimize rumors about children with cancer, parents have the opportunity to provide accurate information to school personnel who can share the information with other children.
- Parents may have concerns about their child being teased, left out, or not fitting in: The return to school is psychologically a very positive event for the vast majority of children, especially when prepared for by interactions between teachers and hospital school or behavioral health personnel.

- Special accommodations might be needed. The majority of schools are open to needed changes using a 504 plan. The "504" refers to Section 504 of the Rehabilitation Act and the Americans with Disabilities Act. A 504 plan lists specific modifications and accommodations that can be used to ensure a child with a physical impairment is not excluded from school, including:
  - Extra sets of books to alleviate carrying heavy backpacks.
  - Use of elevators.
  - Special adjustments/accommodations related to physical education.
  - Extra time to transition between classes (for children in middle or high school).
  - Wearing a hat or scarf.
  - Tape recorder or keyboard for taking notes.
- If parents, children, or teachers believe a child with cancer is beginning to have social problems with peers:
  - Encourage a referral for a comprehensive assessment from the school psychologist to understand why the child is having social problems or is experiencing peer rejection. Treatments vary considerably, dependent upon the cause of the problem. Treatments might include:
    - *Attention problems*—Children with attention problems often have problems with peers.[13] Recommended treatments include stimulant medications for primary attention problems and when co-morbid difficulties are present, use of cognitive behavioral treatments. (See Chapter 18, Cognitive Sequelae.)
    - *Excessive anxiety/depression*—For mild to moderate symptoms, initial treatment should be cognitive behavioral therapy. If this is not effective, adding medications is often helpful. (See Chapter 12, Anxiety and Depression.) We recommend evidence-based behavioral treatments first so children and their parents have an opportunity to learn coping skills that will serve them for the remainder of their lives. Optimally, these services can be provided by a behavioral health specialist within the setting of pediatric oncology to improve access and collaboration.[14]
    - *Poor social skills*—Social-skills training is a form of behavior therapy to help persons who have difficulties relating to other people. A major goal of social-skills training is teaching persons about the verbal as well as nonverbal behaviors involved in social interactions. When social-skills training is not available, many cancer centers have patient groups, and, while they are not social-skills-training programs, they promote social interactions. Similarly, connections with other children with similar conditions can be helpful.
- For children with brain tumors, monitoring of social functioning is encouraged.[11,15] Calls to teachers around re-entry and at least semi-annual calls to teachers can focus on social behavior and social

acceptance/friendship. If problems begin to emerge, careful investigation of why difficulties are occurring (see earlier) can lead to optimal treatment recommendations.

Answers for Clinicians or Parents: When to Seek Help?

Peer relationships tend to be very stable and difficult to influence, although issues with peers can be situational (i.e., a bad year with a particular teacher/class/school; problems with peers on one sporting team). Although some children may "outgrow" social problems with peers, waiting is not recommended.

Children may not be aware they are socially isolated and/or being rejected by peers.[11,16] If teachers, parents, or peers observe social isolation or rejection, intervention in the form of a psychological evaluation is critical even if the child does not seem distressed by their social dysfunction. Social acceptance and friendships are powerful predictors of future success or failure.

References

1. Reiter-Purtill J, Waller J, Noll RB. Empirical and theoretical perspectives on the peer relationships of children with chronic conditions. In: Roberts MC, Steele R, eds., *Handbook of Pediatric Psychology*. 4th ed. New York: Guilford Press; 2009: 672–688.
2. Laird RD, Pettit GS, Dodge KA, Bates JE. Peer relationship antecedents of delinquent behavior in late adolescence: Is there evidence of demographic group differences in developmental processes? *Dev Psychopathol.* 2005;17(1):127–144.
3. Nangle DW, Erdley CA Newman JE, Mason CA, Carpenter EM. Popularity, friendship quantity and friendship quality: Interactive influences on children's loneliness and depression. *J Clin Child Adolesc Psychol.* 2003;32(4):546–555.
4. Hodges EV, Boivin M, Vitaro F, Bukowski WM. The power of friendship: Protection against an escalating cycle of peer victimization. *Dev Psychol.* 1999;35(1):94–101.
5. Conti G, Galeotti A, Mueller G, Pudney S (2009). Popularity. Institute for Social and Economic Research, ISER Working Paper Series, No. 2009-03.
6. Davies WH, Noll RB, DeStefano L., Bukowski WM, Kulkarni R. Differences in the child-rearing practices of parents of children with cancer and controls: The perspectives of parents and professionals. *J Pediatr Psychol.* 1991;16(3):295–306.
7. Noll RB, Gartstein MA, Vannatta K, Correll J, Bukowski WM, Davies WH. Social, emotional, and behavioral functioning of children with cancer. *Pediatrics.* 1999;103(1):71–78.
8. Reiter-Purtill J, Vannatta K, Gerhardt CA, Correll J, Noll RB. A controlled longitudinal study of the social functioning of children who completed treatment of cancer. *J Pediatr Hematol Oncol.* 2003;25(6):467–473.

9. Gartstein MA, Short AD, Vannatta K, Noll, R.B. Psychosocial adjustment of children with chronic illness: An evaluation of three models. *J Dev Behav Pediatr.* 1999;20(3):157–163.

10. Nassau JH, Drotar D. Social competence among children with central nervous system–related chronic health conditions: A review. *J Pediatr Psychol.* 1997;22(6):771–793.

11. Vannatta K, Gartstein MA, Short A, Noll RB. A controlled study of peer relationships of children surviving brain tumors: teacher, peer, and self ratings. *J Pediatr Psychol.* 1998;23(5):279–288.

12. Noll RB, Bukowski WM. Commentary: Social competence in children with chronic illness: the devil is in the details. *J Pediatr Psychol.* 2012;37:959–966.

13. Hoza B, Gerdes AC, Mrug S, et al. Peer-assessed outcomes in the Multimodal Treatment Study of Children with Attention Deficit Hyperactivity Disorder. *J Clin Child Adol Psychol.* 2005; 34:74–86.

14. Kazak A, Noll RB. The integration of psychology in pediatric oncology research and practice: Collaboration to improve care and outcomes for children and families. *Am Psychol.* In press.

15. Vannatta K, Gerhardt CA, Wells RJ, Noll RB. Intensity of CNS treatment for pediatric cancer: prediction of social outcomes in survivors. *Pediatr Blood Cancer.* 2007;49(5):716–722.

16. Noll RB, Reiter-Purtill J, Moore BD, et al. Social, emotional, and behavioral functioning of children with NF1. *Am J Med Genet.* 2007;143A(19):2 261–2273.

Chapter 28

School and Academic Planning

Ernest R. Katz

Introduction

This chapter will review the following topics critical to helping childhood cancer patients and survivors achieve their academic and vocational potential:

1. Hospital and home-based instruction.
2. School re-entry.
3. School risk profiling: identifying patients at-risk for school problems.
   a. Preexisting developmental, learning, or emotional-behavioral difficulties.
   b. Minimally involved or non-English-speaking parents.
   c. Prolonged school absences.
   d. Neurocognitive impairments.
4. Federal laws protecting the educational rights of children with Disabilities: special education services and general education modifications.
5. Getting specialized academic help.
6. Transitions in healthcare status, developmental and school levels: need for ongoing monitoring and vigilance.

During the initial phases of treatment, it is not unusual for a child to miss weeks or months of school. For a child undergoing a bone marrow transplant, the time away from school may be even longer. It is important to the child's overall quality of life and adaptation to illness that school continue during periods of hospitalization or when homebound because of health issues. Both hospital and home instruction are available to help.

Hospital and Home-Based Instruction

Hospital Instruction. What Is It and How Does It Work?

- Under the federal laws known as the Individuals with Disabilities Education Act (IDEA) of 2004 (enacted in 1975, amended in 1997, and reauthorized in 2004), and Section 504 of the Rehabilitation Act of 1973, stipulations are made for the continuation of educational programs for young people who are not able to attend a regular school because of health concerns.

- Each individual state also has educational laws and regulations that follow the federal guidelines to implement these services.
- Hospital teaching is provided by teachers of the school district within which the hospital caring for the ill child is located. Some hospitals generate an automatic referral for a hospital teacher, whereas some hospitals may require the parent or medical team to generate the referral for this service to begin.
- Most children's hospitals and large pediatric departments of general medical centers employ teachers who teach hospitalized children.
- A minimum *projected* hospital stay of 5–10 school days is usually required before a hospital teacher will be assigned, depending on the district. A physician must sign the request for services, attesting to the expected length of stay. If the actual stay is less than the minimum number of days, or a child is in and out of the hospital for multiple short stays, most hospital instruction programs will still provide instructional services even if the minimum days of hospitalization are not precisely met.
- During a hospital stay that meets the minimum criteria for length of stay, a child is technically "transferred" from the regular school to the hospital school for that period of time, after which the student will be transferred back to the school or to home teaching (see next section).
- In larger pediatric hospitals, hospital-based teachers will generally identify a new patient and will automatically meet with the child and parents and initiate the referral process with the medical team to engage hospital teaching.
- Smaller pediatric inpatient programs may not have full-time hospital teachers and referrals to hospital teachers may need to be initiated by the social worker or child-life specialist.
- Hospital teachers begin by collecting information about the child's regular school program and teachers, and/or special needs. The hospital teacher will contact the regular school and coordinate the curriculum.
- Hospital teaching is usually limited to about one hour per day, but that is often all an ill child can tolerate. Hospital teachers accommodate their teaching schedule to the medical needs and hospital schedule of each child. Teachers may not be able to cover every subject, especially for middle and high school students with numerous classes and teachers. However, school credits are still earned during hospital teaching, and this can help children feel a sense of normalcy in their lives.

Home-Based Instruction

- When a child is discharged from the hospital but is unable to return to a regular school campus for three or more weeks due to health concerns (i.e., low blood counts, immunosuppression, severe fatigue), the child's regular school district must provide a home based teacher to go to the home to teach the child on a regular basis.

- States differ in the minimum weekly number of home instruction hours that are provided. The instruction is usually delivered in two or three weekly meetings. Older students in middle school and high school may augment home teaching with online/distance learning provided by the school district or other educational enterprise. There may be fees associated with private online courses, whereas district options do not generally have additional fees.
- The teacher brings the student work, teaches and reviews material, collects homework, and assigns new homework for the next meeting.
- Parents and students need to understand that home teaching provides less teaching time than occurs on a regular campus, but the student is able to earn most of the credits necessary to stay current with their class.
- Larger school districts may have teachers assigned to home-based instruction who have specialized training in teaching young people with health challenges.
- Smaller districts may recruit a teacher to work with a homebound child from their pool of regular or substitute teachers. This takes a longer time. Parents may need to persist to assure finding a teacher is identified as quickly as possible.
- If the child has not been assigned a home teacher within two weeks of the paperwork being filed with the district, the healthcare team may need to intervene.
- For a home-based teacher to effectively provide instruction in the home, she/he will need to understand the child's illness, treatment, and schedule for outpatient medical appointments and/or hospitalizations stays. The child's parent, healthcare team, and/or school liaison (when available) may need to communicate information needed to effectively work with the child (i.e., schedule of chemotherapy administration and clinic or hospital visits, drug interactions with energy and learning ability, attention, or concentration).
- It is the home-based teacher's responsibility to contact the child's regular classroom teachers and coordinate teaching materials and course of instruction to be similar with that covered in the regular classroom. Although home teachers may not cover all the regular class material, they should complete the basic elements of the instructional program. The home teacher will assign grades at regular report card times, and the credits earned will be credited to the child in his cumulative school record.
- Home-based teachers should be experienced in working with the age and grade level of the specific child referred, and they need to be sensitive to unique language needs of parents and children, cultural issues, or religious traditions of the family in order to be respectful and appropriate in dress and interactions during teaching sessions. Non-English-speaking parents may have difficulty comprehending scheduling instructions for home teaching if not presented in their native language through a competent translation service.

- Home teachers need to be notified immediately if the child's schedule for medical appointments or hospitalization changes in a planned or urgent manner. If parents are not aware of their need to notify the home teacher of a change, or the parents cannot easily communicate with the home teacher due to language constraints or difficulty connecting with them, the child might be dropped from home teaching even though it may be greatly needed. Monitoring of the home-teaching situation by a member of the medical team through dialogue with the child and parent can reduce this problem and rectify it quickly if it does actually occur. If a parent or child does not feel comfortable with the home teacher or the teaching provided, parents have the right to discuss this situation with their school district's director of home instruction and explore available options. The medical team and/or school liaison staff may be needed to facilitate this dialogue.

The Child who Fluctuates between Home and the Hospital

- If a child is in and out of the hospital for many short admissions, maintaining a consistent educational program can be challenging.
- When the regular school district is different from the hospital's school district, it may not make sense to transfer the child's school program back and forth between districts, as each transfer requires paperwork and time. In such cases, it may be best to leave the child enrolled in the regular district, and ask the hospital teacher to provide educational supervision and limited assistance, as needed, during relatively brief hospital stays.
- If the hospital and home-school districts are the same, the child can move back and forth between hospital and home teaching. Sometimes a home teacher may come and work with her students during brief hospitalizations.

Special Education and Home Instruction

- If a child was receiving special education services before the cancer diagnosis, the IEP (Individualized Educational Program) team should be reconvened to make sure the home teacher is capable of working with the child, and to determine if special education services beyond academic home teaching are necessary.
- If the child needs additional services like speech therapy, this may not be available at home but could be made available at a local public school campus where the child might be brought for brief periods of time. The IEP team and special education staff can help monitor educational progress during home instruction.
- If the child has special educational needs because of the diagnosis and treatment of cancer (for example, having a brain tumor that effects thinking or communication skills), the special education process should be initiated before the student returns to school. Being eligible for special education may enable the child to take advantage of additional

services during home instruction and will also be helpful when returning to school. See Box 28.1.

Maintaining Friendships and Social Relationships While at Home/Hospital

- It is extremely important that children receiving home or hospital instruction maintain friendships and connections with peers at school. This kind of social support helps children feel more optimistic and hopeful, and will help with the school re-entry process. Unfortunately, it can be challenging for healthy, busy children to continue calling and visiting, and they may need assistance in order to keep up these connections.
- The ill child may also withdraw from normal relationships because of changes in appearance (for example, being bald or skinny) or fear of being ridiculed.
- If a child resists interacting with healthy peers, professional guidance or psychotherapy from hospital staff may be helpful. Some cancer centers have support groups for school age or adolescent patients that can help kids develop their social skills and abilities to reach out and communicate with peers at school and the community. If the child is immunosuppressed and cannot participate in a group meeting, some centers are providing online or virtual group experiences that allow social interactions without increasing risk.
- Classroom teachers may need help reaching out to the homebound child. The home/hospital teacher and hospital staff can help classroom teachers consider different ways to comfortably keep the ill child

Box 28.1 Education in the Hospital and Home

- Continuing education for an ill child is vital to quality of life and long-term adjustment.
- A child is eligible for teaching in the hospital if he or she will be hospitalized for a minimum number of days (depending on State and school district).
- Home Instruction should begin as soon as a child returns home if not medically ready to return to school for a period of weeks or months. The home teacher should be oriented to the child's illness, treatment, schedule, and special family and cultural issues.
- During Hospital and Home Teaching, efforts should be made to help the child maintain connections to peers at school. Visits to the campus or classroom should be encouraged even while on home teaching.
- Hospital staff can be very helpful in supporting home teachers with the information and background they need to be successful.
- Special education services already in place should continue for children who have received them before getting ill. If the child will need special assistance when they return to school, the special education qualifying process (known as the I.E.P.) should be started during this period of home instruction.

connected, through visits of the child to the school campus, visits of friends to the home or hospital, letter writing, and use of social media technology by students in the classroom (e.g., skype, e-mail, texting, and phone).

School Re-entry: Transition from Home Teaching to the Regular School

- The return to regular school attendance when it becomes medically feasible may be a seamless process for parents who are comfortable interacting with their child's school and knowledgeable about the impact of illness and treatment on their child's school participation.
- For the growing number of immigrant children, parents may not possess this knowledge or experience, and they may need more intensive support in re-entering regular school participation.
- Many centers have developed school-liaison positions to coordinate planning and implementation among the child, family, and healthcare team, and school personnel assist with school issues like re-entry or special-educational needs. In the absence of a designated individual or team, other centers rely on social workers, nurse coordinators, or child-life specialists to assist with this type of liaison work. Whichever structure exists in a particular treatment center, it is imperative to plan for the child's return to school and assist those children and families who are not able to negotiate this process on their own.

Preparing Parents

- When a child's medical condition stabilizes and his physician provides approval for returning to school, parents may be reluctant to allow their child to return to school for a variety of reasons, which may include:
  - Difficulty changing their perception of child as extremely medically fragile when that is no longer the case.
  - Desire to protect their child from potential hurt, ridicule, and/or rejection by other children.
  - Feelings of guilt at causing their child discomfort by not "protecting" their child from contracting a life-threatening illness; ongoing parental fears of their ill child being exposed to germs or viruses that may create a life-threatening situation.
- The following parent handbook is an example of readily available Web-based material with useful information on the school re-entry process: http://www.chop.edu/export/download/pdfs/articles/oncology/parent-guide-school-reentry.pdf

Preparing the Patient

- The child and adolescent who has been out of school because of illness and treatment may also be apprehensive about returning to school, looking and feeling differently, being unable to resume all regular activities, and feeling unsupported by peers and staff.

- Children may benefit from individual counseling and preparation to prepare for the emotional and real-world challenges associated with the return to school. They may need help preparing for academic and social challenges, and developing a joint plan for informing and supporting peers and teachers regarding the child's experience and school needs.
- Videos may be very helpful in facilitating the child's cooperation and support for the re-entry process, such as the "Back to School Video" in the *Videos with Attitude Series* of the Starbright Foundation (1999), The Cancervive "Back to School Videos" (1997), or "Why Charlie Brown? Why?" (1986; distributed by the Leukemia/Lymphoma Society). These videos and others similar to them can be used in schools and classrooms to help the other children understand their peer's experience with greater precision.

Preparing School Personnel

- Teachers and school administrators need to be closely apprised and prepared with regard to the child's medical condition and to begin their preparation for the child's return. With the family's consent, the child's teacher and staff should be prepared with basic medical and treatment information that might impact the child's learning and social performance. An example of an excellent handbook for school-support teams assisting students with chronic illness was developed by Carol Kaffenberger: http://www.fcps.edu/cco/prc/resources/events/docs/workshops_2010-11/Handbook_Manual_revised_2010.pdf
- Staff preparation should include information about potential immunosuppression related to chemotherapy and the need for parents of other children to be informed and vigilant regarding communicable diseases.
- As the child progresses academically, year to year, open communication between school personnel and the school liaison needs to occur to keep them apprised of any possible late effects that may be experienced by the child as a result of the medical treatment received. (Please refer to Box 28.2 Neurocognitive Deficits.)

For most teachers, a child with a serious chronic illness or injury returning to the classroom is a new experience. Preconceived notions about certain cancer diagnoses, limited knowledge about cancer, and the vulnerability communicated by the change in a child's appearance or energy level may cause teachers to arrive at the premature or erroneous conclusion that the child is likely to die. Teachers may be overwhelmed, unsure of how to approach the child, and uncomfortable in seeking information from the parents who are already stressed from the illness experience and unable to deal with their own anxieties about the situation.

- Teachers need specific information regarding the illness, treatment, and possible impact on school performance and general development. This information allows teachers to adapt instruction to ensure the child is successful.

Box 28.2 Neurocognitive Deficits

In the classroom setting, these neurocognitive deficits often result in the child or adolescent experiencing specific academic and social difficulties associated with underlying neural pathways, which can include the following:

(1) Variabilities in *attention.*
(2) Difficulties with *memory.*
(3) Difficulties completing tasks quickly due to decreased *processing speed.*
(4) *Poor planning and organizational skills* impacting the ability to self-monitor and complete projects independently.
(5) Difficulty *writing quickly and accurately.*
(6) Difficulty *copying or writing visual information,* such as assignments written on a blackboard.
(7) Difficulty *learning visual information* that is not verbally meaningful.
(8) Problems with *mathematics calculation* skills.
(9) Increased difficulty with *reading comprehension.*
(10) Problems maintaining *social discourse* with peers due to inability to detect and respond to subtle social cues.

- Educators may benefit from the Web-based resource such as that produced by Children's Hospital Philadelphia: http://www.chop.edu/export/download/pdfs/articles/oncology/oncology-teacher-guide-school-reentry.pdf

Preparing Classmates

Classmates and peers may need some basic preparation in order to dispel myths and misconceptions about what has happened to the ill child during their absence.

- After discussion with the child's parents, the teacher or school counselor should inform the class about their classmate's illness in general terms.
- Communication with the hospitalized child may be encouraged through cards, electronic mail, phone calls, weekly newsletters, class meetings conducted with a speakerphone to include the classmate, audio taped class discussions of a high-interest topic with comments from the teacher to include the classmate, and, when possible, visit from classmates to the hospital. If peers stay in close contact with the ill child during protracted absences, the child may feel more connected and supported by their class and find it easier to return to school with less negative affect.
- To ease the transition back into the classroom, if the child and family agree, members of the medical team may visit the school and present information about cancer and its treatment. The child is generally given

the opportunity to provide "expert" information during the presentation to encourage peers to communicate directly with the child or adolescent if they have questions, but the ill child may elect not to do so.

- Components of the classroom presentation, presented in developmentally appropriate terms, include providing a basic understanding of cancer and the specific type involved, basic approaches to cancer treatment, demystification (i.e., cancer is not contagious, it is not caused by bad or inappropriate behavior), adverse side effects of treatment that students might notice in the chronically ill child at school (i.e., hair loss, weight gain, absences), and the critical role of peer support and how peers can help in the process. Classroom presentations help facilitate open communication and peer social support that will likely result in a more reinforcing environment for the child (Cancervive *Teacher's Guide for Kids with Cancer*—www.cancersourcekids.com/parents/schoolintro).

School Risk Profiling: Identifying Patients At-Risk for School Problems

A. *Preexisting developmental, learning, or emotional-behavioral difficulties. Cancer and its treatments may exacerbate premorbid difficulties.*
   - Children and adolescents with preexisting developmental disabilities such as mental retardation, learning disabilities such as reading or math problems, attention deficit hyperactivity disorder, or anxiety and depression are at greater risk for school problems.

B. *Minimally involved or non-English-speaking parents*
   - Children whose parents were only minimally involved with their child's school prior to the illness may also experience educational disadvantages after a cancer diagnosis. These parents may lack the knowledge, communication skills, or experience regarding school procedures to know how to access help when problems are encountered.

C. *Prolonged school absences*
   - Academic difficulties will likely be compounded by gaps in knowledge and classroom experiences sustained during prolonged school absences. For children who were only marginally academically or socially successful prior to the onset of the illness, the effects of prolonged or even brief absences may be especially disruptive to learning and social relationships.

D. *Neurocognitive impairments*
   - The greatest risk for difficulties with school and academic problems is associated with youth who experience cognitive toxicities as a direct consequence of cancer effecting the brain (i.e., a brain tumor) or secondary to treatment, such as surgery, cranial irradiation, whole body radiation, or intrathecal chemotherapy used to prevent infiltration of the leukemia cells into the central nervous system.

- The locus and extent of direct brain damage through disease or treatment will generally correlate with the level of school and functional impairment experienced by the child.
- Females and children who are younger at time of treatment (generally under age 6) tend to have greater neurocognitive deficits.
- The effects of radiation therapy and chemotherapy on cognitive functioning in children treated for brain tumors and leukemia may be global for some children, although typically nonverbal abilities are affected more intensely than verbal abilities.
- The full impact of neurocognitive deficits usually takes several years to completely emerge, and requires ongoing evaluation and advocacy to ensure that proper educational assistance is provided. See Box 28.2.

Federal Laws Protecting the Educational Rights of Children with Disabilities: Special Education and School Program Modifications

- Ensuring successful re-entry and ongoing adjustment to school requires careful understanding and examination of a child's academic needs and available resources through general and special education programs.
- The goal is to meet the child's learning and social needs in the least restrictive educational environment (LRE) that is most like a regular classroom with nondisabled peers.
- Four federal laws protect the educational rights of children who have disabilities that impede their ability to benefit from their educational environment: the Individuals with Disability Education Act (IDEA), the Rehabilitation Act (Section 504), the Americans with Disabilities Act (ADA), and the recently enacted No Child Left Behind Act (NCLB).
- IDEA Part B provides legal protection to students with a disability ages 3 through 21, while IDEA Part C provides legal protection to students from birth to age 2.
- All of these laws apply to every level of education, from early intervention to college and vocational training, and the laws guarantee every child a right to education regardless of physical, mental, or health impairment.

Qualifying for Special Education Services

- To receive special education under the provision of IDEA, children with cancer must qualify for one of 13 special education classifications that delineate criteria for eligibility (please refer to Table 28.1: Eligibilities under IDEA).
- "Other Health Impaired" is the classification commonly applied to youth diagnosed with cancer, when their disease and/or treatment adversely impact their ability to perform in school.

Evaluation

- If a child is suspected of needing special educational services to meet their academic potential, the parent or school must make a formal request. Typically, the parent makes this request by submitting, in writing, a letter requesting that their child be evaluated to determine if the students has a disability that affects his/her learning.
- Parents should submit this letter to the school principal, teacher, administrator or special education department at the school.
- Additionally, the parent should request signed confirmation that the letter has been received.
- The school must then comply with strict guidelines for completing the evaluation (please refer to Box 28.3: Timing of Evaluation and IEP).
- If the child with cancer has received neuropsychological, physical, or occupational therapy evaluations while in the hospital, the parent can provide these reports to the appropriate school personnel.
- A letter from the treating oncologist regarding diagnosis, treatment course, and any illness or treatment-related impairments also is helpful.
- Some school systems require the oncologist to complete a standard form verifying the eligibility to receive services through the classification of Other Health Impaired.

Individualized Education Plan Development

- Once the school agrees to evaluate the student, the parent will be provided with an assessment plan, and if the parent agrees with the plan, the parent must sign and return the assessment within the required time period.
- Once the assessment plan has been returned to the school, the school has an allotted amount of time to conduct the assessment and hold an IEP meeting to review results and determine eligibility for services (please refer to Box 28.3: Timing of Evaluation and IEP).

Table 28.1 Eligibilities under IDEA
Emotional Disturbance
Deaf-Blindness
Deafness
Mental Retardation
Autism
Hearing Impairment
Orthopedic Impairments
Multiple Disabilities
Specific Learning Disabilities
Traumatic Brain Injury
Other Health Impairment
Speech and Language Impairment
Visual Impairment

Box 28.3 Timing of Assessment and IEP

Parent submits a written request for an assessment of their child at any time a disability is suspected.

↓

The school has 15 (fifteen) days to respond in writing to the request. If the school agrees to evaluate the student, the parent will be provided with an assessment plan.

↓

The parent has 15 (fifteen) days to review, sign, and return the assessment plan to the school.

↓

Upon receipt of the assessment plan, the school has 60 (sixty) days to conduct the assessment and hold an Individualized Education Program (IEP) to discuss the results and determine eligibility.

- At a minimum, this meeting should include the parents, the student, if appropriate, the district administrator, the general education and special education teacher, the person who assessed the child, and anyone the parent or school district believes has relevant information about the child, such as someone from the hospital (school liaison).
- Once the IEP is signed by all participants at the meeting, it becomes a legal document that, by law, the school is required to carry out. However, parents should not feel forced to sign the IEP at the meeting and can review it at home or with someone's assistance. The downfall to this is that the plan will not be in effect until it is signed by the parent.
- The plan is evaluated on a yearly basis with a reevaluation of appropriateness of eligibility for special education services performed no less than every three years. The parents can call for an IEP meeting at any time to review their child's educational program.

School Program Modifications: Section 504

- In some cases, a child may not meet criteria for special education services and a Section 504 Plan will be instituted.
- Although Section 504 of the Rehabilitation Act of 1973 (reauthorized in 1998) is not an education law or a federal grant program, it does contain a provision that allows schools to develop intervention plans specific to meeting student needs without necessarily identifying these students as eligible for special education services. Students requiring only minor environmental and instructional accommodations services may be best served through this law.
- Section 504 protects all qualified students with disabilities, defined as those having any "physical or mental impairment that substantially limits one or more major life activities (including learning)".
- Students who meet this definition are covered, even if they do not fall within the IDEA designated categories, and even if they do not participate in specific special education programs. Because the legal

obligations of 504 plans are outside the purview of IDEA 2004, the law governing provision of services in special education programs, the opportunities to develop, prescribe, and obtain such plans are usually not as difficult as when special education services are needed.
- The level and frequency of developing 504 plans is variable across school districts and somewhat dependent on the degree of child advocacy. Since school districts do not view 504 plans as having the full force of legal protections for either the child or the school, many districts do not readily agree to the development and implementation of 504 plans and prefer, instead, to have students identified under the legal mandate of IDEA.

Transition Services

Transitions for children and teens from one stage of treatment to another may have important school ramifications because of more or less demands. Transitions from preschool to elementary to middle school, high school, and college or vocational school may also be filled with challenges to the child who is on or off treatment. Some young people will need assistance at every level of their educational program, and they and their parents or guardians must be empowered with knowledge to identify needs and resources, and advocacy skills to be able to get help and evaluate progress.

- The educational transition from high school to college or vocational training for adolescents with cancer requires intensive consideration for any child with special learning needs.
- Federal law, under the IDEA legislation, requires that schools provide services for the student receiving special education who will be exiting high school that promote the adolescent's transition to post secondary education, work, and community integration.
- These transition services are part of the student's IEP, and are mandated to begin between the ages of 14 and 16 years old.
- The goal of transition is meaningful employment and a quality of adult life for all students with disabilities.
- Critical planning for the adolescent's future usually takes place at the annual school review of each student's IEP, and school districts have identified transition coordinators to ensure that this type of planning occurs.
- Each special education student should have an Individual Transition Plan (ITP) developed for him or her that carefully outlines the plans of the team to prepare the adolescent for college, vocational training, or community support programs, and ensure that any needed support services will be there when the child arrives.
- Transition services should focus on educational and social needs, including preparing the student for independent living (i.e., grooming, mobility, managing finances, recreation, etc.).
- Survivors who have more intensive problems may need alternative learning and vocational options that must be anticipated well in advance of graduation.

- Parents may need assistance from their child's healthcare and school professional teams to advocate for effective transition services to prepare their child for life after high school.

Many long-term survivors with learning disabilities who are college bound may need learning assistance in that setting in order to succeed. Many college-bound students with learning differences may not be clear about their specific educational needs, unaware of the support services available at their future college, and uncertain about how to access such services when they are informed.

- Connecting the student with the disabilities student center may make the transition from high school to college less worrisome. Making actual contact with the college layout and learning about the resources available may allay worries.
- Colleges are likely to make the accommodations necessary to help a student succeed in college and are open to suggestions and information provided by hospital representatives. A student who has survived a life-threatening illness and is college bound need not worry about how to succeed in college. This student can also receive the assistant received when learning to navigate the formal Kindergarten through high school system.

Section VI

Special Issues in Pediatric Oncology

Chapter 29

Ethical Issues in Pediatric Oncology

Julia A. Kearney and Marguerite S. Lederberg

Medical decisions are often fraught with ambiguity, emotion, and conflicting priorities. Understanding the ethical underpinnings of medical practice is essential for good clinical care. In pediatric oncology, where patients are incomparably vulnerable, parental, or other caregivers particularly distressed, and providers deeply dedicated to the search for a cure, the "right" path is not always obvious. Each case presents a unique set of multilayered considerations and may require systematic review to delineate the factors in any ethical dilemma. Attention to ethical principles described below through staff education, case discussions or ethics consultations will help clarify directions, boundaries, goals, processes and, sometimes conflicts, thereby smoothing the illness experience for patients, families, and staff.

Ethical Principles

Box 29.1 defines the guiding principles for moral and ethical human decisions and behavior. In medicine, they represent the highest expectations professionals have of themselves and form the basis of trust in the relationship between the professional and the patient. Many medico-legal precedents uphold these concepts to varying degrees in our society. They can be thought of as useful "shortcuts" to thinking about competing interests or complex factors in medical decision making.

Key Ethical Issues in Childhood Cancer

See Tables 29.1 and 29.2.

Developmental Issues

Every medical scenario in pediatrics is played out on the backdrop of the child's development, making each pediatric case rich, complex, and unique. Each developmental stage brings with it special challenges, and each child

Box 29.1 Ethical Principles Defined[1,2]

Beneficence—The obligation to provide care that improves health or well-being

Nonmaleficence—The obligation to prevent or avoid harm

Respect for Persons (autonomy)—The general duty to respect a person's legal and ethical right of self-determination regarding choices about his or her life and body, for example, the right to refuse treatment

Competence—The legal state of being of sound mind and ability to make autonomous decisions. (Incompetence can only be designated by court adjudication.)[3]

Capacity—A person's ability to understand relevant information and appreciate the reasonably foreseeable consequences of a medical decision.[4] This applies to an individual facing a particular decision at a particular time and is defined by his or her ability to express a consistent, explainable choice even if it is not the recommended course of action. Capacity, or lack thereof, can be determined by a physician or other professionals as needed.

Justice—The duty to avoid discrimination on the basis of irrelevant characteristics in the care of a given patient, even if it conflicts with distributive justice, which is a societal duty to distribute healthcare resources to all in need, in ways that can be defended as fair and equitable and not arbitrary or capricious.

Truth-telling or Honesty—This applies to deliberate or accidental misinformation as well as omissions of information that could effect the patient's decisions. It is especially important within the doctor-patient relationship because of unequal power and seriousness of the consequences of decisions. It is crucial in the relationship that the patient and/or parent tell the truth as well, about issues such as treatment adherence or alternative treatments used. However, the burden of duty is on the physician to inspire the patient to feel safe to tell the truth without fear of abandonment or reprisal.

Confidentiality—An ethical cornerstone for any doctor-patient relationship, confidentiality establishes the basis for the patient's trust. It is especially crucial to establish at the outset of a psychiatric or counseling relationship with a clear explanation of the legal limits to confidentiality that exist when a patient or other person's safety is at risk.[5]

Special issues in pediatric psychiatry—Confidentiality is a complex balancing act when the patient is a child. The goal from the outset is to establish a dual treatment relationship with both parent and child with a common goal of understanding the child's thoughts and feelings and improving the child's well-being. *It is necessary to establish a three-way message of trust.*

- The parents need to trust that the clinician is their ally in caring for the child and relinquish their need to know every detail from the child's shared thoughts.
- The child must come to trust that the clinician will respect his or her wishes and act on the child's behalf with discretion when divulging information to the parent.

Table 29.1 Key Ethical Issues Over the Course of Childhood Cancer

At Diagnosis	
Disclosure	• The issue of disclosure to children about their illness sometimes leads to an ethical dilemma when clinicians are asked not to disclose a diagnosis to a child. Parents wishing to protect their child are often uncertain about how to talk to the child appropriately. This lack of experience in the face of such a severe threat is anxiety-provoking and can lead to parental avoidance of discussion about the illness. • Working with parents on how to disclose at least limited information in a developmentally appropriate manner is essential. (See Chapter 22, Talking to Children and Adolescents about Cancer.)
During Treatment	
Informed Consent	• Informed consent is the process by which the patient or proxy (if patient is under 18 years old or not competent) is informed of the risks and benefits of the treatment in order to give their explicit consent for the proposed treatment. • The ability to give informed consent involves (a) information (b) comprehension, and (c) voluntary choice to accept or refuse treatment. • The amount of information imparted to the patient or proxy during the consent process should be what a "prudent patient" would want to know. The clinician has a limited ability to invoke the "therapeutic privilege"[6] to withhold information that could harm or incapacitate the patient. • Comprehension by a competent patient must be assured for proper informed consent. The Belmont Report and the Nuremberg Code specify populations at risk for impaired comprehension, especially children, the mentally ill, and possibly hospitalized, ill patients. Minors do not have legal decision-making capacity under the law, so the informed consent is given by a proxy.[4,8] The law is less clear about the requirements for parents and surrogates. Given the requirement to respect autonomy, conflicts may arise when a parent denies a child essential treatment. Staff may resort to the courts, which support the rights of the child to protection by the state and usually rule in favor of the child's welfare. • For patients seeking medical treatment, voluntary participation in the treatment is often assumed. Coercion becomes a concern when obtaining consent for clinical trial participation if the treatment is not otherwise available as the standard of care.[9] • Recent oncology literature emphasizes the ongoing role of the entire medical team in the informed consent process, beyond the initial discussion and paperwork. Ongoing assessment of patient and proxy understanding is the job of every provider.

(continued)

Table 29.1 (Continued)

Assent	• Assent is the agreement of the minor patient to participate in the proposed treatment. It includes: helping the patient achieve developmentally appropriate awareness of the nature of his or her condition; telling the patient what they can expect with tests and treatments; making a clinical assessment of the patient's understanding of the situation; and soliciting expression of the patient's willingness to accept the proposed care (as long as the provider is willing to weigh it seriously). • If the treatment is not optional, the patient should be prepared for what is in store and understand the other negotiable options that remain within the treatment plan.[8,10,13,14] • The ethical principle of respect for persons encourages respect for the developing autonomy of minors by genuinely inviting their participation in decisions about their medical care. • Research on children's cognitive capacity to participate in medical decisions suggests that, starting around age 9–10 years, decisions about medical research and treatment should be approached as a family decision, with the child involved at a developmentally appropriate level. *The clinician's assessment of the child's desire and ability to participate in a decision should help determine how much information the child can process.*[13] • Ethical challenges occur when parents and the adolescent disagree on treatment. Such situations can usually be resolved by careful exploration of the issues and concerns with the adolescent and with the parents at first separately and then together. • Assessment of an adolescent's level of decision-making competence may be needed. The goal is to reach consensus and reduce any rift between the adolescent and the parents.
Consent issues in the care of a Jehovah's Witness	• The medical treatment of Jehovah's Witnesses (JW's) is complicated by the religion's ban on receiving blood products. Care of adults and of-age adolescents should be informed of best possible advances in bloodless medicine as well as recent changes in the policies of the Watchtower Bible and Tract Society (WTS). New rulings by the WTS have revised the ban and allow "personal decision" to be the final determinant for the use of many types of fractionated blood products, stem cells, and factors (e.g., Factor VIII).[15] • Minor patients, however, must be treated by best medical practice, independent of their parents' religious beliefs. The American Academy of Pediatrics (AAP) Committee on Bioethics states, "all children deserve effective medical treatment that is likely to prevent substantial harm or suffering or death. In addition, the AAP advocates that all legal interventions apply equally whenever children are endangered or harmed, without exemptions based on parental religious beliefs."[16,17]

(continued)

Table 29.1 (Continued)

	• The most complex cases may be those of "mature minors" who are not of legal age of consent but demonstrate mature decision making and would otherwise be considered to be legally autonomous. Seeking a court order may be the best practice in cases of mature minors.
Participation in Clinical Research Trials	• Seventy percent of children with cancer participate in a clinical trial during treatment.[13] This widespread availability for participation in large, multicentered pediatric oncology trials has led to remarkable advances in evidence-based, standardized treatments for common pediatric cancers. This unique situation has also created a blurring of the line between clinical care and research with ethical issues resulting.[9] Both parents and physicians may struggle with deciding whether the "possible benefits" from research represent the best interests of an individual child. This reality demands high standards for monitoring ethical practices, and provides a model for research with other vulnerable populations. • Institutional Review Boards (IRBs) provide oversight to assure that clinical research is conducted under the highest ethical standards. Advanced communication skills trainings for clinicians around discussions of clinical trials are available and may be useful.[18] • Regulations about whether children's assent is required for a trial take an "all-or-nothing" approach. In oncology trials, the requirement for assent is often waived because the trial offers a "direct benefit" to the child that would not otherwise be available.[13] Despite the regulations, including children in medical decision making is recommended, as long as the child's preferences can be genuinely incorporated into treatment planning.
Use of Complementary and Alternative Medicine (CAM) (See Chapter 21, Integrative Oncology).	• A family-centered approach should include openness to considering CAM, within the best interests of the child.[19] The physician has a responsibility to be willing to review risks and benefits of CAM, to work with CAM practitioners to provide high standard of multidisciplinary care, and to educate parents to make informed decisions. Having basic knowledge about the most accepted and proven CAM practices will provide patients with continuity and trust in the doctor–patient relationship and state of the art care. However, if parents pursue harmful CAM treatments for their minor child, or forgo best medical practice for ineffective CAM, the child is protected under the law and legal action against the parents is warranted.
During Relapse/Progression of Disease	
Prognosticating	• Prognosticating in oncology elicits ethical issues due to the inaccuracy of most prognostic projections and the devastating impact of delivering such predictions.

(continued)

Table 29.1 (Continued)

	• Physicians are typically wrong (less than 20% accurate) about prognosis when predicting quantitative time until end-of-life (overestimating by as much as fivefold).[20] • Studies of prognostic awareness show that parents who are aware of their child's impending death have increased distress, but in the long run may have less complicated bereavement (with less depression and impairment). • Clinicians fear that bad news will "crush the hopes" of the patient and family, but studies show that hope exists independent of prognostic awareness.[21–23] There are many hopes beyond the "hope for cure" for dying patients, even children, including being free from unnecessary suffering, being assured that one lived a meaningful life, and being assured that one will not be abandoned.
During Palliative Care and at End-of-life (See Chapter 30, Integrating Palliative Care)	
Aggressive palliation versus treatment with curative intent	• Termination of curative treatment should not result in abandonment of the patient by the primary doctor. Advances in and awareness of pediatric palliative care can improve end-of-life options for aggressive symptom management. These services should be made available to all children facing end-of-life.
Withholding treatment versus withdrawing supportive treatment	• Legally and ethically there is no distinction between a medical decision to withhold or withdraw a treatment (despite a common feeling from staff and parents that "once we start, we can't stop"). Doctors' daily medical decisions involve stopping treatments that are harmful or no longer beneficial. When supportive care is deemed to be futile, the same principle applies. Helping families arrive at this conclusion for themselves may be more challenging.[1]
Pain medication/ terminal sedation	• It is generally considered ethically acceptable to administer medication with the intent to relieve symptoms (pain, anxiety, delirium, etc.) even if that medication may suppress breathing and hasten the death of the patient (the "double effect"). It is the intent of the act that is judged in ethical and legal decisions—intent to relieve suffering is ethical and legal, but intent to hasten death or end life is not.[24,25]
Barriers to Palliative Care	• Very few children die in hospice care in the United States, whereas many die in ICU settings. Lack of funding and reimbursement for palliative care for children may inhibit access to hospice.[1] • Pediatric practitioners need more education and training, as late referral of patients to palliative care programs (often less than 3 days) leads to underutilization of services.[1]

(continued)

Table 29.1 (Continued)

During Survivorship (See Chapter 33, Pediatric Cancer Survivors)	
Medical Late Effects • Sexuality • Infertility • Neurocognitive • Psychological • Genetic Risk	Patients and proxies need to know the long-term risks of treatment in order to make fully informed decisions and to prepare for "life after cancer," which may include significant health burdens or adjustment to impaired quality of life.

Table 29.2 Special Issues in Stem Cell Transplant (SCT) (See Chapter 16, Psychosocial Issues for Transplant Patients and Donors)

Prognostic Awareness (See Table 29.1 on prognosticating)	Patients are often offered stem cell transplant (SCT) as a high risk "last option" that also holds potential for a possible cure. Situations may arise suddenly where the prognosis rapidly shifts from "hope for cure" to "imminent demise."[26] In these cases it is even more important that an informed consent discussion be meaningfully done in the context of a supportive, open-minded and mutually honest treatment relationship.
Pediatric Donors	• The use of minor siblings as stem cell donors has been heavily scrutinized because donors do not directly benefit from donating stem cells and are exposed to some risk (side effects and possible rare complications during collection). • Due to the relatively small risk to the donor and the potential for great benefit to the recipient, it is generally considered ethical for children to be used as donors for family members. Previously discussed concepts of assent/consent should be applied. Current consensus supports using even children under 6 months of age as donors.[26,27] • Psychosocial evaluations of donors (particularly for solid organs) under age are required in some institutions and in some states to assess the donor's understanding of the procedure and possible outcomes, as well as to assure that coercion is not a factor.[27]
Creating a donor	• Having a baby to create a potential donor has been found to be psychologically and ethically complicated. It is not unethical per se, but clinicians and families need to be aware of the dangers inherent in such a situation: potential traumatic exposure of the donor to the death of a sibling and parental grief; inevitable uncertainty attached to the pregnancy and SCT outcomes; and the dangers of the intrusion of biology on family symbolism and dynamics.[28] • Psychological support should be encouraged for a family considering this option even when good outcomes are predicted. Once such a decision has been made, a family should be supported unequivocally.

traverses these stages in unique and various ways. Box 29.2 gives examples for a few developmental stages; there are many more than listed here. (See Chapter 22, Talking to Children and Adolescents about Cancer, and Chapter 23, Coping with Pediatric Cancer). See Box 29.3 for review of common ethical conflicts encountered in pediatric oncology and Box 29.4 for recommendations for resolution of conflicts.

Box 29.2 Example Ethical Issues by Developmental Stage

Infants/Toddlers

- Parents universally feel guilty for their child's illness, no matter the child's age, but these feelings are often most acute in infancy due to the child's total dependence on the parents. Babies cannot make sense of their own suffering and can seem particularly distressed by procedures and interventions. This perceived betrayal of trust is a burden on parents and staff alike.

School-age Children

- Disclosure of cancer-related information to school age children is complicated. Every effort should be made to understand parents' reasons for not telling a child about a diagnosis or treatment plan and to provide them with developmentally appropriate versions of explanations.
- The goal is to best help the child understand, have a sense of mastery, and to cope with treatment. The child's ability to understand explanations and to develop coping skills will have a reciprocal calming effect on the parents.

Adolescents

- Illness attacks autonomy, an issue of great importance to teens. Regression during illness creates internal conflicts about autonomy and dependency needs. Parental expectations can add to a teen's frustration by expecting "grown-up" skills to prevail when the teen is feeling like a sick child or by indulging in "babying" the adolescent when such attention is unwanted.
- Ethical challenges arise when parents choose not to disclose diagnostic or prognostic information, or allow the teen's participation in decisions about treatment or quality of life.
- Psychiatry, psychology, and clinical social work services may help negotiate these dynamic issues, especially when they involve consent, adherence to treatment, and risky behaviors such as drug use and sexual activity.

Box 29.3 Common Conflicts for Oncology Staff

Staff Values Conflict with Family's Values

Each clinician brings to work his or her own opinions about the burdens of treatment, what makes "good care" and even a "good death." These ideas may conflict with the needs and wishes of a family or patient that are bound to particular religious and cultural values. Staff members have the responsibility to give priority to the patient's needs. They must:

- Convey therapeutic support, not personal judgments.
- Provide clinical care and participate with conflict resolution if necessary.

(continued)

Box 29.3 (Continued)

If conflicts persist, outside experts may assist, including clergy, psychosocial staff, and ethics committees. When staff members feel their clinical judgment is impaired by intense inner conflict, they should request additional consultation and may request reassignment.

Boundary Issues in the Inpatient Setting

Intense relationships may develop between staff and patients in the intimate setting of the inpatient medical unit during extended or repeated stays that blur the regular boundaries of provider and patient. Staff support, education and peer supervision around appropriate boundaries and the dangers of boundary violations may help balance strong feelings for patients in these complicated therapeutic relationships.

Box 29.4 Conflict Resolution

Ethical Conflicts

- There are times when family, patient, or team members have ethical objections to a proposed course of treatment. These may or may not be true "ethical dilemmas." They can be differences of opinion or failures of communication among staff or between staff and family, or lastly, psychiatric problems masked as ethical conflicts (e.g., a patient refusing treatment because of delirium or anxiety).[29] Resolving conflicts may require clinical skills that bridge communication barriers and build consensus. They can be as simple as employing translation services for assisting with a language barrier, or may require more complex solutions.
- The team must make a situational diagnosis by assessing: What are the patient/family issues (psychological, cultural, or other)? What are the staff's issues? Are there relationship issues between the two? What are the legal concerns? And finally, is there a true ethical dilemma?

Institutional Ethics Committees

Joint Commission on Accreditation of Healthcare Organizations has required each hospital to have a designated body for conflict resolution. The Ethics Committee is a board of multidisciplinary members who serve a threefold function in the institution: (1) clinical consultation, available to families or staff to assist in "articulating processes and resolving disputes about clinical care"; (2) development of institutional policies, such as Do Not Resuscitate orders; and (3) education of staff on current ethical practice. They do not have legal jurisdiction to enforce decisions or make rulings (such as withdrawal of treatment.)[1,30] Ethics consultation may be requested by anyone meaningfully involved in the child's care.

References

1. Field MJ, Berman RE, eds. *When Children Die*. Washington DC: The National Academies of Medicine Press; 2003: 690.
2. Fost N. Ethics in pediatric care. In: Behrman RE, R.M. Dliegman RM, and H.B. Jenson HB, *Nelson Textbook of Pediatrics*, eds. 2000, Philadelphia, PA: W.B. Saunders Company; 2000: 5–9.
3. Shaw RJ, DeMaso DR, *Legal and Forensic Issues* in *Clinical Manual of Pediatric Psychosomatic Medicine*. 2006, Washington DC: American Psychiatric Publishing; 2006: 59–74.
4. Etchells E, Darzins P, Silberfeld M, et al. Assessment of patient capacity to consent to treatment. *JGIM*. 1999;14:27–34.
5. American Psychiatric Association. *Ethics Primer of the American Psychiatric Association from the Ethics Committee of the American Psychiatric Association*. Washington DC: APA; 2001.
6. Hendrick J. *Legal Aspects of Child Health Care*. Oxford, UK: Chapman & Hall; 1997.
7. Belmont Report (1979). *The Belmont Report: Ethical principles and guidelines for the protection of human subjects of research*. Retrieved December 13, 2011, from hhs.gov/ohrp/humansubjects/guidance/belmont.html
8. American Academy of Pediatrics Committee on Bioethics Policy Statment: Informed consent, parental permission, and assent in pediatric practice. *Pediatrics*. 1995;95:314–317.
9. de Vries MC, Houtlosser M, Wit J, et al. Ethical issues at the interface of clinical care and research practice in pediatric oncology: a narrative review of parents' and physicians' experiences. *BMC Med Ethics*. 2011;12:18.
10. Spinetta JJ, Masera G, Jankovic M, et al. Valid informed consent and participative decision-making in children with cancer and their parents: a report of the SIOP Working Committee on psychosocial issues in pediatric oncology. *Med Pediatr Oncol*. 2003;40(4):244–246.
11. Berry DL, et al. Informed consent: process and clinical issues. *Oncol Nurs Forum*. 1996;23(3):507–512.
12. Yamokoski AD, Hazen RA, Kodish ED. Anticipatory guidance to improve informed consent: a new application of the concept. *J Pediatr Oncol Nurs*. 2008;25(1):34–43.
13. Joffe S, et al. Involving children with cancer in decision-making about Research participation. *J Pediatrics*. 2006;(December):862–868.
14. Unguru Y, Sill AM, Kamani N. The experiences of children enrolled in pediatric oncology research: implications for assent. *Pediatrics*. 2010;125(4):e876–e883.
15. Muramoto O. Bioethical aspects of the recent changes in the policy of refusal of blood by Jehovah's witnesses. *BMJ*, 2001;322(7277):37–39.
16. American Academy of Pediatrics Committe on Bioethics: Religious Objections to Medical Care. *Pediatrics*. 1997;99(2):279–281.
17. Tenenbaum T, et al. Oncological management of pediatric cancer patients belonging to Jehovah's Witnesses: a two-institutional experience report. *Onkologie*. 2004;27(2):131–137.
18. Brown RF, et al. Seeking informed consent to cancer clinical trials; evaluating the efficacy of doctor communication skills training. *Psychooncol*. 2007;16(6):507–516.

19. Gilmour J, et al. Pediatric use of complementary and alternative medicine: legal, ethical, and clinical issues in decision-making. *Pediatrics*. 2011; 128(Suppl 4):S149–S154.
20. Iwashyna TJ, Christakis NA, Physicians, patients and prognosis. *Western J Med*. 2001;174:253–254.
21. Mack JW, et al. Understanding of prognosis among parents of children with cancer: parental optimism and parent-physician interaction. *J Clin Oncol*. 2006;25(11):1357–1362.
22. Mack JW, et al. Communication about prognosis between parents and physicians of children with cancer: parent preferences and the impact of prognostic information. *J Clin Oncol*. 2006;24(33):5265–5270.
23. Hinds PS, Preparing mothers and fathers for death of their child. *Lancet*. 2007;8:666–667.
24. McIntyre A. The double life of double effect. Theoret Med & Bioeth. 2004;25(1):61–74.
25. Sulmasy DP, Pellegrino ED. The rule of double effect: clearing up the double talk. *Arch Intern Med*. 1999;159(6):545–550.
26. Massimo L. Ethical problems in bone marrow transplant in children. *Bone Marrow Transplant*. 1996;(November):8–12.
27. American Academy of Pediatrics, Committee on Bioethics Children as hematopoietic stem cell donors. *Pediatrics*. 2010;125(2):392–404.
28. Alby N. The child conceived to give life. *Bone Marrow Transplant*. 1992;9(Suppl 1):95–96.
29. Lederberg MS, *Making a situational diagnosis. Psychiatrists at the interface of psychiatry and ethics in the consultation-liaison setting. Psychosomatics*. 1997; 38(4):327–338.
30. Truman JT, van Eys J, Pochedly C, *Human Values in Pediatric Hematology/Oncology*. 1986, New York, NY: Praeger; 1986.

Chapter 30

Integrating Palliative Care

Sarah Friebert, Todd Dalberg, and Lori Wiener

Pediatric palliative care (PPC) is an organized system of holistic care for children with life-threatening conditions and their families. It focuses on relief of symptoms, pain, and stress caused by a serious illness or its treatment, combining aggressive symptom control with provision of timely, accurate information and support in decision making to help families live as normally as possible.[1] Delivered by an interdisciplinary team in partnership with a patient's primary and subspecialty providers, PPC is appropriate at any age and any stage, and should be implemented concurrently with disease- or cure-directed treatment.[2]

Even though modern cure rates assure that most children with cancer will survive,[3] the cancer journey itself is rife with many opportunities for increased support with symptom management (including pain, nausea, agitation, depression, fatigue/sleep issues, appetite changes), decision making, communication, emotional issues of parents and siblings, financial and practical crises, and spiritual and psychosocial/emotional dimensions of healing. These are all core components of PPC. In fact, any cancer-directed treatment or intervention can be seen as palliative, including chemotherapy, radiation, and surgery. Whether a particular treatment is cure directed or palliative (or both) depends on the anticipated goals and purposes of the treatment. The relative focus of cure-directed or care-directed (palliative) interventions may change throughout the illness experience but are almost never mutually exclusive.

Despite increasing evidence to support the benefit of palliative care services for pediatric oncology patients,[4] only 58% of Children's Oncology Group institutions have a dedicated PPC team.[5]

- The utilization of available services early in the child's course of treatment remains low,[6] mainly due to difficulty determining the appropriate time for palliative care referral.[7–10] A recent study found a disparity between physician and nonphysician pediatric oncology providers in terms of perceptions of palliative care; specifically, physicians were concerned that PC would affect the role of the physician, that PC is inconsistent with cure-directed therapy, and that oncologists experience emotions that may bias treatment modalities they provide their patients.[11]
- Additional barriers to palliative care include concerns about uncertain prognosis, role overlap among teams, perceptions that the family

is not ready to acknowledge an incurable disease, language barriers, time constraints, and insufficient education in pain and palliative care.[6]

To help overcome some of these persistent obstacles to effective integration of oncology and PPC services, this chapter reviews the transition to palliative care, advance care planning with children and adolescents, and follow-up with the family following the death of a child.

Referral for Palliative Care Services

Integration of palliative care should occur early in a child's illness trajectory so that the children/adolescents, the family and professional caregivers can derive maximum benefit from all that palliative care services have to offer.

- Provision of high-quality palliative care should not be contingent on families (or providers) switching from "active" to "palliative" treatment. Expecting families to back away from disease-directed therapy prior to palliative care referral restricts access unnecessarily and introduces an artificial breakpoint between the two modes of treatment instead of positioning them as complementary care paths that exist well concurrently.
- A sudden switch from curative to comfort care can feel very much like abandonment or "giving up" to professional caregivers and families alike. Such a shift also creates an unnecessary division between the oncology and palliative care teams rather than allowing families to view both groups as a cohesive, comprehensive entity.
- It is helpful for institutions or programs with dedicated PPC teams to develop organization-specific triggers for automatic palliative care referral, to avoid last-minute transitions in care, crisis-based decision making or perceptions of abandonment. Examples of such triggers are available at www.capc.org.
- Upon determination that PPC services are indicated, referral to PPC should come from the child's provider team, as with other medical subspecialty consultation. Asking families whether they would like to meet PPC may place too much responsibility on them to make decisions about something with which they are not familiar or have misconceptions.
- Adopting a local standard of care within an institution can also remove any stigma a family may experience as a result of receiving palliative care services.[11]

Possible Entry Points for Palliative Care along the Oncology Trajectory

- At time of diagnosis of any malignancy, knowing that the journey will be burdensome and support resources may be limited [which may even include diagnoses with the most favorable outcomes, e.g., standard-risk acute lymphoblastic leukemia (ALL)].

- When a new diagnosis is accompanied by difficult psychosocial concerns.
- At time of diagnosis for malignancies with a poor prognosis (as defined by an event-free survival rate of <40%) even with active treatment or if family chooses not to pursue curative therapy. Some examples are listed next, though it is important to recognize that these considerations may be resource-dependent:
  - Hematopoietic stem cell transplant.
  - Progressive or relapsed malignant disease.
  - Diffuse intrinsic pontine glioma.
  - Stage IV neuroblastoma.
  - Metastatic solid tumors.
- Early in treatment for comprehensive, aggressive symptom management (e.g., severe neuropathic pain, anxiety, and depression in newly diagnosed patient with metastatic Ewing Sarcoma).
- At time of relapse or recurrence for certain malignancies (e.g., Burkitt's lymphoma, T-cell ALL, or rhabdomyosarcoma).
- At time of development of metastatic disease or progression while on therapy.
- Prior to enrollment on a Phase I or II study.

Communication Among Child, Family, and Healthcare Providers

Children should be involved in decisions about their healthcare, and particularly about their end of life, to whatever degree they are cognitively able and wish to participate.

- It is critical that all involved team members (especially members of the oncology team and the home hospice agency) communicate seamlessly and efficiently to avoid providing conflicting information or mixed messages to families.
- Setting the stage early, wherein the primary oncologist includes the child in honest and accurate discussions about the disease trajectory and treatment options, can allow the team to assist families in early planning.
- Spiritual concerns of all immediate family members should also be assessed regularly. (See Chapter 26, Spiritual and Religious Considerations.)
- Communicating prognostic disclosure should be family centered and culturally sensitive.
- Evidence supports parents' desires to receive as much information about prognosis as possible, with 85% of surveyed parents wanting it expressed numerically.[12]
- Treatment teams should regularly assess communication between patients and their families. Limited communication concerning serious illness, dying and death can lead to the development of symptoms of distress or significant later emotional problems for siblings and parents.[13]

- The child's primary care provider (PCP) must also be kept informed. This may involve reconnection if the PCP has not been actively involved during the cancer treatment. The PCP can play an important role in helping the family after the child's death, particularly in terms of care of surviving siblings.
- Whether the child is at home or in the hospital (or, rarely, in an alternate location), oncology teams need to maintain an active role during a child's cancer treatment.
- Skillfully held, goal-directed conversations about end-of-life issues (such as advance directives) can occur in a "preparing for the worst while hoping for the best" mode. The family, and particularly the dying child, should be provided an opportunity to express preferences, and identify goals and closure activities. This helps to avoid crisis-based decision making that can occur at crucial medical turning points or end of life.

When the Child's Treatment Enters a Strictly Comfort-Oriented Phase: Hospice Considerations

Children remaining on oral chemotherapy to keep the disease at bay or those receiving palliative radiation therapy to assist with pain or wound management are usually appropriate for hospice services.

- When (or where) hospice services are not available, close coordination among the oncology team, home-care agency and PPC team can combine to provide hospice-like care for children who are dying at home.
- Hospice programs vary in their ability and comfort level in managing pediatric patients with cancer. Many adult hospices are willing to work with pediatric patients when they are able to receive 24/7 guidance from knowledgeable pediatric practitioners.
- Unlike adults, most children who are nearing their end of life still benefit from interventions such as total parenteral nutrition (TPN), transfusion therapy, and IV pain management. Smaller hospices face significant financial barriers in providing these therapies, which must be incorporated under the modest per diem they are paid when a child is on the hospice benefit; thus, it is often not discomfort with pediatrics that precludes hospice involvement but realistic resource appraisal instead.

Place of Death

Many children with cancer and their families choose to have death occur in the hospital for multiple reasons. Parents should be helped not to feel that this decision lets the child down, but rather, is a way of maximally supporting the child. During prolonged oncology treatment, the hospital often comes to feel like a second home, and this comfort, along with other issues such as sibling and parent fears about being subsequently able to live in the home where the child died, may mean that a hospital death is preferable for a particular family. Most families, however, choose to have their child die at home when they feel adequately supported[14] and may, in fact, regret their decision when that does not occur.[15] Whenever feasible, the child's preference should be given strong consideration.

Advance Care Planning with Children and Adolescents

Although standards in palliative care suggest that discussion of end-of-life issues be routine and commence soon after diagnosis, in actual practice these conversations can be one of the most difficult aspects of cancer treatment and are often postponed.

In a study designed to determine if adolescents and young adults with advanced cancer feel that an advance directive (AD) document would be useful in addressing end-of-life issues, participants reported that an AD workbook was important, appropriate, and potentially helpful to complete.[16] Participants acknowledged that waiting until the time when death was imminent would be too stressful for meaningful reflection on these issues, acknowledged giving considerable thought to end-of-life issues, and expressed concern that if they spoke about these issues with family members, it would be perceived as "giving up" or "losing faith." Some of their thoughts are presented in Box 30.1.

- Children and adolescents living with cancer need to be informed when treatment is no longer curative and that palliative care is available to them. They also need to be provided the opportunity to be involved in decision making and, when developmentally appropriate, about how they will live the life they still have, and how they want to be remembered after their death, if death is inevitable.[17]

Box 30.1 Issues Children and Teens Report Thinking About

Specific treatments and/or procedures I never want to experience again.
Where I want to be when the end of my life is near.
The people I would like to be with me.
How I want my family to treat each other.
How I want to be remembered on my birthday and/or specific holidays.
How I want my school/work to remember me.
Whether I want to be buried or cremated.
Whether I want an open casket, and if so, what clothes I want to be wearing, and specific items I would like in the casket with me.
The people whom I would like to have my specific belongings.
Whether I would like a memorial service or celebration of my life; if so, the people I would like to attend, specific music, readings, etc.

- Having an advance care-planning document could foster discussion with family and friends, and could facilitate communication with the primary healthcare provider regarding personal goals, values, or beliefs.
- Few established resources exist to aid pediatric cancer patients and their families in accepting and understanding their changing physical, emotional, and social needs when treatment is no longer effective.
- One AD document, Five Wishes®, has been particularly successful with the adult population because of the consideration of personal, emotional, and spiritual needs, in addition to medical and legal concerns.
- An advance care-planning guide, known as Voicing My CHOICES™, has been designed to aid adolescents and young adults make decisions about their care and how they wish to be remembered after their death.[18]
- My Wishes®, was developed to help young children communicate their wishes and is available for pediatric use. (Five Wishes®, Voicing My CHOICES™, and My Wishes® can be viewed and obtained at www.agingwithdignity.org).

In addition to facilitating these discussions, the transfer of resources from hospital to community-based services can be challenging and conversations surrounding this topic can provoke anxiety. A model known as FOOTPRINTS helps bridge the relationship between the hospital and community resources.[19]

Team Follow-up with the Family

One of the most significant barriers to early and seamless integration of palliative care into the care of children and adolescents with cancer and their families is the bi-directional fear of abandonment. Families fear that they will lose contact with their primary oncology team, and providers fear that their relationships with the family will be subsumed by a new team. Maintaining a continued active presence during a child's dying and a family's bereavement is one of the most difficult but also most satisfying parts of the practitioner–patient relationship and can go a long way toward dispelling fears of abandonment. The pediatric cancer experience is an intimate, long-term relationship that does not need to be severed with the child's death.

Role of the Oncology Team Immediately after the Child's Death

Most families wish to maintain relationships with their primary oncology team after their child has died. Professional caregivers are often hesitant to contact families, fearing that hearing from the team who was not able to cure the child might be painful for families. More painful is the sudden separation of the child's treatment team from the family, who often feels the lack of contact as a compounded loss.

- When comfortable and feasible for the individual, most mental health professionals recommend practitioners participate in a child's funeral, especially when they have cared for the child for a long time or have been particularly close to the child or family.
- If not able to attend in person, sending a personal (preferably handwritten) letter to the family is appropriate; suggestions about letter content and importance are available from several sources.[20–23]
- Families generally appreciate the opportunity to keep their child's name and memory alive by sharing experiences with those who knew their child well.

Maintaining a Therapeutic Relationship with Families after a Child's Death

Practitioners need to come to terms with their own emotions surrounding the events. Feelings of failure, regrets about decisions made or not made, or personal experiences with death and dying, need to be processed separately from the practitioner–family dynamic. When this does not occur, these issues can significantly interfere with a family's own grieving process and unduly burden survivors. Practitioners' relationships with future patients and parents and even relationships within the practitioner's own family can also be hampered.

- Careful attention to boundary issues is of primary importance. If questions about appropriate boundaries arise, discussion with other colleagues, especially mental health or ethics experts, can help determine a reasonable plan that is respectful of professional roles and family boundaries.

Especially with the increasing presence of social media, the relationship between patient/family and provider can, at times, become blurred. (See Chapter 32, Social Media and Healthcare.)

- All providers should become familiar with their institutions' social media policies and procedures, placing patient privacy as a top priority. A recent Association of Pediatric Hematology/Oncology Nurses (APHON) policy statement addresses social media in the work place, advocating that providers not engage in sites such as Facebook, Twitter, and CaringBridge. (See Chapter 32, Social Media and Healthcare.)[25] Another paper specifically addresses these issues for pediatric oncologists.[24]
- When ready, families should be afforded the opportunity to discuss their child's care and death with the primary oncology team, including the review of autopsy findings if an autopsy was performed. If possible, this meeting should be arranged at an outside site (or at least in another building on the hospital campus) so that the family is not forced to confront difficult memories before they are able/ready.
- A home visit by the primary oncology team following a child's death is often extremely comforting to families and offers an opportunity for staff to achieve closure as well, especially if the child died at home and

the primary oncology team has not seen the family since prior to the child's death.

Beyond the Immediate Bereavement Period

Hospice programs provide, at a minimum, 13 months of bereavement services, which include phone calls, cards at anniversaries and birthdays, and individual, group, or counseling sessions as needed.

- Most PPC and hospice programs recognize that 13 months is too brief a period in the trajectory of grief for families losing a child.
- For many families, the second year after the child's death is more difficult than the first, as the shock wears off and the reality of the child's absence begins to set in. Programs often extend bereavement services to at least 2 years, and some even continue as long as the family wishes to remain in contact. Increasingly, PPC programs continue to remember a child's birthday and death anniversary with cards, reminding families that their children continue to remain alive in the thoughts of those who helped care for them.
- In addition to periodic contact, families and staff alike may benefit from remembrance services, family/sibling grief groups or bereavement camps and opportunities for participation in mentorship or volunteer programs.

Reactions to the death of a child are always complex and painful. However, well-recognized algorithms for differentiating "normal" grief responses in survivors from those that are non-productive or non-resolving and require counseling or other interventions are readily available from mental health colleagues (Table 30.1).

Table 30.1 Expected Grief and Pathological Grief

(All pediatric deaths provoke complicated grief responses almost by definition.)

Expected Grief Responses	Pathological Grief
Usually able to connect depressed feelings to the event	Often do not relate depressed feelings to any life event
Disbelief, denial, shock	Total denial of the reality of the death
Often openly angry	Persistent anger or hostility Frequent complaining or irritability (indirect expressions of anger)
Sense of unreality, withdrawal from others	Persistent withdrawal from friends and family
Disruption of typical behavior or personality	Prolonged behavior or personality changes
Responds to comfort and support	Continual rejection of offers of support or help
Can experience moments of enjoyment in life increasingly frequently with time from the death	Projection of pervasive sense of doom

(continued)

Table 30.1 (Continued)

Expected Grief Responses	Pathological Grief
Feels sad and empty	Projection of hopelessness and emptiness
Often has transient physical complaints	Chronic physical complaints and/or actual medical illness
May express guilt over some aspect of the loss	Expression of prolonged feelings of guilt over the death or generalized feelings of guilt
Self-esteem temporarily impacted, but overall intact	Deep loss of self-esteem Beginning or expanding use of alcohol and drugs Suicidal thoughts and/or actions

Adapted and reprinted with permission from: Wolfelt, Healing the Bereaved Child, © 2007 Companion Press;[26] and Simons & Pardes, Understanding Human Behavior in Health and Illness, © 1981 Williams & Wilkins.[27]

References

1. Institute of Medicine (IOM). *When Children Die: Improving Palliative and End-of-Life Care for Children and Their Families*. Field MJ, Behrman RE, eds. Washington, DC: The National Academies Press; 2002.
2. http://www.capc.org/tools-for-palliative-care-programs/marketing/public-opinion-research/2011-public-opinion-research-on-palliative-care.pdf
3. http://www.childrensoncologygroup.org/index.php/childrens-oncology-group
4. Wolfe J, Hammel J, Edwards K, et al. Easing of suffering in children with cancer at the end of life: Is care changing? *J Clin Oncol*. 2008;26:1717–1723.
5. Johnston D, Nagel K, Friedmam D, et al. Availability and use of palliative care and end-of-life services for pediatric oncology patients. *J Clin Oncol*. 2008;26:4646–4650.
6. Johnston D, Vadeboncoeur C. Palliatve care consultation in pediatric oncology. *Support Care Cancer*. 2012;20:799–803.
7. Davies B, Sehring S, Partridge C, et al. Barriers to palliative care for children: Perceptions of pediatric health care providers. *Pediatrics*. 2008;121:282–288.
8. Thompson L, Knapp C, Madden V, Shenkman E. Pediatricians' perceptions of and preferred timing for pediatric palliative care. *Pediatrics*. 2009;123:777–782.
9. Knapp C, Thompson L. Factors associated with perceived barriers to pediatric palliative care: a survey of pediatricians in Florida and California. *Pall Med*. 2011;26:268–274.
10. Junger S, Vedder A, Milde S, et al. Paediatric palliative care home care by general paediatricians: a multimethod study of perceived barriers and facilitators. *BMC Palliat Care*. 2010;9:11.
11. Dalberg T, Jacob-Files E, Carney P, et al. Pediatric oncology providers perceptions of barriers and facilitators to early integration of pediatric palliative care. *Pediatr Blood Cancer*. 2013;60:1875–1881.
12. Mack J, Wolfe J, Holcombe E, et al. Communication about prognosis between parents and physicians of children with cancer: parent preferences and the impact of prognostic information. *J Clin Oncol*. 2006;24:5265–5270.

13. Tan JS, Docherty SL, Barfield R, Brandon DH. *J Palliat Med*. May 2012, 15(5): 579–584.

14. Vicker J, Carlisle, C. Choices and control: parental experiences in pediatric terminal home care. *J Pediatr Oncol Nurs*. 2000;17:12–21.

15. Meyer E, Burns J, Griffith J, et al. Parental perspectives on end-of-life care in the pediatric intensive care unit. *Crit Care Med*. 2002;30:226–231.

16. Wiener L, Ballard E, Brennan T, Martinez P, Pao M. How I wish to be remembered: the use of an advance care planning document in adolescent and young adult populations. *J Palliat Med*. 2008 December; 11(10):1309–1313.

17. Wiener L, Pao M, Wendler D, et al. An exploratory study of the use of Five Wishes as a tool for advanced care planning in young adults with high-risk cancer [Poster abstract of the APOS 4th Annual Conference]. *Psycho-Oncol*. 2007;16(Suppl. 3):S67–S68.

18. Wiener L, Zadeh S, Battles H, et al. Allowing adolescents and young adults to plan their end-of-life care. *Pediatrics*. 2012;130:891–905.

19. Toce S, Collins MA. The FOOTPRINTSSM model of pediatric palliative care. *J Palliat Med*. 2003;6:989–1000.

20. Zunin LM, Zunin HS. The art of condolence: What to write, what to say, what to do at a time of loss. New York: Harper Perennial; 1992.

21. Bedell SE, Cadenhead K, Graboys TB. The doctor's letter of condolence. *N Engl J Med*. 2001;344(15):1162–1164.

22. Kane GC. A dying art? The doctor's letter of condolence. *Chest*. 2007;131(4):1245–1247.

23. Wolfson R & Menkin E. Writing a condolence letter. *J Palliat Med*. 2003;6(1):77–78.

24. Wiener L, Crum C, Grady C, Merchant M. To friend or not to friend. The use of social media in pediatric oncology. *J Oncol Pract*. 2012;8:103–106.

25. http://www.aphon.org/files/public/socialmediapaper11.pdf

26. Wolfelt A. *Healing the Bereaved Child*. Fort Collins, CO: Companion Press; 2007.

27. Simons RC, Pardes H. *Understanding Human Behavior in Health and Illness*. 2nd ed. Baltimore, MD: Williams & Wilkins; 1981.

Further Reading

Macdonald ME, Liben S, Carnevale FA, et al. Parental perspectives on hospital staff members' acts of kindness and commemoration after a child's death. *Pediatrics*. 2005;116(4):884–890.

Wiener L, Zadeh S, Wexler L, Pao, M. When silence is not golden: engaging adolescents and young adults in discussions around end-of-life care choices. *Pediatric Blood & Cancer*. 2013;60(5):715–718.

Chapter 31

Caring for International Patients

Maria E. Radulovic

An international caregiver who is either a family member or a guardian usually accompanies international pediatric patients. It is important to take into account the issues that affect these patients and caregivers.

Before the Patient's Arrival

Documents to Travel to the United States

B-2 Visa

Patients and caregivers may need a B-2 visa (issued for medical reasons) to enter the United States to receive treatment at a medical center. The medical organization can facilitate the process by sending the patient a letter indicating the appointment time and date. The patient presents the appointment letter at the corresponding U.S. consulate at the time of the consular interview appointment and begins the process of a visa application online at the US consulate website of his/her country. Patients who receive a B-2 visa for medical reasons are usually allowed to stay in the United States for six months. For further information, log onto: www.uscis.gov or call +1 800.375.5283.

Visa Waiver Program

Visitors originating from countries from which citizens have the choice to enter the U.S. under the Visa Waiver Program should be aware of the limited time they are permitted to remain in the United States and the fact that, under no circumstance, can patients who enter the country under this type of visa extend their stay *beyond 90 days*. Currently, citizens of the countries listed in Table 31.1 qualify for the Visa Waiver Program.

If the treatment requires a stay beyond 90 days, it is strongly recommended that the patient and caregiver apply for a B-2 visa. A B-2 visa allows a person to extend his/her stay while remaining in the United States. Persons entering the United States under the Visa Waiver Program who want to re-enter the country to continue receiving medical care, will have to leave the country, and re-enter the United States from a nonborder

Table 31.1 Countries Whose Citizens Qualify for the Visa Waiver Program

Andorra	Finland	Japan	New Zealand	Spain
Australia	France	Latvia	Norway	Sweden
Austria	Germany	Liechtenstein	Portugal	Switzerland
Belgium	Greece	Lithuania	San Marino	Taiwan
Brunei	Hungary	Luxembourg	Singapore	U. Kingdom
Chile				
Czech Republic	Iceland	Malta	Slovakia	
Denmark	Ireland	Monaco	Slovenia	
Estonia	Italy	The Netherlands	South Korea	

country, usually their country of origin. Complete information on foreign nationals who qualify for the Visa Waiver Program should read all instructions found in:

> Travel.state.gov/content/visas/English/visit/visa-waiver-program.html and apply to the Electronic System for Travel Authorization (ESTA) at: http://cbp.gov/xp/cgov/travel/id_visa/esta/

I-94 Form and Extension (I-539)

When international patients arrive at a U.S. port of entry with a B-2 visa, their passports are stamped with an arrival and departure date. The departure date is the last date they may remain legally in the United States, unless they apply for an extension of nonimmigrant stay by submitting an application on United States Customs and Immigration Service (USCIS) Form I-539. *International patients and their caregivers should bring copies of the personal documents presented at the U.S. consulate in their country of origin when they applied for a B2 visa.* Many of these same documents will be needed to attach to their application of extension of stay, and knowing to bring them along when traveling to the United States may avoid the difficulties attached to obtaining them once the patient is here. See Table 31.2.

Custody Documents

If the caregiver of the international patient is not the biological parent, the caregiver must provide translated custody documentation and power of attorney for medical decisions.

Medical Records

Request pertinent medical records from patient's country of origin.

Medical Travel Insurance

Ask the international caregiver to explore and, if possible, obtain medical travel insurance. These insurances usually cover some expenses in case of

Table 31.2 Concise Description of Immigration Documents and Forms. The following table provides a short description of common consular and immigration terms that may be useful to the international patient.	
Visa	Stamped permit in passport issued by U.S. consulate abroad to enter United States. Patient should request a B-2 visa issued for medical reasons in country of origin.
Visa Waiver Program	Specific country nationals may enter United States without a visa stamped in their passport. Must conform to certain requirements.
B-2 status	Status generally given to patients seeking medical treatment in the United States.
USCIS Form I-539	Application to extend nonimmigrant status. Extension document for persons who need to remain in the United States longer than the expiration date stamped in their passports.
I-94	Arrival and Departure Record. Available at: https://i94.cbp.dhs.gov/I94/request.html

accident or emergency treatment while the person is abroad and can only be purchased in the country of origin before departing. The policies can usually be purchased through a travel agent or an insurance agent.

Communicating with the International Patient and the Patient's Caregiver

When the patient and caregiver are not fluent in English, an interpreter should be engaged to help communication. A translator can help write e-mails and other correspondence in the patient's language. Reducing the language barrier helps put the patient and caregiver at ease. Machine translations, such as Google Translate, are notorious for their serious mistakes and distorted meanings. They should never be used for medical purposes.

General Considerations

Setting Up an Interview

Before meeting with the patient in person, the provider should become familiar with the patient and caregiver's country of origin. Know where the country is located. Not confusing it with another location shows respect for and interest in the international family. The Department of State website: http://www.state.gov/ can provide additional information. Once in the website, click on "Countries and Regions" and choose the desired country.

Cultural Diversity

Be familiar with cultural non-Western habits, such as greetings, handshakes, eye contact, clothing worn for religious purposes, family gender roles, and so forth. It is a courtesy toward an international patient to acknowledge their cultural customs. If the provider needs further information, he

Table 31.3 Communication Resources	
Translation and interpretation referrals	American Translators Association Telephone: +1 703.683.6100 Fax: +1 703.683.6122 Website: www.atanet.org
Some remote telephone and video interpretation sources	All remote telephone and video interpretation companies charge a fee for their services and provide special equipment for access to these services. • Language Line: +1 877.886.3885; www.languageline.com • Cyracom: +1 800.481.3293; www.cyracom.com • World Wide Interpreters: +1 866.967.5313; www.e-wwi.com

should address his questions to the Interpreter Services Department or, if available, the International Center at his facility.

Limited English Proficiency

If the patient and caregiver have limited English proficiency or are culturally and linguistically diverse, it is essential to use an interpreter. Unless the provider is completely fluent in the patient's language, always use a qualified interpreter or remote interpretation (a telephone or video service that provides an interpreter through the telephone or on a screen—Table 31.3).

If the provider is only somewhat familiar with the language, it may lead to misunderstandings and medical safety issues. Patients from many parts of the world would consider it rude to tell a provider that they did not understand what had been discussed because of the provider's poor language skills.

Use of Family or Friends as Interpreters

Always use a professional interpreter even if the pediatric patient speaks some English but the caregiver does not. Never use a family member or friend to interpret conversation between the patient or caregiver and the physician. Important information may be misinterpreted and sensitive information may be omitted. If a family friend or family member must be used (this is *not* recommended) speak in extremely short sentences and allow the interpretation to take part after each phrase or sentence. In this way you can control whatever is being said and what is being interpreted.

Psychosocial Considerations During an Interview

Level of Education

Adjust difficulty of explanations according to level of education of caregiver and patient. Be responsive to the possibility that caregivers may not be literate and, therefore, unable to write or sign their names in their own language. Diplomatically ask the caregiver to tell you in their own words the critical information you have given them in order to be sure that the basics have been understood.

Reading Skills

If a consent or instruction is translated into the patient's language, ask if the caregiver prefers to read the document or have it read to him. If the latter is chosen, be sensitive that the person may have no, or very basic, reading skills.

Questions by the Patient

International patients may feel intimidated or embarrassed to ask questions of the provider. Explain that in the United States questions from a patient and/or family members are welcomed and a well-informed patient is preferable to one who is not.

Unrealistic Medical Expectations

Patients who come from abroad may have unrealistic expectations about the success of treatments in the United States. It is important to assess patient and caregiver expectations.

Suggestions to Improve Communication with International Patients

Bilingual Staff

Whenever possible, assign bilingual staff to the patient.

Remote Interpretation Equipment

If possible, install equipment for remote telephone interpretation in the patient's room or the physician's office. This will allow the patient to communicate with staff at all times in the absence of an interpreter (Table 31.3).

Rapport and Trust

It takes a longer time to build a rapport and earn the patient's trust when using an interpreter and communicating via a third person. Suggestions for building a rapport with the child include playing with child, drawing, and utilizing child-life services. Caregivers need time to share their concerns and experiences.

Translations

All-important documents should be translated (including consents, side effects, use of medications, discharge summary, etc.) for better understanding, compliance, and patient safety. Do not use computer translations; the integrity of the original concept may be distorted (Table 31.3).

Topics to Address with the International Patient and Caregiver

Signing Consents

The international family needs to understand the importance of signing informed consents, HIPAA forms, release forms, and other documents that require a signature. Be sure that the accompanying person has custody and power-of-attorney documents. It is not common practice in many countries to have the physician explain, in great detail, all the side effects of a treatment or medication, including death. Malpractice suits are rare in other countries, and U.S. medical privacy laws may seem strange to those from other countries.

Role of Primary Physician

In many countries, the primary physician, rarely a specialist, presents medical findings. Frequent provider changes may be unfamiliar and disconcerting. Explain to the patient and the caregiver who will be responsible for their daily care, the function and role of that person, the roles of other key members of the medical team, and whom they should address when questions arise.

Explanation of Procedures

Additional explanations may be necessary due to lack of similar treatments, procedures, testing and equipment in the country of origin.

Adherence

Emphasize the need for strict adherence to the treatment plan. Many cultures do not emphasize compliance.

Over-the-Counter Medications (OTC) and Complementary/Alternative Medicine (CAM)

Medications sold under prescription in the United States may be sold OTC abroad. Alternative medicine treatments are widespread in Europe, Asia, Africa, and Latin America. These include homeopathy, herbal supplements, and indigenous potions. It is recommended that the provider specifically ask about using these alternative/complementary/holistic treatment approaches and that the patient does not use them unless first discussed with the medical provider.

Names of Medications

Patients may not know the names of their current medications and dosages. They may identify them by color or size. Encourage patients to bring all their current medications to their appointments.

Punctuality

Emphasize the importance of appointment punctuality. Many cultures are less concerned with this issue and will arrive late with the expectation that they will be served at the time of arrival.

Different Measurements and Scales

Measurements and scales may vary from country to country. These differences can be confusing to patients and their family members. For example: Fahrenheit versus Celsius; pounds versus kilograms; yards, feet, and inches versus the metric system.

Do Not Resuscitate (DNR)

International caregivers may not be familiar with a Do Not Resuscitate (DNR) document. DNR needs to be explained at the appropriate time.

911

Providers should explain to the patient and the caregiver what 911 stands for and under what circumstances it is appropriate to use this service. The provider should also explain that there is a cost associated with this service.

Stressors for International Patients and their Caregivers

Giving the patient resource information prior to or upon arrival can minimize stressors and concerns associated with being treated in the United

States. If the medical center has information on resources available to all patients that can be translated into the appropriate language, sharing these with the international family would be helpful. Support groups for caregivers can also be very useful.

Language

If the patient and/or caregiver does not speak English, inform them about the availability of interpreter services and remote interpretation equipment.

Loss of School Time

If the international patient of school age brings his school books along in order to do homework while on treatment, try to provide tutoring in the patient's language at the medical facility. Patients who visit the United States on a B-2 visa violate immigration laws if they attend public or private schools in the US on this particular type of visa. Violating these immigration laws may prohibit them from extending their stay or of returning to the United States in the future. If the patient intends to go to elementary, high school or college (public or private) while receiving medical treatment in the US, the patient must apply for a different type of visa at the US consulate in his native country before entering the US and before attending school.

Loss of Connection with Family and Friends

Provide Internet access so the patient and/or caregiver can e-mail, instant message, Skype, text, or use a webcam to stay in touch with friends and relatives for emotional support. It is important to discuss with whom the child has a close rapport back at home and to find a way to facilitate such contact. This can be achieved by asking the patient about whom he or she is missing most or with whom he or she wants to stay in touch. In addition, talk to the advocate for the patient, stressing the importance of such support.

Nutrition

International patients generally need some time to become adjusted to U.S. meal schedules (light lunches and earlier heavier, if possible, dinners). Pediatric patients are particularly "picky" when presented with unfamiliar food fare. Allow the caregiver to prepare "home-cooked" meals to assure adequate nutritional intake. Help identify the availability of local markets where the spices, vegetables, and other foods they are familiar with can be found.

Additional Stressors for Caregivers of International Pediatric Patients

Language

Frustration is often experienced when a parent is unable to communicate directly with the medical staff about one's child due to a language barrier. This can be reduced by making sure of the availability of an interpreter.

Finances: Medical, Housing, and Daily Living Expenses

International patients usually do not have insurance that will cover the medical expenses incurred in the United States. Expenses should be discussed before the arrival of the patient from abroad. If free medical care is provided, inform the caregiver of its precise limitations. Housing and daily living expenses, including free housing, if available, should also be addressed prior to arrival, if possible.

I-539 Application to Extend Nonimmigrant Status before the Date Stamped in the Passport Expires

Care should be taken that the patient and caregiver maintain valid legal immigration status at all times. Form I-539 from the USCIS website (www.uscis.gov) should be completed about 45 days before expiration of the date stamped in the passport when the patient arrived at port of entry. Do not confuse this date with the expiration date of the visa that is typed on the visa issued at the U.S. consulate abroad. The visa, stamped in the passport, is a document that permits the patient to enter the United States and has no other function (such as establishing length of stay).

Filling Out Form I-539

Pediatric patients older than 14 years can fill out their own Form I-539. However, it is easier if patients under 21 years of age have the caregiver (only if he or she is the biological parent) fill out the form in the caregiver's name and list the pediatric patient as a dependent.

- All patients over 21 years of age must fill out an individual Form I-539 separate from their caregiver.
- For specific instructions not found on Form I-539, call USCIS at +1 800.375.5283.
- If the medical facility is located in a large urban area, search for the ethnic community or religious groups who can provide assistance with the completion of Form I-539. One such agency is Catholic Charities, which serves clients of all countries and religions.

Respite

International pediatric patients usually have only one caregiver. If the patient is admitted for a long treatment, the caregiver will need respite time. Arrange for volunteers to offer respite care several times a week.

Hospice

Hospice services are available for international patients. Consult with the hospice of your area to find out if a patient qualifies to receive care. Some hospices have charitable funds to cover expenses for those families without medical insurance or sufficient income to pay for the cost of these services.

Coping and Support Systems for International Pediatric Patients

The support systems used by international patients may vary based on culture, distance from home, and proficiency in English.

Suggestions

- Linkage to a local community group, church, or cultural organization.
- Recreational activities.
- Psychological/emotional support for patient and caregiver.

- Availability of long-distance telephone calls, e-mail, and videoconferencing, such as Skype.
- Accessibility to interact with other pediatric patients who speak the same language.
- Special care and reassurances must be given at the time of discharge. International patients often develop an unusually strong attachment to those who have offered treatment and can be frightened to return to their country of origin when they know that they will not have access to the same kind of medical care offered in the United States. Fear of being medically abandoned by the U.S. team and not taken care of by the home- country team is a commonly expressed concern.

Chapter 32

Social Media and Health Care

Rachel A. Tunick and Sarah R. Brand

Social Media

The digital age has irrevocably transformed the landscape of healthcare. With the advent and ever-growing popularity and pervasiveness of social media, those practicing within the field of pediatric oncology regularly encounter a wide range of potential opportunities and possible adverse consequences related to its' use. These may range from mundane and innocuous to ethically challenging and provocative situations.

Social media (SM) are defined as the myriad of Internet-based applications in which contents are user generated and interactive, and which provide a forum for the dissemination and sharing of ideas and information.

- Forms of SM technologies include:
    - Weblogs or "blogs" (some of which are designed specifically for patients and families experiencing medical illness; e.g., CaringBridge, CarePages).
    - Social networks (e.g., Twitter, Facebook, LinkedIn).
    - Wikis.
    - Podcasts, Internet forums or message boards.
    - Multimedia sharing (e.g., Pinterest, Instagram, YouTube).
- Although the pervasiveness of SM is associated with far-reaching and multifaceted benefits for professionals as well as patients and families, associated ethical and professional dilemmas may arise. Practitioners may face potentially problematic situations involving SM use by patients and families, as well as with regard to their own online presence and activity.
- Across each of these domains, it is advisable that practitioners stay informed about SM resources relevant to one's patients and/or professional practice; remain thoughtful, vigilant and self-aware about how use of these technologies may intersect with their work and their relationships with patients and parents; and anticipate dilemmas that may arise and plan accordingly.

Use of Social Media by Patients and Families

Searching for Health-Related Information

The Internet is now a major source of health-related information, and growing numbers of patients and families turn to SM and other online tools to search for guidance, treatment options, and hope when facing a pediatric oncology diagnosis.[1] The amount of available health information on the Web, however, can be overwhelming to parents and teen users. An August 2013 Google search yielded over 2 billion hits for "health information," 774 million hits for "cancer information," and 7.5 million hits for "pediatric cancer information." Both parents and adolescents who have grown up in the online era and are typically familiar and comfortable with this medium often seek out health information via the Internet, and report benefits to the availability of both general and targeted online health information (diagnosis, treatment, and treatment side-effects).[3] Patients and families may utilize SM and the Internet to seek out a range of health-related information, such as:

- Uncovering opportunities for treatment trials (e.g., through websites such as TrialX.com or clinicaltrials.gov).
- Accessing contacts for second opinions.
- Reading relevant scientific abstracts.

Seeking information can:

- Promote a sense of control and empowerment in the context of a highly stressful situation in which parents report feeling otherwise helpless.[4]
- Facilitate coping by providing a deeper understanding of their disease.[5]
- Decrease levels of anxiety, depression, and negative self-esteem in children and adolescents undergoing treatment for cancer.[6]

Information Dissemination/Fundraising/Memory Preservation

In recent years many patients and families have turned to the Internet as a way to share and disseminate information about their (or their child's) illness to a large support network without having to contact each person individually, thus circumventing a time-consuming and emotionally exhausting task.

- CaringBridge and CarePages are specialized sites that allow users to set up a personal page to regularly update extended family and friends about the patient's medical journey.
- Special Facebook pages or personal blogs can serve an analogous function, allowing readers to leave messages of their own and thus providing opportunities for families to receive ongoing emotional backing, practical support, and "virtual" visitation by loved ones.
- Fundraising purposes may be served by such sites as well, for example, families may include information on their site about how to donate to

a healthcare fund for the child, or announce details around upcoming fundraisers, blood, and bone marrow drives.
- Bereaved families (or those anticipating the death of their child) may use SM to provide poignant therapeutic means to document and preserve priceless memories of the child's last days or weeks and to celebrate and honor them.

Development of Virtual Support Networks and Communities

The Internet in general, and SM in particular, allows for the creation of virtual communities of pediatric oncology patients and families. Because many types of childhood cancer are quite rare, there may be very few families whose children share similar diagnoses within a local geographic region. Online support communities may:

- Connect families of children with similar diagnoses from around the country and even the world.
- Create an expansive community who understands what the cancer experience, especially when face-to-face interactions are not possible or when it is felt that those in their own natural social network may not understand their situation.[7]
- Discuss and share health and resource information, in their own timeframe and at their own pace. This is especially important for stressed parents who may only find time for social contact late at night or early in the morning.
  - Provide opportunities for parents to receive social support from others facing similar experiences so that they feel less isolated in their journeys.

In addition to the peer-to-peer support groups that evolve through virtual communities, there has been an interest in developing more formal online support groups. Benefits of such groups include:

- Increased flexibility and convenience.
- Removal of geographical restrictions and other physical limitations.
- Cost-effectiveness.
- Increased likelihood of finding others with similar diseases, allowing for the creation of groups that target specific demographics, and providing anonymity while still offering support.[8,9]

Considerations Regarding Adolescent and Young Adult Cancer Patients

Benefits of use of SM by adolescent and young adult (AYA) cancer patients are especially important for providers to consider and include:

- Providing an avenue for teens, especially those with limited opportunity for in-person interactions with same-age peers, to engage in developmentally appropriate and salient activities, including staying connected to friends and family and maintaining their pre-illness connections and identity.

- Helping AYA cancer patients make online contact with peers facing similar experiences. These virtual connections, including the exchange of information and advice about medical issues such as procedures and treatments, can be as valuable for AYA patients as receiving direct support from family and friends.[10]
- Offering AYA patients an opportunity to share their experiences and provide a sense of group belonging.

Some well-regarded SM resources for AYA cancer patients include lookgoodfeelbetter.org, teenslivingwithcancer.org and stupidcancer.org.

Beyond connecting AYA patients through virtual communities, SM may offer a platform for more formal interventions. For example, McLaughlin and colleagues developed a video-sharing social networking intervention for young adult cancer survivors that provides participants with the ability to interact with other survivors through sharing videos and pictures, creating blogs, group discussions, and private messages. Pilot data indicated that participants used the site as a way of fulfilling social needs that were not being met in their offline lives.[11]

Potential Risks Associated with SM Use by Patients and Families

Notwithstanding the significant benefits already reviewed, the use of SM by oncology patients and families may be associated with various risks.[12] It is important for providers to recognize and understand the potential perils and threats that may accompany SM use by patients and parents, and to communicate openly within their practices about these matters in order to best anticipate and manage challenging situations. These include:

- *Threats to privacy/confidentiality of the patient and/or family.* Patients/families may not appreciate the degree to which
  - Privacy on their SM site is uncontrolled (strangers may easily have access).
  - Permanency of online information (e.g., medical information could be accessed by future prospective employers).
- *Threats around content and scope of SM and online material.*
  - Unsolicited advice and opinions posted on a family's site (such as advice regarding medical decisions) may be upsetting for SM users.
  - The nearly inexhaustible supply of online medical information may be overwhelming or frightening to viewers.
  - Lay people may lack requisite knowledge to identify inaccurate material.
- *Threats regarding information about other patients.* Patients/families may include identifying information about other patients on their SM sites (e.g., mention other children who are hospitalized at the same time as their own child), often without the consent or knowledge of those individuals. This may lead to difficult situations around privacy

and confidentiality matters, particularly in the context of medical setbacks or deaths of other patients.

- Related to this, the death of a child within one's online support community can be tremendously difficult for parents and patients. These communities often develop based on similarities across disease, treatment, and other demographic characteristics, and, therefore, a death within the network may strike painfully close to home. Also of note, SM sites of well-known or otherwise inspirational youth may have the potential to negatively affect self-esteem of viewers.
- *Risks/disadvantages associated with online support groups* include:
  - The restriction of benefits of such groups to those who have regular access to a computer and the Internet.
  - Limited access for those who are less fluent in written English language.
  - Potential for "aggressive" online behavior due to lack of face-to-face interaction or trained facilitator/leader.
  - Difficulty interpreting tone or emotion.
  - Ethical issues such as the role of the moderator and privacy of participants.[8,9]

Guidelines, Recommendations, and Considerations for Practitioners Regarding SM Use by Patients and Parents

- Provide psychoeducation to patients/families about potential uses, benefits, and risks of SM in the context of their oncology treatment.
- Encourage ongoing discussion about the use of SM with parents and patients. Remind parents to talk regularly with their children about SM benefits and risks, perhaps encouraging the development of a family online-use plan that includes regular family meetings to discuss online and related topics (such as establishing household rules limiting permitted time spent online; for more details see recommendations by O'Keeffe and Clarke-Pearson).[13]
- Remain informed about accurate and trustworthy websites and SM resources. Connect with colleagues to share and disseminate information about reliable and reputable resources and those which are not, and check them out yourself in order to become familiar with their content and usage.[14] Then, SM may be viewed as an important opportunity for patient and family engagement, education, and support.
- Initiate discussions about the use of online resources with patients, reminding them to be cautious and careful in their interpretations of the material that they encounter online. Ask about the specific illness-related SM sites on which they participate and visit, and use these discussions as a platform for patient education. Guide them toward well-reputed, legitimate sites (e.g., curesearch.org, cure4kids.org, and childrensoncologygroup.org). Encourage patients and families to discuss information they find online with their medical provider.

- Remember that differences exist in information-seeking style and preferences, and reassure patients and families that there is not a one-size-fits-all approach to SM use.
- Be mindful regarding the substantial emotional trauma that may be associated with the death of another patient within a patient/family's online community and offer compassionate support and guidance as needed.

SM Use by Practitioners

Social media is increasingly a significant part of daily personal (and professional) life for healthcare providers. A recent survey indicated that 93.5% of medical students, 79.4% of medical residents, and 41.6% of practicing physicians regularly use SM,[15] and the vast majority of students across a range of health-related professions (e.g., medicine, nursing, occupational therapy, physical therapy, pharmacy) report a preference for online media as their primary source of information.[16] Social media and related online activity often intersect with professional work and responsibilities, and this is especially true within the field of oncology; for example, compared with physicians overall, oncologists are three times more likely to communicate with patients online.[17]

Social media affords practitioners a range of opportunities for professional growth, development, and connectivity including:

- Continuing education (both formally, and via more informal contacts with others who have similar professional backgrounds, interests, and experiences).
- Promoting e-gathering of up-to-the-minute medical information (e.g., via "tweets" about newly published articles).
- Supporting the acquisition of general information regarding conference updates in real time.[18] Twitter usage at the American Society of Clinical Oncology (ASCO) Annual Conference grew significantly from 2010 to 2011 and is viewed as a professional resource for both on-site conference attendees and nonattendees.[19]
- Serving as a "method of mass communication" with colleagues and healthcare organizations.
- Public health messaging and education.
- Professional consultation and collaboration.
- Facilitating communication with team members.
- Direct engagement with patients for purposes of clinical care.[14]

SM provides new avenues for medical professionals to engage in dialogue with the pharmaceutical industry, promotes the growth of virtual collaborations such as within a "Community of Practice" (e.g., McKenna & D'Alessandro),[20] and affords opportunities for more seasoned providers to connect in meaningful ways with a younger professional generation.

In the personal realm, SM provides oncology practitioners with opportunities for connection with friends and family outside of one's professional sphere, and in this regard may support the maintenance of a healthy work–life balance. Engaging in SM may promote the development of hobbies and non-work-related interests, and may thus afford a healthy distraction from a busy and stressful career. Used in this manner, SM may potentially help to offset burnout, compassion fatigue, and stressors experienced by those who regularly work with children facing substantial medical challenges.

Virtual Encounters with Patients and Families

As patient and family use of SM continues to grow, providers become more likely to encounter online circumstances in which traditional patient–provider boundaries become increasingly blurred. The possibilities for "virtual encounters" are limitless and include scenarios such as the following:

- Providers may cross paths with their patients "virtually" on message boards or other SM sites dedicated to specific oncology-related topics.
- Parents may e-mail their child's physician after hours with time-sensitive questions about medication dosing or other treatment-related matters.
- A provider may be invited to follow along on the CaringBridge site of a current patient, or may learn about information viewed therein by a colleague.
- Parents of a deceased former patient may extend a "friend" invitation, through their personal Facebook account, to their child's beloved physician or to a nurse who cared for their child during his or her final hospital course.
- Practitioners, motivated by an authentic sense of interest in building rapport, may Google a patient in order to learn more about his or her background and outside interests. Patients and families, in turn, may learn personal details about their child's practitioner via a Google search of their own.
- Providers who maintain blogs about their lives and careers may inadvertently violate the privacy of youngsters under their care by posting matters regarding protected health information on their website.

Potential Risks Associated with SM Use by Practitioners

Practitioner usage may also be associated with a range of potential risks.

- *Threats regarding professional/therapeutic boundaries.* Interacting with patients and families outside the more traditional treatment context substantially raises the potential for professional boundary violations. For example, when patients or families learn personal information about their providers in an online context (such as via a Google search or by viewing their Facebook page), this may lead to uncomfortable interactions in subsequent professional interactions.[21] Of related concern is the case in which information about a patient (or family) is obtained by a provider online, but would not otherwise have been known (or is discrepant from information presented in real-life conversations). This is especially worrisome when the information obtained requires urgent or immediate clinical response (e.g., suicidal ideation, adherence issues, breaking contact precautions, other risky behavior), or when the family was unaware that the provider was following their SM activity.

- *Threats to patient care.* If patients are accustomed to communicating with their providers via SM, they may use this method to share clinically urgent or time-sensitive information (e.g., suicidal ideation, child's fever). In this circumstance, in which a delay in response could be harmful or even life-threatening, practitioners are placed in a challenging ethical (and potentially legal) dilemma if they are not continually accessible.
- *Threats to professional reputations and reactions.* Many clinicians have encountered situations in which they learn of (or view) material about themselves on the SM sites of patients/families. Often, such material is favorable in nature. However, this is not always the case, and reading disparaging information about oneself in such a forum may place the practitioner in an uncomfortable and challenging dilemma regarding the working relationship with the patient or parent and may also compromise patient care.[12]
- *Threats to work–life balance.* Communicating with patients via SM outside the usual work environment (such as via after-hours e-mail) may take a toll on one's work–life balance, and ultimately contribute to compassion fatigue or burnout.[21]
- *Threats to privacy/confidentiality of the patient and/or family.* When providers post material online regarding particulars of their professional world (for example, as in the case of those who maintain blogs, or in the context of comments on one's personal Facebook page), this may inadvertently violate the confidentiality of patients under their care. It is not too far-fetched to imagine that such actions might trigger legal actions as well as raise ethical concerns.

Guidelines, Recommendations, and Considerations for Practitioners Regarding Their Personal and Professional Use of SM

- Be mindful, aware, and proactive with regard to use of SM.
- Weigh the benefits and risks associated with online activity.
- If not already available, create one's own SM policy.[22]
- Consult with policies at home institutions (many have established SM guidelines for employees), as well as those put forth by professional organizations with which one maintains affiliations.
- Remain transparent and proactive with patients and families about one's and institution's SM policy.
- Initiate conversations about SM use; informing families up front about own policies and practices (e.g., not accepting friend requests from current or former patients; establishing and documenting clear parameters regarding the expected timeframe for responses to clinical questions posed online).
- Provide explicit guidance that this is not an appropriate forum for contact regarding more urgent matters (as well as accompanying

instruction about appropriate channels of communication for emergency situations).
- Use your own clinical judgment and experience but seek consultation from trusted colleagues if you perceive a concern or conflict pertaining to SM use.
- Practitioners who choose to communicate online with patients and families should create SM accounts for professional use only.
- Maintain clear separations between personal and professional use of SM.
- Remain knowledgeable and diligent about privacy settings associated with accounts designated for personal use; carefully select conservative privacy settings for such accounts in order to minimize the likelihood that personal information could be easily accessed.
- Engage in conversations with trainees about these matters, encouraging them to make thoughtful decisions about their own SM policy and practice.
- Periodically review and monitor the online material associated with one's name (e.g., "Google" oneself to see what patients or families will encounter when one's name is entered in a search).
- Create a "Google profile" and/or a "Google alert" to help monitor information about self, receive notification about new personal data, and remove unwanted content (for more information about monitoring one's online reputation in this manner, see: https://support.google.com/accounts/answer/1228138?hl=en).
- Consider finding a mentor within the field if not yet well-versed in the language of SM.

Other Related Considerations in the Digital Age

Institutional Considerations

In addition to providing support and guidance in the context of establishing one's professional SM policy (as discussed earlier), home institutions may also be helpful in the context of efforts to offer accurate and helpful medical information online.

- Institutionally based SM may provide a platform for the dissemination of evidence-based information, and can serve as a starting point for patients and families in their online search for information about their disease.
- Practitioners should involve themselves in efforts both to develop institutional guidelines regarding employee use of SM, as well as initiatives aimed at developing up-to-date, accessible and informative websites for patient and family use. It is important for such sites to contain clear and explicit guidance for patients and families (which should be underscored in face-to-face interactions) about the inadvisability of using such material as a substitute for direct care.

- Consider creating specific sites for AYA patients. Beyond presenting information in a developmentally appropriate manner, these sites should be engaging to the AYA user and address questions and concerns specific to these populations.

eHealth Services

Beyond SM, other relevant forms of eHealth technologies include cybermedicine and using the Internet to deliver interventions, communication between patients and providers via email, and the use of electronic medical records.

- Children, adolescents, and parents who are the potential consumers of eHealth interventions are interested in using this medium for health promotion[23] and preliminary data have shown efficacious results for self-management online interventions for youth with chronic health conditions.[24]
- Electronic medical records, which allow patients to access their medical information through a secure online portal and to communicate electronically with their healthcare providers, are also becoming more common.
- Within one large healthcare group, the use of secure online messaging between patients and providers was associated with a decrease in office visits and significant increase in patient satisfaction.[25]
- Many researchers are turning to online applications within their study methodology, including subject recruitment and assessment.

Technology use in medicine will only increase in future years and, as reviewed earlier, brings both benefits and the potential for pitfalls (e.g., around privacy/confidentiality matters and professional boundaries).

Other Mobile Devices

With the ever-growing popularity and universality of smartphones, tablet computers, and other mobile devices, mobile applications (or "apps") represent another related form of relevant digital technology.

- There are apps available for a wide range of professional uses including:
    - Accessing clinical information.
    - Connecting and collaborating with colleagues.
    - Viewing conference presentations.
    - Retrieving journal articles and abstracts. ASCO offers a range of downloadable such apps on their website (http://www.asco.org/mobile-applications).
- There are a host of apps suitable for patients and families, with a range of clinical and related uses including:
    - Monitoring and tracking (e.g., adherence, mood, nutritional intake, chemotherapy side effects, blood cell count).
    - Stress management and relaxation (e.g., biofeedback, breathing exercises, mindfulness, imagery, hypnosis).

- Augmentative and alternative communication (AAC) to facilitate communication with patients who are unable to speak.
- Connecting with other patients with similar diagnoses, and fundraising.

As with other forms of SM and related technology, practitioners are advised to remain educated and aware about apps that may be beneficial for their patients, to openly engage in dialogue with patients/families about apps that they are using, and to be mindful of the potential for concern or harm (e.g., apps promoting potentially erroneous or misleading clinical information, or the use of apps as a substitute for actual clinical care).

Summary

For patients, families, and providers alike, SM affords opportunities for community development and interpersonal connection, clinical trial recruitment, dissemination of health-related information, professional education, and a host of other related benefits. However, with these advantages come a host of associated challenges and risks about which practitioners are advised to remain mindful and proactive. In today's digital age there will undoubtedly continue to evolve new developments in SM and related technology that will offer further applications and benefits, and it is certain that these will also be accompanied by new potential risks and ethical and/or professional challenges. We encourage providers to remain informed and educated about the changing landscape of SM, particularly as it intersects with their professional lives.

References

1. Emond Y, de Groot J, Wetzels W, van Osch L. Internet guidance in oncology practice: determinants of health professionals' Internet referral behavior. *Psycho-oncol.* Jan 2013;22(1):74–82.
2. Fox S, Duggan M. Health online 2013. *Pew Internet and American Life Project.* 2013. www.pewinternet.org/reports/2013/Health-Online. Accessed August 8, 2013.
3. Hamm MP, Chisholm A, Shulhan J, et al. Social media use among patients and caregivers: a scoping review. *BMJ open.* 2013;3(5):e002819. doi:10.1136/bmjopen-2013-002819.
4. Penson RT, Benson RC, Parles K, Chabner BA, Lynch TJ. Virtual connections: Internet health care. *Oncologist.* 2002;7(6):555–568.
5. Kyngäs H, Mikkonen R, Nousiainen EM, et al. Coping with the onset of cancer: coping strategies and resources of young people with cancer. *Euro J Cancer Care.* 2001;10(1):6–11.
6. Last B, Van Veldhuizen A. Information about diagnosis and prognosis related to anxiety and depression in children with cancer aged 8–16 years. *Euro J Cancer.* 1996;32(2):290–294.
7. Colineau N, Paris C. Talking about your health to strangers: understanding the use of online social networks by patients. *New Rev Hypermedia & Multimedia.* 2010;16(1-2):141–160.

8. Treadgold CL, Kuperberg A. Been there, done that, wrote the blog: the choices and challenges of supporting adolescents and young adults with cancer. *J Clin Oncol.* 2010;28(32):4842–4849.

9. Winzelberg AJ, Classen C, Alpers GW, et al. Evaluation of an internet support group for women with primary breast cancer. *Cancer.* 2003;97(5):1164–1173.

10. Suzuki LK, Beale IL. Personal Web home pages of adolescents with cancer: self-presentation, information dissemination, and interpersonal connection. *J Pediatr Oncol Nurs.* May-Jun 2006;23(3):152–161.

11. McLaughlin M, Nam Y, Gould J, et al. A videosharing social networking intervention for young adult cancer survivors. *Comput Hum Behav.* 2012;28(2):631–641.

12. Tunick R, Mednick L. Commentary: electronic communication in the pediatric setting—dilemmas associated with patient blogs. *J Pediatr Psychol.* Jun 2009;34(5):585–587.

13. O'Keeffe GS, Clarke-Pearson K. The impact of social media on children, adolescents, and families. *Pediatr.* Apr 2011;127(4):800–804.

14. Dizon DS, Graham D, Thompson MA, et al. Practical guidance: the use of social media in oncology practice. *J Oncol Pract/Am Soc Clin Oncol.* Sep 2012;8(5):e114–124.

15. Bosslet GT, Torke AM, Terry CL, Helft PR. The patient–doctor relationship and online social networks: results of a national survey. *J Gen Intern Med.* 2011;26(10):1168–1174.

16. Giordano C, Giordano C. Health professions students' use of social media. *J Allied Health.* 2011;40(2):78–81.

17. Hede K. Online Networks Present Challenges, Opportunities for Oncology. *J National Cancer Instit.* 2012;104(15):1115–1116.

18. Terry M. Twittering healthcare: social media and medicine. *Telemed J & e-Health.* Jul-Aug 2009;15(6):507–510.

19. Chaudhry A, Glode LM, Gillman M, Miller RS. Trends in twitter use by physicians at the american society of clinical oncology annual meeting, 2010 and 2011. *J Oncol Pract/Am Soc Clinic Oncol.* May 2012;8(3):173–178.

20. McKenna MP, D'Alessandro D. Social networks and the practice of medicine: harnessing powerful opportunities. *J Pediatr.* Jan 2011;158(1):1–2.

21. Wiener L, Crum C, Grady C, Merchant M. To friend or not to friend: the use of social media in clinical oncology. *J Oncol Pract/Am Soc Clin Oncol.* Mar 2012;8(2):103–106.

22. Tunick R, Mednick L, Conroy C. A snapshot of child psychologists' social media activity: professional and ethical practice implications and recommendations. *Prof Psychol: Res & Pract.* 2011;42(6):440.

23. Ritterband LM, Palermo TM. Introduction to the special issue: eHealth in pediatric psychology. *J Ped Psychol.* 2009;34(5):453–456.

24. Stinson J, Wilson R, Gill N, Yamada J, Holt J. A systematic review of internet-based self-management interventions for youth with health conditions. *J Pediatr Psychol.* 2009;34(5):495–510.

25. Baer D. Patient-physician e-mail communication: the Kaiser Permanente experience. *J Oncol Pract.* 2011;7(4):230–233.

Chapter 33

Pediatric Cancer Survivors

Moving Beyond Cure

Lisa A. Schwartz, Julia H. Rowland, and Aziza Shad

Advances in cancer diagnosis, treatment, and supportive care have turned previously fatal diseases of childhood into conditions that can be largely cured or controlled. It is currently estimated that over 80% of children diagnosed with cancer today will be alive at 5 years, and 10-year survival has surpassed 75%.[1] There are already over 329,600 childhood cancer survivors in the U.S. alone, 24% of whom were diagnosed over 30 years ago.[2] A reversal of comparable magnitude in survival outcomes for any of the adult cancers with high lethality (e.g., lung, pancreatic, liver, gastric) has yet to be achieved. As a consequence, pediatric cancer survivors are often considered the "vanguard" of the survivorship movement in the United States.

Adverse Sequelae of Cancer: An Overview

As children live beyond their initial cancer diagnosis, they often experience and are troubled by the adverse sequelae of cancer and its therapy upon entering adolescence and young and older adulthood. Many of the treatments used to cure childhood malignancies are themselves carcinogenic (e.g., radiation, specific classes of chemotherapeutic agents) and/or have the capacity to damage tissue and cell growth and alter the current and future function of developing organs.[3] These outcomes can be of varying duration (Boxes 33.1 and 33.2) and can affect all aspects of a survivor's life (Box 33.3). Consequently, longer-term survival has resulted in a chronic state of uncertainty for the lives of both pediatric cancer survivors and those of their loved ones. In the past decade, survivorship issues have become a focus of national attention.

A major source of current information on childhood cancer survivors' posttreatment health, functioning and quality of life has been and continues to be generated by the Childhood Cancer Survivor Study (CCSS, www.stjude.org/ccss). CCSS includes longitudinal data on two large, consecutively treated cohorts of children initially diagnosed under the age of 21 and treated between the years 1970 and 1986 (original cohort) or between 1987 and 1999 (second cohort).

Box 33.1 Duration of Cancer's Effects

- Acute Effects—Occur during and often in reaction to cancer or its treatment (e.g., nausea and vomiting, hair loss, anemia) and generally go away after treatment ends.
- Long-Term Effects—Also referred to as chronic or persistent, start before or during treatment and persist after treatment ends (e.g., fatigue, problems with memory or concentration); sometimes become permanent (e.g., disability related to amputation, cognitive dysfunction)
- Late Effects—Occur months or even years after treatment ends (e.g., cardiac failure, infertility, second malignancies)

Box 33.2 Characteristics of Long-Term and Late Effects

- Pediatric survivors of all ages can be affected.
- Some survivors have few effects, while others experience many late effects.
- Degree of risk to individual patients is often difficult to predict.
- Adverse sequelae contribute to the physical, psychological, and social burden of illness, and can result in decreased length and quality of survival.
- There can be long latencies in the development of some effects; alternatively some effects can persist for months or years and then remit.
- Second cancers are the most life-threatening late effect, but other disabling and potentially serious health conditions can occur and need to be monitored for, and their impact addressed.
- Early interventions hold the best potential to reduce adverse outcomes.
- Continued surveillance over a lifetime is needed.

As we attempt to care for the psychological needs of childhood cancer survivors, it is important to consider a model proposed by the IOM in its report, Cancer Care for the Whole Patient: Meeting Psychosocial Healthcare Needs.[4] (See Introduction.) This model may need to be adapted when dealing with the whole family in the case of caring for an adolescent population.

Psychosocial Impact of Childhood Cancer[5–7]

- Long-term survivors of childhood cancer are generally psychologically resilient, although having had pediatric cancer is a risk factor for distress, somatic symptoms, cognitive impairment, and deficits or delays of normative developmental tasks.

Box 33.3 Domains of Cancer's Effects

- Physical/medical—second cancers, cardiovascular disease, renal dysfunction, severe musculoskeletal problems, cognitive dysfunction, endocrine disorders, cardio-respiratory-system problems, pain, infertility/sexual impairment, hearing loss, blindness, dental problems, scarring and disfigurement, and sleep disturbances.
- Psychosocial—depression, anxiety, posttraumatic stress, guilt, uncertainty, isolation, poor self-esteem, altered body image, changes in interpersonal relationships (family and peers).
- Academic/Employment/Insurance—problems with return to school, concerns regarding health or life insurance, job lock[a]/loss, employment challenges, financial burden.
- Existential and spiritual—questions about justice and faith, meaning of illness, sense of purpose or worth, appreciation of life, benefit finding

[a] Inability to change jobs for fear of losing health benefits.

- Challenges associated with survivorship include medical and psychological late effects, continuous appraisal of future cancer threat, physical and environmental reminders of cancer, discrimination when seeking employment or insurance, isolation from peers, and mourning of lost self.
- Survivors may experience positive outcomes related to resilience, enhanced coping abilities, and posttraumatic growth.
- Children and adolescents treated for cancer may miss normal age-appropriate activities (e.g. attending school, spending time with family/friends, playing sports).
- When treatment ends, youth may have difficulty re-engaging in such activities.
- Some face the challenge of repeating a grade or losing their circle of friends.
- Due to perceived or actual vulnerability, parents may be more protective of and less likely to promote independence, autonomy, or encourage activities away from home.
- Development during emerging adulthood may be affected due to earlier missed experiences.
- Negative outcomes are more likely for survivors with cognitive or physical late effects that impair social functioning and/or the ability to live independently. (See Chapter 27, School and Peer Relationships.)

Table 33.1 summarizes specific developmental sequelae.

Table 33.1 Potential Adolescent and Young Adult Developmental Sequelae

<table>
<tr><th>Potential Developmental Sequelae</th><th>Implications for Providers</th></tr>
<tr><td>Hindered identity development</td><td rowspan="8">Be aware of developmental level of patients. Patients may be less likely to have close relationships with same-age peers and may be more likely than healthy children to live with and/or rely on their parents for basic, emotional, and healthcare needs. This is more likely for patients who had cancers or treatment with CNS involvement and who currently have late effects. Include parents in care when they are present, but work to facilitate patients' healthcare self-management skills and confidence. Encourage activities that involve normative developmental tasks related to peer socialization and education/employment.</td></tr>
<tr><td>Difficulty forming relationships with same-age peers and/or less satisfaction with relationships</td></tr>
<tr><td>Difficulty forming and/or less satisfaction with romantic or sexual relationships (see Chapter 13, Fertility and Sexuality)</td></tr>
<tr><td>More likely to live at home and be less independent from parents</td></tr>
<tr><td>Reduced marriage rates in young adulthood</td></tr>
<tr><td>Deficits in cognitive ability related to cancer late effects (see Chapter 18, Cognitive Sequelae).</td></tr>
<tr><td>Difficulty with educational/career attainment</td></tr>
<tr><td>Dissatisfaction with self-concept and body image</td></tr>
</table>

Psychological Distress in Survivors[5–11]

- Compared to siblings and controls, survivors are at elevated risk for psychological distress including suicidal ideation, depressive symptoms, anxiety, somatic complaints (pain and fatigue) and posttraumatic stress symptoms (PTSS).
- Studies examining treatment- and disease-related predictors of survivor distress are mixed, but some results suggest that survivors who experienced more intense treatments and who were treated as adolescents are more at risk for later distress.
- Distress is also associated with survivors' perceptions of current health and life threat, perception that cancer treatment was intense, and demographic factors such as female gender, lower socioeconomic status, lack of employment, lower educational achievement, and single status.
- Thus, it is important to assess the patient's perceptions of their health and life threat (in addition to understanding "objective" criteria of disease severity or treatment intensity) when exploring psychosocial issues and predictors of distress.

Table 33.2 summarizes markers of distress.

Symptoms require intervention if they impact important health-related behaviors and optimal quality of life and functioning. It is important to rule out any potential medical etiologies. See Chapter 12 on Anxiety and Depression.

Table 33.2 Markers of Distress

Markers of distress	Symptoms to assess which may require intervention
General distress including symptoms of depression and anxiety	Withdrawal from people or activities of prior interest, flat or sad affect, suicidal ideation, sleeping less or more than usual, eating less or more than usual, excessive worry
Somatic complaints including pain and fatigue	Pain and aches, often out of proportion to what would be expected posttreatment; fatigue; physiological arousal related to anxiety/worry
Posttraumatic stress	Rumination/intrusive thoughts/frequent nightmares about cancer or related experiences, hyperarousal when thinking or talking about cancer, avoidance of thinking or talking about cancer, avoidance of healthcare settings or doing things to take care of health, hypervigilance of body and symptoms, feeling life is prematurely shortened.

Posttraumatic Stress[10]

- The experience of cancer can be traumatic in terms of threat of future cancers or late effects; current late effects; reminders of the cancer; and losses such as diminished social, cognitive and reproductive capacity.
- Up to 50% of survivors experience the posttraumatic stress symptoms of intrusive thoughts, avoidance, and arousal symptoms. Up to 20% of adult survivors meet criteria for posttraumatic stress disorder (PTSD), which is associated with functional impairment, representing a rate up 4 to 5 times higher than siblings or unrelated controls.
- Maturity and enhanced awareness of the implications of cancer, in conjunction with newly identified late effects in early adulthood, may "re-expose" young adults to the trauma of cancer.
- Those who meet diagnostic criteria for PTSD are more likely to be depressed, functionally impaired, and to have a lower quality of life than those who experience posttraumatic stress symptoms (PTSS) but do not meet formal criteria for a psychiatric diagnosis.
- PTSD among survivors is also associated with lower income, unemployment, single status, and intense treatment.
- Other members of the patient's family, particularly parents and also siblings, may experience PTSS, often at higher rates than the survivor.

Resilience, Posttraumatic Growth, and Positive Sequelae[11]

- With increasing cognitive maturity, adolescent and young adult survivors may experience positive benefits or perceived positive impact as a result of their cancer experience. Parents and siblings are also likely to experience positive benefits. These include:
    - Enhanced coping abilities.
    - Motivation in various life domains.

- Positive consequences in the domains of self, relationships, and future plans.
- Posttraumatic growth, which is defined as the process of applying positive interpretations and finding meaning in a traumatic event. Self-awareness of inner resources and available social support may facilitate positive changes related to self-concept, relationships, and life philosophy.
- Survivors are more likely than siblings to report perceived positive impact. Predictors include: female gender, nonwhite race, exposure to at least one intense therapy, a second malignancy or relapse, older age at diagnosis, and fewer years since diagnosis.

Employment Status after Childhood Cancer[12,13]

The health and behavioral consequences of cancer may significantly affect long-term vocational and employment opportunities. Although not all studies have demonstrated deficits in employment, many report employment difficulties in adult childhood cancer survivors, with survivors being nearly twice as likely to be unemployed compared to healthy controls. In addition to poor physical health, the most important risk factor for unemployment, a number of specific factors may increase risk for employment-related problems (Table 33.3).

- Individuals with CNS tumors and survivors of childhood ALL treated with cranial radiation have been identified as the most vulnerable for unemployment due to well-documented difficulties with executive and visual spatial functions, and expressive language and verbal memory resulting from cognitive impairment from CNS disease or CNS-directed therapy.
- Survivors of bone and soft tissue sarcomas such as Ewing's sarcoma are less likely to be employed full-time compared to sibling controls due to physical limitations that can restrict activity and job performance.
- Adult survivors of certain sarcomas, including rhabdomyosarcoma are significantly more likely to report physical impairment characterized by one or more chronic health conditions, cancer-related pain, performance limitations of routine activities, and health-related inability to work, compared to sibling controls.

Table 33.3 Factors Predicting Employment Difficulties

Diagnosis of CNS or bone tumor	**Treatment with cranial radiation > 30 Gy**
Younger age at diagnosis (<4 years)	Lower educational attainment (less than high school)
Female sex	History of motor impairment or epilepsy
Depression	

Table 33.4 Insurance Issues	
General Difficulties with Insurance	**Factors Predicting Insurance Deficits**
Inability to obtain affordable health insurance with a preexisting condition	Younger than 4 years at diagnosis
Lack of comprehensive healthcare coverage	Male sex
Cost-prohibitive premiums	Educational attainment less than high school
Restrictions on health care plans	Household income below $20,000
	Widowed/divorced/separated marital status

- Individuals treated with amputation have been shown to exhibit significant deficits in education, employment and insurance access compared to sibling controls.

Insurance Status after Childhood Cancer[14]

In the United States, where, historically, health insurance is provided largely through employers, restricted employment opportunities affect healthcare access. In the past, long-term childhood cancer survivors were significantly less likely to have health insurance, have more difficulty obtaining insurance (report restrictive policies excluding preexisting medical conditions), and more likely to be denied health insurance because of their cancer history (Table 33.4). However, there has been significant improvement in recent years in the disparity of insurance access between childhood cancer survivors and sibling or population controls, due to legislation prohibiting employment discrimination and facilitating insurance access and portability (Table 33.5). In particular, with the introduction of the Affordable Care Act in 2010, it is expected that more childhood cancer survivors will retain or have access to health insurance, either through longer-term coverage (up to age 27) under parental health insurance policies, or the ability to purchase affordable state or federal health insurance plans.

Protecting Employment and Insurance Access in Childhood Cancer Survivors

Given that a substantial body of evidence confirms that childhood cancer may negatively affect vocational and employment opportunities and insurance access, providers should be aware of legislation that facilitates survivor employment and insurance access (Table 33.5).

- Appropriate vocational planning or rehabilitation and aggressive symptom management is important to promote survivor success in the workplace.
- Employer education and "reasonable" workplace accommodations should be provided for individuals with disabilities as mandated by the Americans with Disabilities Act (ADA) of 1990; these also represent methods to enhance vocational achievement and social competence.

Table 33.5 Legislation Protecting Survivor Employment and Insurance Access

Americans with Disabilities Act (ADA) of 1990	Requires employers to make reasonable accommodations for individuals with a disability who can perform essential job functions
Family Medical Leave Act (FMLA)	Provides 12 weeks per 12 months medical leave for employee or family if the employer has more than 50 employees
Consolidated Omnibus Reconciliation Act (COBRA)	Requires employers or larger businesses to make insurance benefits available for a limited time to employees (and their dependents) who are fired or laid off
Health Insurance Portability and Accountability Act of 1996 (HIPAA)	Allows people with preexisting conditions to keep comprehensive insurance coverage when they are changing insurance plans or jobs
Affordable Care Act of 2010 (ACA)	Extends coverage of children up to age 27 under parents' health insurance policies; prohibits caps on medical expenses over a lifetime; requires all adults to have healthcare insurance and states (through state- or federally based exchanges) to provide access to affordable health care insurance plans

- Despite legislation promoting insurance portability, concerns regarding potential loss of insurance may still limit employment choices.
- Survivors should be encouraged to be proactive in obtaining and maintaining health coverage.
    - Avoiding lapses in coverage will preclude limitations in insurance coverage of preexisting conditions or other related penalties.
    - Planning for transitions that occur with high school, college graduations, job changes, or other life changes are critical to avoid lapses in coverage.
- The development of interventions that help survivors with chronic health conditions obtain and maintain employment will be important in facilitating their social competence and healthcare access.
- Survivors also lack knowledge about insurance issues, yet express interest in being better informed in this area.
- Healthcare providers should initiate conversations about healthcare coverage, especially regarding future transitions.

Health Care Behaviors[15]

Risk-Based Care

Risk-based care incorporates the previous cancer, cancer therapy, genetic predispositions, lifestyle behaviors, age, and co-morbid health conditions. Quality care for cancer survivorship has been defined as "a risk based approach to health care and a systematic plan for life-long screening, surveillance and prevention." Childhood cancer survivors continue to demonstrate significant lack of knowledge and misperceptions about their cancer diagnosis, treatment, and cancer-related health risks following completion of therapy; therefore, healthcare providers must focus on health maintenance and promotion along with surveillance for the early identification of late effects. With many pediatric cancer survivors continuing to engage in high risk-taking behaviors at a rate similar to their peers, it falls on the clinicians to educate these youth to focus on modifiable risk factors (diet, exercise, smoking, drinking alcohol) and to undergo routine surveillance. Potentially, a healthy lifestyle can help minimize the negative physical and psychological effects of cancer and its treatment.

Developing an Individual Risk Profile

This can be accomplished by putting together an "off-therapy summary" with all the information listed:

- Cancer diagnosis and treatment.
- Complications during treatment.
- Posttreatment complications.
- Family history.
- Current problems and medications.
- Physical examination findings.
- Labs and scans to date.
- Health maintenance/screening behaviors.
- Psychosocial health.
- Neuro-cognitive function status.

Modifiable Risk Factors

Educating young adult survivors of childhood cancer on the importance of the below-mentioned modifiable risk factors and prevention cannot be overemphasized.

Primary Prevention

- Eating a balanced diet.
- Exercising regularly.
- Smoking cessation.
- Limiting alcohol intake.
- Sun protection.
- Mimimizing environmental/industrial exposures.
- Safe sex practices: Human Papilloma Virus (HPV) vaccine.
- Health maintenance.

Secondary Prevention

- Breast self-examination (BSE) (females).
- Testicular self-examination (TSE) (males).
- Mammography (females).
- Skin examination (by dermatologist).
- Eye examination.
- Audiogram (in selected cases).
- Regular dental check-up.
- Prostate specific antigen (PSA)-blood test (males).
- Colonoscopy.
- DEXA scan (Bone Mineral Density).
- Other screening tests and labs.

Medical Follow-Up Guidelines[16–18]

Pediatric cancer survivors generally receive follow-up care from a wide variety of healthcare professionals. Many providers lack familiarity with pediatric cancer-related health risks and risk-reduction methods relevant for this population. To implement appropriate risk-based care, survivors and providers must have accurate information about cancer diagnosis, treatment modalities, and potential cancer-related health risks to guide screening and risk-reducing interventions. Several groups have organized clinical practice guidelines:

- Children's Cancer and Leukemia Group's Therapy Based Long-Term Follow-Up: Practice Statement.
- Long term follow-up of survivors of childhood cancer. A national clinical guideline—Scottish Inter-collegiate Guidelines Network (SIGN).[16a]
- The Children's Oncology Group's Long-Term Follow-Up Guidelines for Survivors of Childhood, Adolescent and Young Adult Cancers (COG Guidelines) represent the most comprehensive resource of exposure-based screening recommendations available to healthcare providers supervising the care of childhood cancer survivors. They are also the most widely used guidelines in the United States and Canada.
- Patient educational materials called "Health Links" accompany the COG Guidelines and can be accessed along with the guidelines at http://www.survivorshipguidelines.org.

Table 33.6 Recommended Frequency of Echocardiogram or MUGA scan as per COG Guidelines

Age at Treatment*	Radiation with Potential Impact to the Heart	Anthracycline Dose	Recommended Frequency
<1 year old	Yes	Any	Every year
	No	<200 mg/m^2	Every 2 years
		≥ 200 mg/m^2	Every year
1–4 years old	Yes	Any	Every year
	No	<100 mg/m^2	Every 5 years
		≥ 100 to <300 mg/m^2	Every 2 years
		≥ 300 mg/m^2	Every year
>5 years old	Yes	<300 mg/m^2	Every 2 years
		≥ 300 mg/m^2	Every year
	No	<200 mg/m^2	Every 5 years
		≥ 200 to <300 mg/m^2	Every 2 years
		≥ 300 mg/m^2	Every year
Any age with decrease in serial function			Every year

*Age at time of first cardiotoxic therapy (Anthracycline or radiation, whichever was given first).

*Reproduced from COG Guidelines with permission.

Both survivors and healthcare providers should be educated about potential cancer-related effects, since pediatric cancer survivors may receive follow-up care from a wide variety of healthcare professionals. Table 33.6 is an example of guidelines for monitoring of heart function in survivors who have received anthracyclines as part of their cancer treatment. They take into consideration age, dose of anthracycline, and any associated radiation, providing guidance for frequency of follow-up with echocardiograms or multigated acquisition (MUGA) nuclear medicine scans.

Health Care Summary[19,20]

At the end of therapy, all treating oncologists should provide survivors with a clinical summary that details cancer-treatment exposures, potential cancer-related health risks, and recommendations for health screening and risk-reducing behaviors. Having a complete record of cancer-related events is essential to the development of an appropriate health-monitoring plan. The summary should include:

- Date of diagnosis, cancer histology, and stage.
- Specific treatment modalities (surgery, chemotherapy, and radiation therapy).
- Cumulative chemotherapy dose and radiation-treatment volumes and dose permit more accurate risk assessment to guide screening recommendations.

Table 33.7 shows an example of how COG Guidelines can be used for long-term follow-up and screening. (Example taken from the COG Long Term Follow-up (LTFU) Study Newsletter).

For survivors who have not been provided with this information, several templates from different COG institutions are provided in Appendix I of the COG LTFU Guidelines that can be used by survivors to organize a personal treatment summary. They can be accessed at http://www.survivorshipguidelines.org

Figure 33.1 is an example of the off-therapy summary provided by the Childhood Cancer Survivorship Program, Lombardi Comprehensive Cancer Center to all patients at the end of treatment.

Long-Term Follow-up[21–31]

The Beginning of Long-Term Follow-Up[21,22]

Increasing awareness of the previously described late effects and the need to provide better care to childhood cancer survivors resulted in the establishment of the first long-term follow-up programs (LTFU) in various cancer centers and children's hospitals in the late 1980s and 1990s. Though most of these programs logistically existed within a pediatric oncology clinic, they were separate and distinct, and their sole purpose was to address survivorship issues. By 1997, there were LTFU programs in 96 institutions, nationally and internationally, that were a part of the Pediatric Oncology

Table 33.7 Using the Children's Oncology Group Guidelines

As an example of using the COG Guidelines for long-term follow-up screening, let's assume that a woman was diagnosed in 1988 at age 15 with Hodgkin's disease involving lymph nodes in her neck and chest. The table below shows the possible health risks associated with her treatment history. Screening recommendations for all of these treatments can be found in the CureSearch Children's Oncology Group Long-Term Follow-Up Guidelines at: http://www.survivorshipguidelines.org.

Treatment history	Long-term health risks
Staging surgery with spleen removal (splenectomy)	Removal of the spleen results in a lifelong risk of a serious blood infection with certain bacteria that are handled by the spleen. Survivors who have had their spleens removed are advised to seek prompt medical attention if they develop a fever (101°F or greater) for blood culture and antibiotics.
ABVD Chemotherapy Adriamycin Bleomycin Vinblastine Dacarbazine	Survivors who were treated with ABVD chemotherapy are at risk of heart problems related to the Adriamycin and for lung problems related to the Bleomycin in the combination. The risk is related to the dose of these medicines, which can be estimated by the months of treatment. Most survivors do not have long-term problems after Vinblastine and Dacarbazine therapy.
Radiation to lymph nodes in the neck and chest	Radiation to the lymph nodes in the neck and chest may have long-term effects on the salivary glands, thyroid gland, heart, and lungs. The risk is related to the dose of radiation, which can be estimated by the days of treatment. Radiation to any tissues also increases the risk of developing a second (different) cancer. Girls who had radiation to the chest for a childhood cancer are especially at risk for breast cancer.
Blood transfusion in 1988	A survivor who received a blood transfusion before 1992, when blood banks did not have a reliable way to test if blood donors were infected with hepatitis C, carries a risk of chronic infection with hepatitis C. Individuals with chronic hepatitis C have a higher risk of liver problems, including liver cancer.

Adapted and reproduced with permission from the LTFU Newsletter, Spring 2006.

OFF THERAPY SUMMARY

Georgetown University Hospital

MedStar Health

Childhood Cancer Survivorship Program

Lombardi Comprehensive Cancer Center
Georgetown University Hospital
3800 Reservoir Road NW ▪ Washington DC 20007-2197
Telephone: 202-444-7599

Lombardi
COMPREHENSIVE CANCER CENTER
AT GEORGETOWN UNIVERSITY

Name: ______________________ DOB: ______________________

Medical Record #: ______________________ Treatment Center: ______________________

Primary Oncologist: ______________________ Primary Nurse Practitioner: ______________________

Patient Contact Information:

Address: ____

Email Address: ____

Home Phone: ______________________ Cell Phone: ______________________

Diagnosis: ____

Date of Diagnosis: ______________________ Age at Diagnosis: ______________________

Clinical Trial:

Title: ______________________ Protocol #: ______________________

On Study: ☐ Yes ☐ No

Therapy:

Date Therapy Began: ______________________ Date Therapy Ended: ______________________

Disease Status at end of therapy: ______________________

Remission: ☐ Complete ☐ Partial

Relapse: ☐ Yes ☐ No Date: ______________________ Site: ______________________

Initial Presentation:

____

____

____

____

Figure 33.1 Off Therapy Summary Template. Reproduced with permission from 'The Next Step—Crossing the Bridge to Survivorship'. Published 2008, Lombardi Comprehensive Cancer Center, Georgetown University.

Pre-treatment Evaluation:

1. Labs:

____
____
____
____
____

2. Radiology:

Date: ______ Test: ______________ Result: ______________
Date: ______ Test: ______________ Result: ______________
Date: ______ Test: ______________ Result: ______________
Date: ______ Test: ______________ Result: ______________

3. Pathology:

Date: ______ Source: ______________ Result: ______________
Date: ______ Source: ______________ Result: ______________
Date: ______ Source: ______________ Result: ______________
Date: ______ Source: ______________ Result: ______________

4. ECHO/EKG:

Date: ______ Ejection Fraction: __________ Shortening Fraction: __________
____

5. Pulmonary Function Tests (PFTs):

Date: ______ Result: ____________________________
____

6. Audiology (Hearing test):

Date: ______ Result: ____________________________
____

7. Other:

Sperm Banking ☐ Yes ☐ No Ovarian Cryopreservation ☐ Yes ☐ No
____
____

Figure 33.1 (Continued)

Treatment Summary:

1. Surgery:

Date: ________ Procedure: ____

Date: ________ Procedure: ____

Date: ________ Procedure: ____

2. Chemotherapy:

Drug: ______________________ Total Doses: ______ Dose/m²: ______ Route: ______

Drug: ______________________ Total Doses: ______ Dose/m²: ______ Route: ______

Drug: ______________________ Total Doses: ______ Dose/m²: ______ Route: ______

Drug: ______________________ Total Doses: ______ Dose/m²: ______ Route: ______

Drug: ______________________ Total Doses: ______ Dose/m²: ______ Route: ______

3. Radiation Therapy:

Start Date: ______ Stop Date: ______ Site: ________________ Total Dose cGy: ______

Start Date: ______ Stop Date: ______ Site: ________________ Total Dose cGy: ______

4. Biological Therapy:

Date: ______ Name: ____________________________ Dose: ____________

Date: ______ Name: ____________________________ Dose: ____________

5. Bone Marrow/Stem Cell Transplantation:

Date: ______ Type: ____

BMT/SCT Chemotherapy:

Drug: ______________________ Total Doses: ______ Dose/m²: ______ Route: ______

Drug: ______________________ Total Doses: ______ Dose/m²: ______ Route: ______

Drug: ______________________ Total Doses: ______ Dose/m²: ______ Route: ______

Drug: ______________________ Total Doses: ______ Dose/m²: ______ Route: ______

BMT/SCT Radiation Therapy:

Date: ______ Site: ______________________________ Total Dose cGy: ______

Date: ______ Site: ______________________________ Total Dose cGy: ______

Figure 33.1 (Continued)

Post-treatment Evaluation:

1. Labs:

____

____

____

2. Radiology:

Date: ______ Test: ______________ Result: ______________

Date: ______ Test: ______________ Result: ______________

Date: ______ Test: ______________ Result: ______________

Date: ______ Test: ______________ Result: ______________

3. Pathology:

Date: ______ Source: ______________ Result: ______________

Date: ______ Source: ______________ Result: ______________

4. ECHO/EKG:

Date: ______ Ejection Fraction: __________ Shortening Fraction: __________

____

5. Pulmonary Function Tests (PFTs):

Date: ______ Result: ______________________________

____

6. Audiology (Hearing test):

Date: ______ Result: ______________________________

____

7. Other:

____

____

Figure 33.1 (Continued)

Major Medical Events/Complications:

1. Auditory/Hearing: ☐ Yes ☐ No Describe: ____________________

2. Cardiovascular: ☐ Yes ☐ No Describe: ____________________

3. Dental: ☐ Yes ☐ No Describe: ____________________

4. Drug Reaction: ☐ Yes ☐ No Describe: ____________________

5. Gastrointestinal: ☐ Yes ☐ No Describe: ____________________

6. Hepatic: ☐ Yes ☐ No Describe: ____________________

7. Hematology: ☐ Yes ☐ No Describe: ____________________

8. Infections/F&N: ☐ Yes ☐ No Describe: ____________________

9. Musculoskeletal: ☐ Yes ☐ No Describe: ____________________

10. Neurological: ☐ Yes ☐ No Describe: ____________________

11. Neuropsychological: ☐ Yes ☐ No Describe: ____________________

12. Ocular/Visual: ☐ Yes ☐ No Describe: ____________________

13. Pain: ☐ Yes ☐ No Describe: ____________________

14. Psychosocial: ☐ Yes ☐ No Describe: ____________________

15. Pulmonary: ☐ Yes ☐ No Describe: ____________________

16. Renal/GU: ☐ Yes ☐ No Describe: ____________________

17. Reproductive: ☐ Yes ☐ No Describe: ____________________

Figure 33.1 (Continued)

Health Maintenance after Completion of Therapy (cont.):

2. Pneumocystis carinii (PCP) Prophylaxis:

- Continue on Bactrim 2–3days/week until off therapy for 6 months
  OR
- Pentamadine (aerosolized or IV) once a month until off therapy for 6 months
  OR
- Dapsone daily until off therapy for 6 months

3. Chickenpox Exposure:

- If patient is exposed to chickenpox during the first year off chemotherapy and has no antibodies to varicella, it is recommended that VZIG (varicella zoster immune globulin) be given within 72 hours of exposure.
- Varicella/zoster status: Pre Rx: ☐ Pos ☐ Neg Post Rx: ☐ Pos ☐ Neg

Visits to the Pediatric Oncology Clinic:

- Monthly for first year off therapy, every two to three months for second year off therapy, every three to six months for the third year off therapy, and yearly thereafter.
- All patients qualify for an annual visit to the Long Term Follow-up Clinic, Cancer Survivorship Program, once they are two years off therapy. This visit does not substitute for your regular visit with your oncologist.
- Vital signs, monitoring of growth (may include standing height, sitting height, and arm span yearly until growth has ceased), and Tanner staging at each visit.

Figure 33.1 (Continued)

Potential Concerns for Late Effects:

____

Health Care Recommendations:

____

Signature: ____________________ Date: ____________

Figure 33.1 (Continued)

Group (POG) and Children's Oncology Group (COG). Today, the majority of pediatric oncology programs in the United States provide some form of follow-up for survivors.

Barriers to Care[23–31]

In spite of increasing awareness of survivorship issues, many challenges still remain. There is great variability among programs related to resources, staffing, and needs of each clinic. Some institutions do not have the facilities to follow pediatric survivors as they enter young adulthood. Most do not have a *comprehensive* program that requires at least an oncologist and nurse practitioner (NP) with experience in survivorship issues. This, in most cases, is due to tight department budgets and poor reimbursement.

There is a lack of clinicians who are specifically trained in survivorship issues, and additional education for oncologists and oncology nurses is needed. As the number of survivors is expected to increase by another 100,000 in the next 10 years, this then raises the concerning issue of who will provide the necessary care to this high-risk population.

Reports show that less than 20% of adults who are childhood cancer survivors are followed at a cancer center or by an oncologist, and the likelihood of this type of follow-up decreases with time. Creative solutions are, therefore, needed to deliver optimal evidence based care for survivors of childhood cancer.

In 2005, The Institute of Medicine (IOM) published the report "*From Cancer Patient to Cancer Survivor: Lost in Transition,*" which identified primary-care providers (PCPs) as an integral part of the healthcare team. However, studies have shown that although PCPs have expressed interest in caring for this population of patients, they are uncomfortable with their lack of knowledge on late effects of cancer therapies. Specifically, they are concerned with having the responsibility for cancer surveillance and complicated co-morbidities, and tend to focus on preventative care.

Another key barrier to appropriate follow-up survivorship care is a lack of knowledge on the part of the survivor regarding the potential long-term risks of cancer treatment, and the essential need for life-long follow-up. This is especially true for survivors who were treated at very young ages and have little to no recollection of their cancer experience. It is not unusual for teens or young adults to be unaware of the names of the chemotherapy agents they received because it was always a parent who navigated them through medical situations.

Transition from Pediatric to Adult Health Care[32–36]

Survivors of childhood cancer are a population at risk for morbidity and mortality secondary to the treatment of their primary disease. In most cases, the risk of these effects increases with age and often results in

Table 33.8 Models of Transitional Care

	Advantages	Disadvantages
Cancer-center-based model	• Continuity of care • Survivorship expertise and familiarity with risk-adapted care • Patient familiarity with system and care providers • Ready access to medical specialists • Resources suited for providing comprehensive services • Potential for resource-sharing with adult survivorship program • Existing infrastructure conducive to research • Context facilitates professional training in survivorship	• Resource-intensity unnecessary for many survivors • Specialty-based and potentially excessively disease-oriented • May foster mentality of medical dependence • Geographically fixed and possibly inconveniently located • Care not portable • Potentially difficult to integrate into life as a survivor
Community-based model	• Level of available resources suitable for majority of survivors • Primary care based and wellness oriented • Congruent with sense of empowerment and medical independence • Geographically convenient • Care portable • Likely cost-effective	• Greater potential for discontinuity of care • Patient anxiety due to separation from oncology team • Appropriate survivorship care dependent on patient and provider initiative • Difficult to provide breadth of survivorship expertise and resources • Infrastructure lacking for research studies
Hybrid model	• Advantages of community-based model • Provider and patient access to survivorship expertise and resources readily available • More amenable to conducting longitudinal research	• Relative lack of experience with model currently • Requires establishment of systems to support interactions between center and provider

Freyer DR, "Transition of care for young adult survivors of childhood and adolescent cancer: rationale and approaches," *J Clin Oncol*. 2010;28(32):4810–8. Used with permission.

chronic illness. As survivors age into adulthood and the risk of late effects for these survivors increases, they often must be transitioned to medically and developmentally appropriate adult care.

The transition process is challenging, and many survivors are often lost to follow-up during the transfer of care. Some potential reasons for this include:

- Survivors may be asymptomatic and unfocused on their future health risks.
- Transfer of care occurs at a time of other developmental challenges such as attending college and living independently, moving away from family of origin, pursuing life goals, and changing social networks.
- Lack of communication between cancer centers and PCPs, and between cancer centers and adult survivorship providers, may hinder successful transfer.
- Perceived or actual inadequacies of adult care based on limited knowledge of disease and survivorship issues of adult providers and different healthcare-delivery models. (There is limited formal training available for PCPs in medical school or residency, and most PCPs are not familiar with the needs of adult survivors of pediatric cancer.)

Models of Care[34,35]

Four models of transitional care were defined in 1994 at the working conference, "Moving On: Transition from Pediatric to Adult Health Care." Each had its advantages and drawbacks as it related to adolescents and young adults and their providers:

Disease specific model.
Generic model.
Primary care model.
Single site model.

More recently, the following three models of transitional care have emerged. Table 33.8 describes some of the unique qualities and disadvantages of each model.

a. Cancer-center-based model—This model is located at the pediatric treatment center or within its larger governing institution (university or healthsystem). Transitional care is delivered within the same system as treatment was given and involves direct on-site collaboration of the pediatric and adult teams.
b. Community-based model—This model is located in the office or clinic of the care provider, typically the primary care physician. It requires a coordinated transition of care that includes transfer of all pertinent clinical information and follow-up responsibility from the treatment center to the primary care provider.
c. Hybrid model—With this model, care is transferred to the office or clinic of the primary care provider but relies on an ongoing interaction with the cancer treatment center. This is also called the "Shared Care Model."

Each of these models can result in successful programs. The particular model utilized will be determined by the healthcare system in which the program is being established. An assessment of the system is imperative prior to determining which model will be most successful. Regardless of the program used to assist with transition, the commitment of the concept of transition by the multidisciplinary providers and leadership on both the pediatric and adult teams is essential.

Principles of Successful Transition[24,34,36]

- Transition process should be initiated in early to mid-adolescence; much sooner than age 18.
- Common concerns of young adulthood and specialty care needs must be addressed.
- Transition should promote autonomy, personal responsibility, and disease self-management, with survivors having greater participation in medical decision making over time.
- Flexibility is imperative within the transition program to meet the needs of young adults.
- The transition process is a shared responsibility among providers and the survivor and their family.
- The patient, parent, and provider must have similar transition-related goals and be able to "let go."
- A specific transition plan should be developed beginning at least 12–18 months before the planned event, including identifying and initiating communication with the patient's posttransitional medical provider.
- Future health insurance coverage should be explored.

Summary

Survivors of childhood cancer are a medically and psychosocially vulnerable population in need of ongoing care. Many forces challenge the provision of optimal care to this population including the increasing numbers of survivors, disengagement in care from many long-term survivors, changes and increasing demands on the healthcare system, and shortages within the healthcare workforce with the appropriate knowledge and expertise. Education and training of survivors and caregivers, multidisciplinary services and approaches to care, established guidelines, clear identification of roles and responsibilities, involving the PCP early, and ongoing evaluations of practice are essential components needed to provide this population of patients with the care required for long-term quality of life.

References

1. American Cancer Society. *Cancer Treatment and Survivorship Facts and Figures, 2014–2015*. Atlanta, GA: American Cancer Society, 2014. Available at: http://www.cancer.org/acs/groups/content/@research/documents/document/acspc-042801.pdf

2. Mariotto AB, Rowland JH, Yabroff KR, et al. Long-term survivors of childhood cancer in the United States. *Cancer Epidemiol Biomarkers Prev.* 2009; 18(4):1033–40.
3. Hudson MM, Ness KK, Gurney JG, et al. Clinical ascertainment of health outcomes among adults treated for childhood cancer *JAMA.* 2013;309(22):2371–2381.
4. A model for delivering psychosocial health services. In: Adler NE, Page AEK, eds., *Institute of Medicine (IOM). Cancer Care for the Whole Patient: Meeting Psychosocial Health Needs.* Washington, DC: The National Academies Press; 2008: 153–218.
5. Zebrack BJ. Psychological, social, and behavioral issues for young adults with cancer. Cancer. 2011;117(10):2289–2294.
6. Kazak AE, Derosa BW, Schwartz LA, et al. Psychological outcomes and health beliefs in adolescent and young adult survivors of childhood cancer and controls. *J Clin Oncol.* 2010;28(12):2002–2007.
7. Kirchhoff AC, Krull KR, Ness KK, et al. Physical, mental, and neurocognitive status and employment outcomes in the childhood cancer survivor study cohort. *Cancer Epidemiol Biomarkers Prev.* 2011;20(9):1838–1849.
8. Brinkman TM, Zhu L, Zeltzer LK, et al. Longitudinal patterns of psychological distress in adult survivors of childhood cancer." *Brit J Cancer.* 2013;109(5):1373–1381.
9. Recklitis C, Diller LR, Li X, et al. Suicide ideation in adult survivors of childhood cancer: a report from the Childhood Cancer Survivor Study. *J Clin Oncol.* 2010;28(4):655–661.
10. Stuber M, Meeske KA, Krull KR, et al. Prevalence and predictors of posttraumatic stress disorder in adult survivors of childhood cancer. *Pediatrics.* 2010;125(5):1124–1134.
11. Zebrack BJ, Stuber ML, Meeske KA, et al. Perceived positive impact of cancer among long-term survivors of childhood cancer: a report from the childhood cancer survivor study. *Psychooncol.* 2012;21(6):630–639.
12. Kirchhoff AC, Krull KR, Ness KK, et al. Occupational outcomes of adult childhood cancer survivors: A report from the childhood cancer survivor study. *Cancer.* 2011;117(13):3033–3044.
13. Kirchhoff AC, Leisenring W, Krull KR, et al. Unemployment among adult survivors of childhood cancer: a report from the childhood cancer survivor study. *Med Care.* 2010;48(11):1015–1025.
14. Park ER, Kirchhoff AC, Zallen JP, et al. Childhood Cancer Survivor Study participants' perceptions and knowledge of health insurance coverage: implications for the Affordable Care Act. *J Cancer Surviv.* 2012;6(3):251–259.
15. Oeffinger KC, Wallace WH. Barriers to follow-up care of survivors in the United States and the United Kingdom. *Pediatr Blood Cancer.* 2006;46(2):135–142.
16. Children's Cancer and Leukemia Group. *Therapy Based Long-term Follow up: Practice Statement.* 2nd ed. Leicester, UK: CCLG; 2005, April. http://www.cclg.org.uk/dynamic_files/LTFU-full.pdf. Accessed Nov 25, 2013.

16a. Scottish Intercollegiate Guidelines Network (SIGN). Long term follow up of survivors of childhood cancer. Edinburgh: SIGN; 2013. (SIGN publication no. 132). [March 2013]. Available from URL: http://www.sign.ac.uk

17. Children's Oncology Group. *Long-term Follow-up Guidelines for Survivors of Childhood, Adolescent and Young Adult Cancer* (version 2.0). Arcadia, CA: COG; 2006, March. http://www.survivorshipguidelines.org.

18. Landier W, Bhatia S, Eshelman DA, et al. Development of risk-based guidelines for pediatric cancer survivors: the Children's Oncology Group long-term follow-up guidelines from the Children's Oncology Group Late Effects Committee and Nursing Discipline. *J Clin Oncol.* 2004;22(24):4979–4990.

19. Children's Oncology Group. Summary of cancer treatment (abbreviated). In: *Long-term Follow-up Guidelines for Survivors of Childhood, Adolescent and Young Adult Cancer: Appendix I, Materials for Clinical Application of LTFU Guidelines*. Arcadia, CA: COG; 2006, March: 12. http://www.survivorshipguidelines.org.

20. Long-Term Follow-Up Study (LTFU). *Using the COG Screening Guidelines. Long-Term Follow-Up Study Newsletter, Spring 2006*. Memphis, TN:LTFU; 2006, March:4. http://www.stjude.org/stjude/v/index.

21. Zeltzer LK, Recklitis C, Buchbinder D, et al. Psychological status in childhood cancer survivors: a report from the Childhood Cancer Survivor Study. *J Clin Oncol.* 2009;27:2396–24.

22. Aziz N, Oeffinger K, Brooks S, Turoff A. Comprehensive long-term follow-up programs for pediatric cancer survivors. *Cancer.* 2006;107:841–848.

23. Ganz PA, Casillas J, Hahn EE. Ensuring quality care for cancer survivors: implementing the survivorship care plan. *Semin Oncol Nurs.* 2008;24:208–217.

24. Freyer D. Transition of care for young adult survivors of childhood and adolescent cancer: rationale and approaches. *J Clin Oncol.* 2010;28:4810–4818.

25. Oeffinger KC, Hudson MM. Long-term complications following childhood and adolescent cancer: foundations for providing risk-based health care for survivors. *CA Cancer J Clin.* Jui-Aug 2004; 54(4):208–236.

26. Oeffinger KC, Eshelman DA, Tomlinson GE, Buchanan GR. Programs for adult survivors of childhood cancer. *J Clin Oncol.* 1998;16:2864–2867.

27. Nissen MJ, et al. Views of primary care providers on follow-up care of cancer patients. *Fam Med.* 2007;39:477–482.

28. Snyder CF, et al. Prevention, screening, and surveillance care for breast cancer survivors compared with controls: changes from 1998-2002. *J Clin Oncol.* 2009;27:1054–1061.

29. Nathan P, Greenberg M, et al. Medical care on long-term survivors of childhood cancer: a report from the Childhood Cancer Survivor Study. *J Clin Oncol.* 2008;26:4401–4409.

30. Nathan P, Ford J, Henderson TO, et al. Health behaviors, medical care, and interventions to promote healthy living in the Childhood Cancer Survivor Study Cohort. *J Clin Oncol.* 2009;27:2663–2673.

31. Nathan P, Hayes-Lattine B, Sisler J, Hudson M. Critical issues in transition and survivorship for adolescents and young adults with cancer. *Cancer.* 2011;117:2335–2341.

32. Oeffinger KC, Mertens AC, Sklar CA, et al. Chronic health conditions in adult survivors of childhood cancer. *N Engl J Med.* 2006;355(15):1572–1582.

33. Schwartz CL, Hobbie WL, Ruccione K, Constine LS. *Survivors of Childhood and Adolescent Cancer: A Multidisciplinary Approach*. Berlin, Germany: Springer; 2005.

34. Summary of conference recommendations. *J Adolesc Health*. 1995;17(1):6–9. [This paper was commissioned for the working conference "Moving On: Transition from Pediatric to Adult Health Care" presented by the Center for Children with Chronic Illness and Disability, National Center for Youth with Disability, and the Keland Endowment Fund of the Johnson Foundation, September 9–11, 1994.]

35. Shad A, Myers SN, Hennessy K. Late effects in cancer survivors: "the shared care model. *Curr Oncol Rep*. 2012 Apr;14(2):182–190.

36. Schwartz LA, Brumley LD, Tuchman LK, et al. Stakeholder validation of a model of readiness for transition to adult care. *JAMA Pediatr.* 2013;67(10): 939–946.

Appendix

Health-related Quality of Life in Pediatric Oncology

Diana E. Nora, Rebecca A. Prengler, and Lisa M. Horowitz

Pediatric-health-related quality of life (HRQOL) refers to the impact of a physical illness, such as cancer, on a child's social, psychological, and physical well-being.[1, 2] Assessing quality of life is particularly helpful for monitoring patients' functional status as they progress through diagnosis, treatment, and remission or life after treatment.[3] Furthermore, HRQOL measures can provide clinicians and families with insight into how cancer may affect a child's physical, social, academic, and emotional development.[4] Pediatric HRQOL tools should be multidimensional, developmentally appropriate, and nonburdensome to complete. If a patient is too young or too sick to complete the self-administered form, HRQOL tools should be flexible enough to allow for a parent or caregiver to respond on behalf of the child. Obtaining permission from a parent or guardian to share results with the patient's clinical-care team may be a valuable approach in ensuring that the comprehensive needs of children with cancer are met.

Scales are applicable to patients of all ages and may be available in several different languages. The following measures have reliability and validity data within an acceptable range, and several were designed specifically for a pediatric oncology setting. See Table A.1.

Table A.1 Suggested Measures of HRQOL

Instrument	Age range (years)	Domains (Type of report)	No. of items	Languages
Pediatric Oncology Quality of Life Scale (POQOLS)	4–18	Physical functioning, emotional distress, adjustment to medical treatment (Parent report)	21	English,[6] Dutch[7]
Pediatric Quality of Life Inventory 4.0 (PedsQL 4.0)	2–18	Physical, emotional, school, and social functioning (Parent report & child self- report)	23	English,[8,9] Argentinean Spanish,[10] Arabic (ages 8–18),[11] Chinese,[12] German,[13] Greek,[14]* Indonesian,[15] Japanese (SF-15, ages 5–18),[16] Norwegian[17]* (ages 13–15), Persian,[18] Sinhala,[19]* Swedish,[20]* Thai,[21]* UK-English[22]
Pediatric Quality of Life Inventory 3.0 Cancer Module (PedsQL 3.0)	2–18	Pain, nausea, procedural anxiety, worry, cognition, perceived physical appearance, communication (Parent report & child self-report)	27	English,[9] Brazilian,[23] Chinese,[24] German,[13] Indonesian,[15] Japanese,[25] Turkish (ages 8–12)[26]
Pediatric Quality of Life Inventory Brain Tumor Module	2–18	Cognitive problems, pain and hurt, movement and balance, procedural anxiety, nausea, and worry (Parent report & child self-report)	24	English,[27] Japanese[28]
Pediatric Functional Assessment of Cancer Therapy—Childhood Brain Tumor Survivor Version 2.0—Youth Form (Peds-FACT-Brs)	7–12	Physical well-being, emotional well-being and illness experiences, social/family well-being, and brain tumor survivor specific concerns (Child self-report)	34	Korean[29]

Pediatric Functional Assessment of Cancer Therapy-Childhood Brain Tumor Survivor Version 2-Adolescent Form (Peds-FACT-Brs)	13–18	Physical well-being, emotional well-being and illness experiences, social/family well-being, and brain-tumor survivor specific concerns (Parent form & adolescent self-report)	37	Korean[30,31]
Pediatric Cancer Quality of Life Inventory—32 (PCQL–32)	8–18	Disease & treatment related symptoms, physical, psychological, social and cognitive functioning (Parent report & child self-report)	32	English[32]
The Miami Pediatric Quality of Life Questionnaire (MPQOLQ)	1–18	Social competence, self competence, emotional stability (Parent report)	56	English[33]
SF-36[]	≥14	Physical functioning, role limitation–physical, role limitation–emotional, social functioning, mental health, energy and vitality, bodily pain, general health perception (Adolescent self-report)	36	English,[34] Persian[35]*
Minneapolis-Manchester Quality of Life Questionnaire—Youth Form (MMQL-YF)[]	8–12	Outlook on life, physical symptoms, physical functioning, psychological functioning (Interview-based child report)	32	English,[36] Swedish[37]*

(continued)

Table A.1 (Continued)

Instrument	Age range (years)	Domains (Type of report)	No. of items	Languages
Minneapolis-Manchester Quality of Life Adolescent Form (MMQL-AF)	13–20	Physical, cognitive, psychological, and social functioning, body image, outlook on life, intimate relations (Adolescent self-report)	46	English,[38] Swedish[37]*
Minneapolis-Manchester Quality of Life-Child Form and Parent Form (MMQL-UK(CF and PF))	8–18	Physical appearance, school, social, emotional, and physical functioning (Child self-report and parent report)	29	UK-English[39,40]
Child Health Questionnaire—Child Form 87 (CHQ-CF87)	5–18	Physical functioning, physical role limitations, general health perceptions, body pain, change in health, impact on family, behavioral role limitations, self-esteem, mental health, general behavior (Child self-report)	87	English,[41] UK,[42]* Canadian-French[42]*

Child Health Questionnaire—Parent Form 50 (CHQ-PF50)	N/A	In addition to CHQ-CF87 domains, emotional impact on parent, impact of child health on parent personal time (Parent report)	50	English,[40] German[43]
Child Health Ratings Inventory—General Module (CHRIs)	5–18	Physical function, role function, emotional well-being, energy, global HRQOL (adolescent and parent report) (Parent report & child self-report)	20	English[44–47]
Disease-Specific Impairment Inventory- Hematopoietic Stem Cell Transplantation (DSII-HSCT)	5–18	Hassles, body image, worry (Parent report & child self-report)	10	English[44–46]

*Validated in healthy or other chronically ill populations.

References

1. Ware JE, Jr. Conceptualizing disease impact and treatment outcomes. *Cancer.* 1984;15S:2316–2323.
2. Palermo TM, Long AC, Lewandowski AS, et al. Evidence-based assessment of health-related quality of life and impairment in pediatric psychology. *J Pediatr Psychol.* 2008:33:983–996.
3. Nathan PC, Furlong W, Barr RD. Challenges to the measurement of health-related quality of life in children receiving cancer therapy. *Pediatr Blood Cancer.* 2004;43:215–223.
4. Drotar D, ed. *Measuring Health-related Quality of Life in Children and Adolescents: Implications for Research and Practice.* Mahwah, NJ: Erlbaum; 1998.
5. Klassen AF, Strohm SJ, Maurice-Stam H, et al. Quality of life questionnaires for children with cancer and childhood cancer survivors: a review of the development of available measures. *Support Care Cancer.* 2010;18:1207–1217.
6. Goodwin DAJ, Boggs SR, Graham-Pole J. Development and validation of the pediatric oncology and quality of life scale. *Psychol Assess.* 1994;6:321–328.
7. Bijttebier P, Bercruysse T, Vertommen H, et al. New evidence on the reliability and validity of the Pediatric Oncology Quality of Life Scale. *Psychol Health.* 2001;16:461–469.
8. Varni JW, Seid M, Kurtin PS. PedsQL 4.0: reliability and validity of the Pediatric Quality of Life Inventory version 4.0 general core scales in healthy and patient populations. *Med Care.* 2001;39:800–812.
9. Varni JW, Burwinkle TM, Katz ER, et al. The PedsQL in pediatric cancer: reliability and validity of the Pediatric Quality of Life Inventory Generic Core Scales, Multidimensional Fatigue Scale, and Cancer Module. *Cancer.* 2002;94:2090–2106.
10. Roizen M, Rodríguez S, Bauer G, et al. Initial validation of the Argentinean Spanish version of the PedsQL™ 4.0 Generic Core Scales in children and adolescents with chronic diseases: acceptability and comprehensibility in low income settings. *Health Qual Life Outcomes.* 2008;6:59.
11. Arabiat D, Elliott B, Draper P, et al. Cross-cultural validation of the Pediatric Quality of Life Inventory™ 4.0 (PedsQL™) generic core scale into Arabic Language. *Scand J Caring Sci.* 2011;25:828–833.
12. Hao Y, Tian Q, Yiyun L, et al. Psychometric properties of the Chinese version of the Pediatric Quality of Life Inventory™ 4.0 generic core scales. *Qual Life Res.* 2010;19:1229–1233.
13. Felder-Puig R, Frey E, Proksch K, et al. Validation of the German version of the Pediatric Quality of Life Inventory™ (PedsQL™) in childhood cancer patients off treatment and children with epilepsy. *Qual Life Res.* 2004;13:223–224.
14. Gkoltsiou K, Dimitrakaki C, Tzavara C, et al. Measuring health-related quality of life in Greek children: psychometric properties of the Greek version of the Pediatric Quality of Life Inventory. *Qual Life Res.* 2008;17:299–305.
15. Sitaresmi MN, Mostert S, Gundy CM, et al. Health-related quality of life assessment in Indonesian childhood acute lymphoblastic leukemia. *Health Qual Life Outcomes.* 2008;6:96.

16. Chen X, Origasa H, Ichida F, et al. Reliability and validity of the Pediatric Quality of Life Inventory™ (PedsQL™) Short Form 15 generic core scales in Japan. *Qual Life Res.* 2007;16:1239–1249.

17. Reinfjell T, Diseth TH, Veenstra M, et al. Measuring health-related quality of life in young adolescents: reliability and validity in the Norwegian version of the Pediatric Quality of Life Inventory™ 4.0 (PedsQL) generic core scales. *Health Qual Life Outcomes.* 2006;4:61.

18. Amiri P, Ardekani EM, Jalali-Farahani S, et al. Reliability and validity of the Iranian version of the Pediatric Quality of Life Inventory™ 4.0 generic core scales in adolescents. *Qual Life Res.* 2010;19:1501–1508.

19. Danansuriya MN, Rajapaksa LC. Psychometric properties of the Sinhala version of the PedsQL™ 4.0 Generic Core Scales in early adolescents in Sri Lanka. *Health Qual Life Outcomes.* 2012;10:105.

20. Petersen S, Hägglöf B, Stenlund H, et al. Psychometric properties of the Swedish PedsQL, Pediatric Quality of Life Inventory 4.0 generic core scales. *Acta Paediatrica.* 2009;98:1504–1512.

21. Sritipsukho P, Wisai M. Reliability and validity of the Thai version of the Pediatric Quality of Life Inventory 4.0. *Qual Life Res.* 2013;22:551–557.

22. Upton P, Eiser C, Cheung I, et al. Measurement properties of the UK-English version of the Pediatric Quality of Life Inventory™ 4.0 (PedsQL™) generic core scales. *Health Qual Life Outcomes.* 2005;3:22.

23. Scarpelli AC, Paiva SM, Pordeus IA, et al. Measurement properties of the Brazilian version of the Pediatric Quality of Life Inventory (PedsQL) cancer module scale. *Health Qual Life Outcomes.* 2008;6:7.

24. Li HCW, Williams PD, Williams AR, et al. Confirmatory factor analysis of the Chinese version of the Pediatric Quality-of-Life Inventory Cancer Module. *Cancer Nursing.* 2013;00:1–7.

25. Tsuji N, Kakee N, Ishida Y, et al.Validation of the Japanese version of the Pediatric Quality of Life Inventory (PedsQL) Cancer Module. *Health Qual Life Outcomes.* 2011;9:22.

26. Tanir MK, Kuguoglu S. Turkish validity and reliability of a pediatric quality of life cancer module for children aged 8–12 and parents. *Asian Pacific J Cancer Prevention.* 2011;12:125–130.

27. Palmer SN, Meeske KA, Katz ER, et al. The PedsQLTM Brain Tumor Module: initial reliability and validity. *Pediatr Blood Cancer.* 2007;49;287–293.

28. Sato I, Higuchi A, Yanagisawa T, et al. Development of the Japanese version of the Pediatric Quality of Life Inventory™ Brain Tumor Module. *Health Qual Life Outcomes.* 2010;8:38.

29. Yoo H, Ra Y, Park H, et al. Validation of pediatric Functional Assessment of Cancer Therapy: patient version 2 of "brain tumor survivor" for grade school patients aged 7–12 years. *Qual Life Res.* 2011;20:529–535.

30. Yoo H, Kim D, Shin H, et al. Validation of the Pediatric Functional Assessment of Cancer Therapy Questionnaire (Version 2.0) in brain tumor survivors aged 13 years and older. *J Pain Symp Manage.* 2010;40:559–565.

31. Yoo H, Kim D, Lai J, et al. Validation of Pediatric Fuctional Assessment of Cancer Therapy Questionnaire (Version 2.0) in brain tumor survivor aged 13 years and older (parent form) (PedsFACT-BrS Parent of Adolescent). *J Korean Neurosurg Soc.* 2011;49:147–152.

32. Varni JW, Katz ER, Rode CA. The Pediatric Cancer Quality of Life Inventory–32 (PCQL–32). 1: Reliability and validity. *Cancer.* 1998:82:1184–1196.

33. Armstrong FD, Toledano SR, Miloslavich K, et al. The Miami Pediatric Quality of Life Questionnaire: parent scale. *Int J Cancer.* 1999;12(Suppl.):11–17.

34. Ware JE, Jr., Sherbourne CD. The MOS 36-item short-form health survey (SF-36). I. Conceptual framework and item selection. *Med Care.* 1992;30:473–483.

35. Montazeri A, Goshtasebi A, Vahdaninia M et al. The Short Form Health Survery (SF-36): translation and validation study of the Iranian verison. *Qual Life Res.* 2005;14:875–882.

36. Bhatia S, Jenney ME, Bogue MK, et al. The Minneapolis-Manchester Quality of Life Instrument: reliability and validity of the youth form. *J Pediatr.* 2004;145:39–46.

37. Einberg E, Kadrija I, Brunt D et al. Psychometric evaluation of a Swedish version of Minneapolis-Manchester quality of life-youth form and adolescent form. *Health Qual Life Outcomes.* 2013;11:79.

38. Bhatia S, Jenney ME, Bogue MK, et al. The Minneapolis-Manchester Quality of Life Instrument: Reliability and validity of the Adolescent Form. *J Clin Oncol.* 2002;20:4692–4698.

39. Hutchings HA, Upton P, Cheung W et al. Adaptation of the Manchester-Minneapolis Quality of Life instrument for use in the UK population. *Arch Dis Child.* 2007;92:855–860.

40. Hutchings HA, Upton P, Cheung W et al. Development of a parent version of the Manchester-Minneapolis quality of life survey for use by parents and carers of UK children: MMQL-UK (PF). *Health Qual Life.* 2008;6:19.

41. Landgraf JM, Abetz L, Ware JE. *The Child Health Questionnaire (CHQ): A Users Manual.* Boston, MA: HealthAct; 1996.

42. Landgraf JM, Maunsell K, Speechley N, et al. Canadian-French, German and UK versions of Child Health Questionnaire: methodology and preliminary item scaling results. *Qual Life Research.* 1998;7:433–445.

43. Warschburger P, Landgraf J, Petermann F, et al. Health-related quality of life in children assessed by their parents: Evaluation of the psychometric properties of the CHQ-PF50 in two German clinical samples. *Qual Life Research.* 2003;12:291–301.

44. Parsons, SK, Shih, MC, Mayer DK, et al. Preliminary psychometric evaluation of the Child Health Ratings Inventories (CHRIs) and Disease-Specific Impairment Inventory-HSCt in parents and children. *Qual Life Res.* 2005;14:1613–1625.

45. Parsons, SK, Shih, MC, DuHamel, KN et al. Maternal perspectives on children's health-related quality of life during the first year after pediatric hematopoietic stem cell transplant. *J Pediatric Psychology.* 2006;31:1100–1115.

46. Kaplan SH, Barlow S, Spetter D, et al. Assessing functional status and health-related quality of life among school-aged children: reliability and validity of a new self-reported measure. *Qual Life Res.* 1995;4:444.

47. Rodday AM, Terrin N, Parsons SK, et al. Measuring global health-related quality of life in children undergoing hematopoietic stem cell transplant: a longitudinal study. *Health Qual Life Outcomes.* 2013;11:26.

Index

Q

R